AF688819

Diagnosis and Treatment in Family Medicine

Diagnosis and Treatment in Family Medicine

Editor: Nora Ortega

AMERICAN
MEDICAL PUBLISHERS
www.americanmedicalpublishers.com

AMERICAN
MEDICAL PUBLISHERS
www.americanmedicalpublishers.com

Cataloging-in-Publication Data

Diagnosis and treatment in family medicine / edited by Nora Ortega.
p. cm.
Includes bibliographical references and index.
ISBN 978-1-63927-446-8
1. Family medicine. 2. Medicine. 3. Physicians (General practice). I. Ortega, Nora.
R729.5.G4 F36 2022
610--dc23

© American Medical Publishers, 2022

American Medical Publishers,
41 Flatbush Avenue,
1st Floor, New York,
NY 11217, USA

ISBN 978-1-63927-446-8 (Hardback)

This book contains information obtained from authentic and highly regarded sources. Copyright for all individual chapters remain with the respective authors as indicated. All chapters are published with permission under the Creative Commons Attribution License or equivalent. A wide variety of references are listed. Permission and sources are indicated; for detailed attributions, please refer to the permissions page and list of contributors. Reasonable efforts have been made to publish reliable data and information, but the authors, editors and publisher cannot assume any responsibility for the validity of all materials or the consequences of their use.

Trademark Notice: Registered trademark of products or corporate names are used only for explanation and identification without intent to infringe.

Contents

Preface

Over the recent decade, advancements and applications have progressed exponentially. This has led to the increased interest in this field and projects are being conducted to enhance knowledge. The main objective of this book is to present some of the critical challenges and provide insights into possible solutions. This book will answer the varied questions that arise in the field and also provide an increased scope for furthering studies.

The medical specialty that is concerned with the comprehensive health care for people of all ages is known as family medicine. It is a sub-division of primary care that is based on the knowledge of the patient's cultural and family background. It primarily focuses on preventing diseases and promoting health. It also aims at providing continuous and comprehensive health care to individuals and families over all diseases, ages, genders and parts of the body. Various chronic, acute and preventive medical care services are provided under family medicine. It includes routine check-ups, immunization, health-risk assessments, personalized counseling and screening tests for maintaining a healthy lifestyle. This book contains some path-breaking studies in the field of family medicine. It traces the progress of this field and highlights some of its key concepts and applications. The extensive content of this book provides the readers with a thorough understanding of the subject.

I hope that this book, with its visionary approach, will be a valuable addition and will promote interest among readers. Each of the authors has provided their extraordinary competence in their specific fields by providing different perspectives as they come from diverse nations and regions. I thank them for their contributions.

Editor

1

Patient-centeredness to anticipate and organize an end-of-life project for patients receiving at-home palliative care

Agnès Oude Engberink[1,2,3,8*], Mélanie Badin[1], Philippe Serayet[1], Sylvain Pavageau[1], François Lucas[1], Gérard Bourrel[1,2,3], Joanna Norton[4,5], Grégory Ninot[2,3,6] and Pierre Senesse[3,6,7]

Abstract

Background: The development of end-of-life primary care is a socio-medical and ethical challenge. However, general practitioners (GPs) face many difficulties when initiating appropriate discussion on proactive shared palliative care. Anticipating palliative care is increasingly important given the ageing population and is an aim shared by many countries.

We aimed to examine how French GPs approached and provided at-home palliative care. We inquired about their strategy for delivering care, and the skills and resources they used to devise new care strategies.

Methods: Twenty-one GPs from the South of France recruited by phone according to their various experiences of palliative care agreed to participate. Semi-structured interview transcripts were examined using a phenomenological approach inspired by Grounded theory, and further studied with semiopragmatic analysis.

Results: Offering palliative care was perceived by GPs as a moral obligation. They felt vindicated in a process rooted in the paradigm values of their profession. This study results in two key findings: firstly, their patient-centred approach facilitated the anticipatory discussions of any potential event or intervention, which the GPs openly discussed with patients and their relatives; secondly, this approach contributed to build an "end-of-life project" meeting patients' wishes and needs. The GPs all shared the idea that the end-of-life process required human presence and recommended that at-home care be coordinated and shared by multi-professional referring teams.

Conclusions: The main tenets of palliative care as provided by GPs are a patient-centred approach in the anticipatory discussion of potential events, personalized follow-up with referring multi-professional teams, and the collaborative design of an end-of-life project meeting the aspirations of the patient and his or her family. Consequently, coordination strategies involving specialized teams, GPs and families should be modelled according to the specificities of each care system.

Keywords: General practice, Palliative care, Patient-centred approach, Qualitative phenomenological study, Semiopragmatic analysis

* Correspondence: agnesisambert@wanadoo.fr
[1]Department of General Medicine, University of Montpellier, Montpellier, France
[2]CEPS Platform, University of Montpellier, Montpellier, France
Full list of author information is available at the end of the article

Background

According to a 2013 ONFV report (*Observatoire National de la Fin de Vie*, French National End-of-Life Observatory) [1], 25% of French people died at home; professionals lack adequate training. In its recommendations, this report notes that end-of-life conditions should be improved. Regardless of the WHO (World Health Organization) recommendations palliative care is often restricted to a reactive approach and to the relief of physical symptoms in the terminal phase [2].

During the 2015 MASCC (Multinational Association of Supportive Care in Cancer) conference, LH Einhorn reminded attendees that "early palliative care" and "symptoms relief" were two of the five main challenges in oncology [3]. Meeussen [4] revealed that many patients die in places they had not chosen, with often unwanted interventions.

To facilitate identification of patients in need of palliative care several sets of indicators have been developed [2] such as the Supportive and Palliative Care Indicators Tool (SPICT) in Scotland, The Prognostic Indicator Guide (PIG) in England, and the Radboud Indicators for Palliative Care needs (RADPAC) in the Netherlands. In a Dutch RCT [5] GPs in the intervention group were trained in identifying patients in need of palliative care and anticipatory care planning. Next, for each identified patient, they were offered a coaching session with a specialist in palliative care. The control group did not receive any training or coaching. The study did not find any difference between the intervention and control groups in out-of-hour contacts, contacts with their own GP, hospitalizations or place of death. However, the authors conclude that better adapted tools and training programmes may be necessary to show an improvement on identification of patients in need of palliative care and providing adequate care.

In Europe, GPs have difficulties identifying at the right time the need for palliative care, as shown in Belgium [6]. GPs found it difficult to determine the right moment to implement palliative care and to interpret patient aspirations; they reported that they could only help patients in their last year of life.

An Australian systematic review [7] surveyed 66 studies published between 1966 and 2000 relevant to GP provision of palliative care. They corroborate to show that GPs value this area of their work, and patients appreciate their involvement when their physicians are available, make time to listen to them, allow them to express their feelings and make efforts to alleviate their symptoms. In the Netherlands, where GPs have historically been involved in palliative care, a qualitative study [8] of 22 GPs used 3 focus groups to examine their perceptions. The GPs described their palliative care tasks as satisfactory but burdensome. The challenges they faced were categorized according to three levels: 1) personal (knowledge, skills, emotions), 2) relational (communication and collaboration), and 3) organizational (organization of care and compartmentalization in healthcare).

Major barriers to effective home palliative care and end-of-life appear to be lack of medical training and health organization. In two studies surveying 62 medical schools, Sullivan et al. [9, 10] showed that students were critical of their training: they felt it lacked educational expertise and role-models, and that it focused more on cure-driven practices than on care-driven ones. Slort [11] identified the main barriers for GP-patient communication in a systematic review (fifteen qualitative studies and seven quantitative questionnaire studies): lack of availability and GPs' ambivalence to discuss palliative prognosis. Also, in a recent French study [12] 87 GPs reported on their involvement in the decision-making process for assigning patients to palliative care. Seventy percent of these GPs felt that their involvement in the care strategy was practically nil, and 83% reported that they had not been consulted on decisions regarding the limitation or cessation of therapeutics by hospital staff. In addition, a specialist doctor usually becomes the primary caregiver for patients in their final stage of life.

Taken collectively, the above-mentioned studies stress the importance of structuring organized palliative care in coordination with primary care. They also raise the issue of adequate GP-patient communication training for students and practicing GPs, as well as other relevant skills to develop.

Thus, exploring the lived experience of GPs providing at-home palliative care is a relevant topic in many countries; a better understanding of their approaches and practices would likely allow us to formulate improvements which could impact the quality of the palliative care received by patients.

Methods

Aim

We performed a qualitative study to determine how French GPs provide palliative care in at-home settings, what their needs may be, and what skills and resources they mobilize for these interventions.

Design

We used a phenomenological approach to analyse the semi-structured in-depth interviews of GPs regarding their palliative care lived experience. Subsequently, we carried out a semiopragmatic analysis of the data.

The study's design met COREQ criteria [13] (COnsolidated criteria for REporting Qualitative research).

Setting

Characteristics of participants

GPs were selected from the *French Regional College of General Practitioners* in the Languedoc-Roussillon region, and contacted by telephone by the investigator (FL). We used purposive sampling to obtain a diversity of GP experiences across various characteristics such as age, sex, work setting (alone or in a team, urban or rural), and years of practice. We applied the principle of data saturation without pre-defining the number of interviews.

Data collection

An interview guide (Table 1) including phenomenological questioning focused on lived experience was developed by the methodology team. Two qualitative methodology experts (AOE, MD; GB, MD) verified the appropriateness, as well as the intelligibility, of the questions in two initial test sessions administered by the investigator. Follow-up prompts were designed to lead participants to recount their personal experience.

The semi-structured interviews were carried out in the workplaces of participants. The investigator introduced himself as a general medicine intern working on a thesis on palliative care. The interviews were recorded with a Philips digital recorder. The sound quality was sufficient to produce audible and understandable voice files. The interviewer made sure to create an atmosphere of confidence such that answers would be spontaneous and truthful. The respondents were informed that their responses would remain confidential and anonymized as they would not be aggregated with their personal identification details. They were made aware of the possibility to stop the interview at any time without any reason. The recordings were transcribed completely and faithfully. We did not plan to collect non-verbal data.

Table 1 Semi-structured in-depth interview guide (phenomenological approach)

What does the palliative care process mean to you, and where does it fit within the practice of general medicine? Prompt: How do you feel about Palliative Care in general medicine?
How do you feel about providing at-home palliative care to patients? Prompt: How do you feel about providing care to end-of-life patients?
Think about one of your palliative care experiences (the most recent one or one which made a mark – positive or negative – on you). Tell me about it. Prompt: How did it go? Do you remember what your thoughts were then? What your feelings were? What you did? How did you feel about it? Why? Do you recall another experience, a "different" one?
What challenges do you face when providing palliative care? Prompt: What type of skills would you like to improve to be better prepared?
In your opinion, can at-home palliative care be implemented, and what are the requirements for it to be provided under good conditions?

Ethical considerations

The study was conducted in accordance with all French regulations. Participants provided written consent for the publication. Approval from the French Ethical Research Committee (Comité de Protection des Personnes, CPP) was sought but deemed unnecessary because of the non-pharmaceutical bio-medical nature of the research [14].

Data analysis

Phenomenology is a descriptive method for categorizing lived experience recorded in interview transcripts. The various steps of this analysis were performed according to a method similar to that of grounded theory [15, 16] and completed by a semiopragmatic data interpretation procedure inspired by C. S. Peirce [17, 18]. In this method, the analyst takes into account all the semiotic elements of a text, including linguistic clues, as well as contextual ones. Categories emerge by constant comparison. In our study, semiopragmatic analysis allowed the logical ordering of these empirical categories according to Peirce's classes of signs. Typically, as a result of this ordering, the conceptually densest category (i.e., of highest level in the hierarchy of signs) commanded the meaning of the phenomenon at play.

The steps of our analytical process are described in Table 2.

Reliability criteria

This work hypothesized an internal methodological consistency between the researched object (lived experience), the phenomenological approach to data collection, and the data analysis favouring a logic of emergence.

The investigator received preliminary training on phenomenological reformulation (prompts) in order to carry out in-depth interviews. He reported his involvement after each interview. Investigator triangulation was achieved by compiling the analyses of the two qualitative research experts and the trained investigator. The interviews were stopped upon reaching data saturation, without the need to add more participants.

Table 2 Semiopragmatic analysis steps

Accurate transcription of the recordings (French: verbatims).
Identifying the most relevant elements of contextual anchoring.
General reading, followed by targeted reading.
Dividing text in meaning sections.
Identifying all indexical, textual and contextual elements informing the construction of a category (categorizing by continuous comparison).
Semiopragmatic characterization of emergent categories according to their semiotic level.
Arranging those categories according to their logical inter-relationships.
Constructing the meaning of an emerging phenomenon via a general proposition.

Semiopragmatic analysis uses a priori sign classes and adds precision to the logical constructs of a studied phenomenon by limiting investigator-related interpretation bias in the final summary.

Results

Participant characteristics (Table 3)

Of the 30 GPs contacted, 21 agreed to participate in the study. The interviews were carried out between April 1, 2013 and February 28, 2014. Saturation was achieved after 15 interviews, since no new pertinent information was gathered thereafter. Six GPs were not interviewed.

Transcription and punctuation were completed by the investigator, who played the audio files multiple times. The transcripts were numbered from P1 to P15. Triangulation was achieved with the investigator and two semiopragmatic analysis experts. The first two transcripts were analysed jointly; the other records were rigorously compared in vivo until an agreement was reached on conceptual categories.

Emergent categories

We identified four emergent categories. They are presented here in general present-tense propositions (phenomenological statements) comprising all meaningful elements.

Palliative care represents another dimension of care: the transition from a disease-centred curative paradigm to a patient-centred multi-dimensional support and end-of-life quality paradigm

For most GPs, the palliative phase corresponded to the end of the curative pharmacological approach. *"You forget the curing part."* P1,2,3,4,7,13.. *"We're there to provide care to people, not to diseases."* P3. All of them implemented palliative steps towards a comfortable and qualitative end-of-life for their patients. For most GPs, palliative care was provided *"within a different care dimension"*(P6): It was empathetic, multidimensional, and based on patient's preferences; it took into account the entire spectrum of suffering as well as existential dimensions. *"What remains is psychological management, rather; comfort, quality of life."* P1,2, 3, 6, 9, 11. *"And then, maybe, there can also be a spiritual dimension, with religious beliefs, and the question of the meaning of life and of what it is to exist."* P4, P12, P13, P15. *"Trying to listen to them, it's important to be available"* P3. *"Since we don't have much else to offer, we give time."* P1

GPs' patient-centered approach combines duty as a human being with professional and personal values

GPs found that palliative care made them face their own human condition and its limits. *"We're just Men... and death is part of life."* P3. Emotionally, several GPs suffered from this confrontation with end-of-life issues affecting patients to whom they were attached. *"I have a real tough time with it, because I get very close to them, and when they start going, it's very difficult for me...that's that."* P10, P12. P8 and P15 saw end-of-life caregiving as a moral duty.

> *"I've never abandoned any of my patients in any such situations. Er... I feel that it's part of my job, of my duty as a Man"* P8.

Table 3 Characteristics of the 15 GPs respondents

GP	Sexe	Age ranges	location	Practice	Years of Practice	Duration (minutes)
P1	F	30–40	Semi rural	Group (2 GPs)	5	30
P2	F	30–40	Semi rural	Group (2 GPs)	4	49
P3	M	50–60	Rural	Solo	24	48
P4	F	50–60	Rural	Group (2 GPs)	24	52
P5	F	50–60	Urban	Group (3 GPs)	22	33
P6[a]	F	40–50	Urban	Group (3 GPs)	9	28
P7	F	40–50	Urban	Group (3 GPs)	14	46
P8	M	60–70	Urban	Solo	30	37
P9	F	40–50	Semi rural	Solo	17	35
P10	M	60–70	Rural	Solo	33	32
P11	F	30–40	Urban	Group (3 GPs)	3	37
P12	F	30–40	Semi rural	Group (4 GPs)	1,5	34
P13	F	30–40	Semi rural	Solo	6	28
P14	M	50–60	Urban	Group (5 GPs)	29	64
P15	F	30–40	Urban	Group (3 GPs)	9	58

[a]had a palliative care training

The GPs' palliative care process integrated the values of their profession and their own values. P2 deemed his involvement *"natural"* and *"authentic"*. P3, P7 and P9 talked about *"birth-to-death care"* as a tenet of general medicine. GPs found they were *"in their legitimate place"* when providing palliative care. P3 thought that *"the job is fabulous when you give yourself the means for it"*. P5 and P8 insisted on the need for drug therapy training, and regretted the lack of resources. Others had received complementary training *"relaxation and psychosomatics training"*P9. Only P8 admitted to being "ignorant in palliative care" and relieved by end-of-life hospital care.

The GPs stated that they also tapped into their personal experiences, or in that of their friends and families, to develop palliative care approaches.

> *"I think that this type of caregiving can be provided from a personal experience perspective... I mean, the wisdom of [...] knowing yourself."* P7, P3.

Discussing and anticipating potential events allows GPs to collaboratively devise "end-of-life projects" with their patients

The GPs reported that this process was initiated by an early discussion (upon diagnosis) to anticipate potential intercurrent events and patient wishes. *"For me, anticipating is key, for everything."* P9. Anticipating potential events allows the creation of space for discussion where the patient may verbalize his or her lived experience. *"I try to discuss things with them on the basis of their emotions, about how things might evolve, how they feel about it..."* P9, P15.

For P4, *"anticipating means leaving options open for patients, so they may change their mind at any time."* Though the GPs did not point to a "perfect moment" at which this discussion may be started, they reported seizing opportunities created by intercurrent events, such as when patients left the hospital (P 2). Anticipating also means designing an "end-of-life project" with patients and families, which helps confirm and validate their status as a living person with "time left to live", allowing them to exercise free will, up to the choice of place of death. *"And you're still within life, there is time left to live, still... there're so many things to do, so much stuff to take care of"* (P5). P1, P7 and P8 stressed that *"the decision-making process must be shared with the patient."*

Organizing human presence around the patient by sharing the caregiving amongst a multi-disciplinary team

The physicians sought support from referring hospital doctors, existing networks, and French home care system options (UMSP, Unité Mobile de Soins Palliatifs). *"It feels comfortable to share the caregiving with others."* P2

Depending on location, GPs have to set up an informal operational network dedicated to patients. *"The first thing is a solid inpatient-outpatient network; generally, I try to surround myself and have relationships with surgeons and oncologists whom I trust."* P14.

This takes time, and requires significant personal resources. Furthermore, they stressed the need to share the caregiving (with unit, at-home hospital doctors, for example), to develop at-home nursing care with social workers, and to organize informal discussions with peers and nurses. *"Bedside meetings with everyone, caregivers and helpers."* P7.

All GPs shared the idea that the end-of-life requires human presence, and that it was their mission to organize it around the patient. *"You can't do anything without the entourage, whether it's relatives or neighbors."* P4, P9. Such coordination requires that the physician remain a permanent link available by telephone (P2, P7, P14). *"At any rate, even end-of-life patients have my mobile phone number, or nurses with whom I've worked."* P1.

Comprehensive statement according to semiopragmatic analysis (Fig. 1) : the GP's patient centered approach combining duty as a human being, professional and personal values is the core category.

Discussing, anticipating and organizing are the operations of the Patient-Centered Approach in practice, implementing an end-of-life project. These operations mobilize suffering or pleasure, compassionate presence, phenomenological attitude and availability.

Discussion

Our study showed that, when GPs provided palliative care, they moved from a disease-centred curative paradigm to a patient-centred multi-dimensional paradigm. To them, palliative care was first and foremost their duty as a human being. The experiences reported by the participants showed they felt in their "rightful place" in the palliative care process, tapping into the values of their profession based on GP-patient communication while listening to patients, spending time with them, making time to answer their questions, using their knowledge of the patient's medical and personal background to do so. In spite of their skillsets (only one GP stated that he felt "incompetent"), they expressed the need for additional support from referring specialists or dedicated infrastructures (networks and socio-medical systems). Moreover, they estimated that, without support from specialists, natural and other care providers, the implementation of the at-home palliative care process was difficult.

For these reasons, and in accordance with results published by Bruera et al. [19], an Integrated Care Model, in which physicians routinely refer patients to palliative

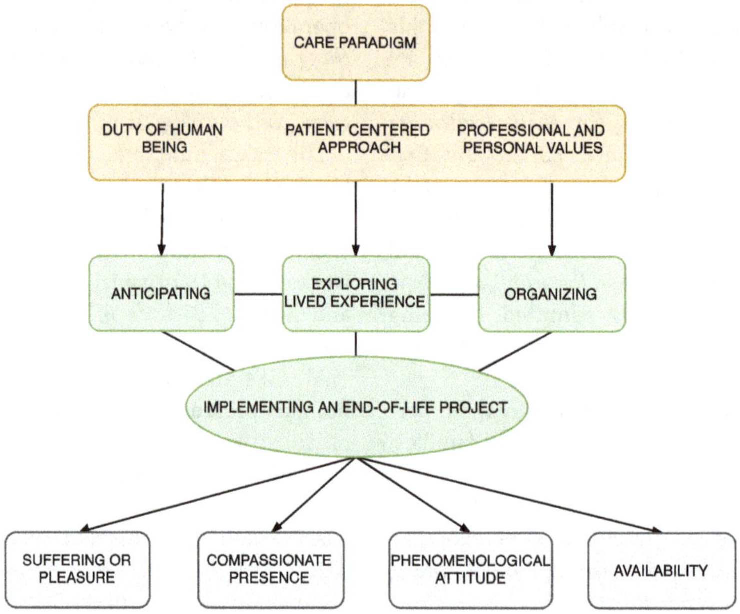

Fig. 1 GP's patient centered approach model in at-home palliative care

care, could help GPs and ensure patients receive comprehensive and integrated care. Most interestingly, in our study, at the core of the GP process is the patient-centred approach which allowed them to anticipate discussion with the patient and their family – of all potential events associated with the disease, its evolution and its psychosocial impact as strongly as recommended [3, 20, 21]. Contrary to the conclusions of Beernaert's study [5], the GPs in our sample deemed these discussions necessary, emphasizing the importance of their being held early, clearly and truthfully with patients and families, in order to explore their feelings and aspirations from diagnosis to treatment cessation, and even to place of death. Moreover, our study focused on the necessity to include GPs in these new programs. For example, in our study, the GPs could not define the most adequate moment for these discussions to be prompted and held; in practice they tried to seize the most suitable time, such as when patients left the hospital, or when asked a question from the family.

Our study showed that anticipating potential events allowed GPs to devise end-of-life projects which met the aspirations of patients and their families. For these physicians, respecting patient choices was critical to designing a suitable end-of-life project. Their underlying objective was to ensure the highest quality of life possible during the "time their patients had left to live". Our phenomenological analysis of the lived experiences GPs reported led us to identify the 3 categories of Slort et al.'s ACA training model (Availability, Current issues, Anticipation) [11, 22] as well as the criteria associated with these categories, such as GP availability (listening to patients, spending time with them, contacting them by phone, the multi-dimensional management of issues, and the anticipation of events (end-of-life project, respecting choices). Though GPs found this model valuable, a study comparing an ACA-trained group of GPs and a control group using the Roter Interaction Analysis System (RIAS) did not find any significant difference in palliative care management efficacy [23]. Even though our purposive-selected GPs had not received specialized palliative care training (except one), they were able to muster and implement a patient-centred professional approach.

For these reasons, our study allows us to hypothesise that patient-centred approach training could improve the quality of communication with patients about end-of-life issues, particularly developing lived experience interview skills using phenomenological attitudes [24].

Beyond applying the many available disease-specific indicators, this person-centred approach could be a useful skill to identify patients in need of palliative care. Similarly to the Thoonsen study design [5], it would be interesting to conduct a RCT with GPs in the intervention group trained to develop a phenomenological patient-centred approach.

Strengths and limitations

Our approach to this work allowed us to meet our objective of a better understanding of how French GPs provide palliative care in at-home end-of-life settings, what their needs may be, and what skills and resources they mobilize for these interventions. The strength of our study lies in our choice to use phenomenological analysis, which enabled the emergence of unexpected categories. Also, we chose to further examine these categories with semiopragmatic analysis in order to highlight the most relevant ones: the patient-centred approach paradigm which enables anticipation— and collaborative discussion — of potential events to facilitate the design and implementation of an end-of-life project which meets the aspirations of the palliative care patient. Our study did suffer from a minor limitation. In spite of having received training on comprehensive interviews, our investigator initially lacked the experience to carry out phenomenological interviews, which should include timely prompts (the key to sound data collection). However, the investigator's technique quickly improved under the supervision of the experts. Nonverbal data was not collected. Triangulation was properly achieved with the investigator and two transcript analysis experts. To our knowledge, no other such study using semiopragmatic analysis has been performed; the fact that the categories were then organized hierarchically and logically — as planned — did assign meaning to the phenomena studied while limiting investigator bias.

Practical consequences and perspectives

The findings from this study highlight the need for specific palliative training for GPs and for setting up palliative care coordinating teams; also, suggestions are made regarding strategies to improve GPs' palliative care practices.

- In addition to the development of palliative care identification indicators, specific training programs based on an interview centered on a patient-lived experience for dealing with human suffering and the caregiving relationship (two central issues in palliative care) should be offered to GP trainees so they may hone relationship, communication and emotional skills. This is essential given the central role expected of GPs as experts in discussing end-of-life questions.
- Anticipating and eliciting all possible events is essential and concerns all the dimensions of care (physical, psychosocial, spiritual and emotional). Discussions must be held early at home between patients, their families and the physician (the "family conference" in Bruera's model [25]), and multidisciplinary evaluations must be conducted regularly.
- A "shared care" process, developed jointly with the family, and other primary and palliative referring care providers, should be validated and coordinated institutionally. Today, in France, such coordination remains informal and the workload proves to be too heavy for a single GP providing at-home care. The coordination of primary care and hospital care services could be centralized within organizations dedicated to supportive care and possessing the entire array of necessary resources (physicians, nurses, physiotherapists, psychologists, nutritionists, spiritual care, and social workers). An approach such as a coordinated comprehensive care program, would meet the expectations of GPs and correspond to what they attempt to achieve informally.
- Future perspectives are to carry out additional research and experiments on the development of supportive care and on the coordination between primary care and hospital care.

Conclusion

In summary, our study showed that, despite a relative lack of specialized specific end-of-life training, the GPs in our sample devised a patient-centred approach to palliative care based on their professional values. This process allowed them to anticipate all potential events and discuss them with patients and families. These discussions generated opportunities for GPs to design personalized palliative care projects for the remaining time left to live hand in hand with their patients. Nevertheless, GPs cannot be expected to individually provide comprehensive care. The development and organization of coordinating structures, whether institutional or within primary care facilities and networks, has become critical to provide coordinated and diversified care to patients from a multi-disciplinary team, integrating and complementing the activities of GPs.

Abbreviations

ACA: Availability current issues anticipation; COREQ: COnsolidated criteria for reporting qualitative research; CPP: Comité de protection des personnes; GP: General practice or general practitioner; MASCC: Multinational association of supportive care in cancer; PIG: Prognostic indicator guide; RADPAC: Radboud indicators for palliative care needs; RCT: Randomised control trial; RIAS: Roter interaction analysis system; SPICT: Supportive and palliative care indicators tool; WHO: World health organization

Acknowledgements

We would like to thank the 15 GPs who participated and Sylvain Billere (French Comptoir) for translation work.

Funding

This study had no funding.

Authors' contributions

AOE, GB, FL designed the study. FL collected the data. AOE, FL, GB analyzed and interpreted the data. AOE, GB, MB, PS1, SP, GN, PS2, JN (native English speaker) were major contributors in writing the manuscript and all authors read and approved the final manuscript. PS1 corresponding to Philippe Serayet, PS2 to Pierre Senesse.

Competing interests

"The authors declare that they have no competing interests".

Consent for publication

Participants have provided written consent for publication of the information contained in Table 3.

Author details

[1]Department of General Medicine, University of Montpellier, Montpellier, France. [2]CEPS Platform, University of Montpellier, Montpellier, France. [3]Epsylon EA4556, Dynamic of Human Abilities and Health Behaviors, University of Montpellier, Montpellier, France. [4]Inserm U1061, Montpellier, France. [5]Université de Montpellier, U1061, Montpellier, France. [6]SIRIC Montpellier Cancer, Institut Régional du Cancer de Montpellier (ICM), Montpellier, France. [7]Department of Clinical Nutrition and Gastroenterology and supportive Care, Institut Régional du Cancer de Montpellier (ICM), Montpellier, France. [8]Centre de Médecine Générale, 2 rue IBN Sinai dit AVICENNE, Cabestany 66330, France.

References

1. ONFV Observatoire national de la Fin de Vie. Rapport annuel : fin de vie des personnes agées. http://www.soin-palliatif.org/actualites/nouveau-rapport-lobservatoire-national (décembre 2013). Accessed 10 Oct 2016.
2. Thoonsen B, Vissers K, Verhagen S, Prins J, van Weel C, Groot M, et al. Training general practitionners in early identification and anticipatory palliative care planning: a randomized controlled trial. BMC Fam Pract. 2015. doi:10.1186/s12875-015-0342-6.
3. Scotté F. Aprés-cancer et soins palliatifs précoces. La lettre du cancérologue. 2015;28 Suppl 8:4–5.
4. Meeussen K, Van den Block L, Bossuyt N, Bilsen J, Echteld M, Van Casteren V, et al. GPs' awareness of patients' preference for place of death. Br J Gen Pract. 2009. doi:10.3399/bjgp09X454124.
5. Thoonsen B, Engels Y, van Rijswijk E, Verhagen S, van Weel C, Groot M, et al. Early identification of palliative care patients in general practice: development of RADboud indicators for PAlliative care needs (RADPAC). Br J Gen Pract. 2012. doi:10.3399/bjgp12X654597.
6. Beernaert K, et al. Early identification of palliative care needs by family physicians: A qualitative study of barriers and facilitators from the perspective of family physicians, community nurses and patients. Palliat Med. 2014;28(6):480–90.
7. Mitchell GK. How well do general practitioners deliver palliative care? A systematic review. Palliat Med. 2002;16(6):457–64.
8. Groot MM, Vernooij-Dassen MJ, Crul BJ, Grol RP. General practitioners (GPs) and palliative care: perceived tasks and barriers in daily practice. Palliat Med. 2005;19(2):111–8.
9. Sullivan AM, Lakoma MD, Block SD. The status of medical education in End-of-life care. A national report. J Gen Intern Med. 2003;18(9):685–95.
10. Sullivan AM, Warren AG, Lakoma MD, Liaw KR, Hwang D, Block SD. End-of-life care in the curriculum: a national study of medical education deans. Acad Med. 2004;79(8):760–8.
11. Slort W, Blankestein AH, Deliens L, Van der Horst HE. Facilitators and barriers for GP- patient communication in palliative care: a qualitative study among GPs, patients, and-of-life consultants. Br J Gen Pract. 2011. doi:10.3399/bjgp11X567081.
12. Nicourt A. Evaluation de l'implication du médecin généraliste dans la prise de décision d'entrée en soins palliatifs lors d'une hospitalisation. Human health and pathology (2014). http://dumas.ccsd.cnrs.fr/dumas-01075483/document. Accessed 10 Oct 2016.
13. Tong A, Sainsbury P, Craig J. Consolidated criteria for reporting qualitative research (COREQ): a 32-item checklist for interviews and focus groups. Int J for Quality in Health Care. 2007;19(6):349.
14. Article du Code de Santé publique L 1123–7 Protection des personnes en matière de santé. Legifrance (2015). https://www.legifrance.gouv.fr/affichCodeArticle.do?cidTexte=LEGITEXT000006072665&idArticle=LEGIARTI000006685880&dateTexte=&categorieLien=cid. Accessed 10 Oct 2016.
15. Glaser BG, Strauss AA. La découverte de la théorie ancrée. Stratégies pour la recherche qualitative. Paris: Armand Colin; 2010.
16. Guillemette F. L'approche de la Grounded Theory; pour innover? Recherches Qualitatives. 2006;26(1):32–50. http://www.recherche-qualitative.qc.ca/documents/files/revue/edition_reguliere/numero26(1)/fguillemette_ch.pdf. Accessed 5 Feb 2017.
17. Peirce CS. Pragmatisme et pragmaticisme. Tiercelin C et Trabaud P editors. Paris: Les éditions du cerf; 2002.
18. Oude Engberink A, Carbonnel F, David M, Norton J, Bourrel G, Boulenger JP, et al. Management of current psychiatric disorders : a French qualitative study. Can J Psychiatry. 2016;61(7):413–21. doi:10.1177/0706743716639922.
19. Bruera E, Hui D. Conceptual models for integrating palliative care at cancer centers. J Palliat Med. 2012;15(11):1260–9.
20. Temel JS, Greer JA, Muzikansky A, Gallagher ER, Admane S, Jackson VA, et al. Early palliative care for patients with metastatic Non–small-cell lung cancer. N Engl J Med. 2010. doi:10.1056/NEJMoa1000678.
21. Greer JA, Jackson VA, Meier DE, Temel JS. Early integration of palliative services with standard oncology care for patients with advanced cancer. CA Cancer J Clin. 2013. doi:10.3322/caac.21192.
22. Slort W, Blankenstein AH, Wanrooij BS, van der Horst HE, Deliens L. The ACA training programme to improve communication between general practitioners and their palliative care patients: development and applicability. BMC Palliat Care. 2012. doi:10.1186/1472-684X-11-9.
23. Kumar SP, Goyal M, Sisodia V, Kumar VK. Availability, current issues, and anticipation training for clinician-patient communication in palliative care: learning and doing or learning by doing? Indian J Palliat Care. 2014. doi:10.4103/0973-1075.138405.
24. Stewart M, Brown JB, Weston WW, McWhinney IR, McWilliam CL, Freeman TR. Patient-centered medicine: transforming the clinical method. 2nd ed. Abingdon: Radcliffe Medical Press; 2003.
25. Bruera E, Hui D. Conceptual models for integrating palliative care at cancer centers. J Palliat Med. 2012. doi:10.1089/jpm.2012.0147.

2

Primary health care organizational characteristics associated with better accessibility: data from the QUALICO-PC survey in Quebec

Andrée-Anne Paré-Plante[1,2*], Antoine Boivin[3,4,5], Djamal Berbiche[2,6], Mylaine Breton[2,6] and Maryse Guay[2,6,7]

Abstract

Background: First-contact accessibility remains an important problem in Canada, with this indicator staying the worst of all Organization for Economic Co-operation and Development countries. In the province of Quebec, a number of primary healthcare (PHC) organizations have adopted measures to improve access (e.g. advance access scheduling, expanded nursing role, electronic medical record, financial incentives). The impact of those changes is unknown. The goal of this study is to assess which PHC organizations' characteristics are associated with improved first-contact accessibility.

Methods: We conducted a secondary data analysis of the Quebec survey, conducted as part of the QUALICO-PC study on primary care performance. QUALICO-PC is a cross-sectional study to assess quality, costs and equity in PHC across 35 countries and jurisdictions. Organizational characteristics were measured from the family practitioners' questionnaire. First-contact accessibility was measured from the patient questionnaire filled by patients who received care in the participating PHC organizations. Multi-level logistic regression was used to assess the association of organizational characteristics as predictors of patient-reported accessibility.

Results: A total of 218 family practitioners participated in the study with 1798 of their patients. PHC organizations characteristics associated with increased first-contact accessibility included the possibility to have a same-day appointment or to walk in the clinic without an appointment, higher number of physicians per clinic and higher number of hours worked by the family physician. Electronic medical record and expanded nursing role were not associated with increased accessibility.

Conclusions: Same-day access and higher family physician working hours are associated with improved patient-reported accessibility. Other PHC organizations characteristics targeted by recent reforms were not associated with improved accessibility.

Keywords: Primary health care, Quebec, Survey, Secondary data analysis, First-contact accessibility

* Correspondence: andree-anne.pare-plante@usherbrooke.ca
[1]Département de Médecine de Famille et de Médecine d'Urgence de l'Université de Sherbrooke, Campus de Longueuil, 150 place Charles-Le Moyne, 9e étage, Longueuil J4K 0A8, Canada
[2]Centre de recherche Charles-Le Moyne - Saguenay–Lac-Saint-Jean sur les innovations en santé, Campus de Longueuil, 150 place Charles-Le Moyne, 9e étage, Longueuil J4K 0A8, Canada
Full list of author information is available at the end of the article

Background

Primary health care (PHC) is the first level of care for the patient, his family and his community as defined by WHO [1]. PHC serves four main functions: accessibility, continuity, comprehensiveness and coordination [2]. Accessibility is a dimension of the patient's experience of care that can be measured to assess the performance of PHC. One of the indicators frequently used to measure accessibility is first-contact accessibility, defined by the ease to have a timely appointment with a PHC provider [3].

Different levels of PHC characteristics influence its performance [4]. The system level is where the government policies, the funding of health care and the provider remuneration act as factors on PHC. The context level is where the practice setting and its community integration affect PHC performance. Finally, the practice level is where specific characteristics of clinics influence their performance on care delivery. This study will look at organizational characteristics of PHC organizations, specifically resources and types and scope of services, and their effect on first-contact accessibility.

First-contact accessibility remains an important concern in Canada, with this indicator staying among the worst of all countries participating in international surveys on PHC performance [5, 6]. During the past decade, primary care reforms in the Canadian province of Quebec have sought to improve access to PHC [7, 8] and other dimensions of PHC performance [9]. It started with the implementation of Family Medicine Groups in 2002 and integration of the interdisciplinary team into these Family Medicine Groups in 2013 [10] with expanded nursing roles (nurse practitioners and clinical nurses in chronic disease prevention and management). Family Medicine Groups are family practitioners working in a clinic with other health professionals to dispense health services to a population of registered patients [11]. The electronic medical records were progressively used in a majority of organizations with incentives for PHC organizations to adopt them between 2002 and 2017 [10]. Since 2010, advanced access, a scheduling method designed to offer same-day appointments and meet the demand for care without a waiting-list, has been highly recommended through financial incentives and policies to be implemented across PHC organizations. All of these innovations were adopted with variation between practices. The actual impact of these changes in PHC practices on access, on which this article is focusing, is not well known.

In Quebec, prior to PHC reforms, attributes of PHC organizations associated with increased first-contact accessibility included the presence of a nurse and the number of family practitioners in the clinic being greater than 5 [9]. In a recent study conducted in Ontario (Canada), the number of years of practice of a family practitioner was the sole practice characteristic associated with increased first-contact accessibility [12]. However, the association between practice characteristics and first-contact accessibility has not been studied after PHC reforms in Quebec.

The **objective** of this study is to identify organizational characteristics of PHC practices associated with better first-contact accessibility.

Methods

Study design

This study is based on a secondary analysis of the Quebec survey data collected in a larger international cross-sectional study on PHC performance: the Quality and Costs of Primary Care in Europe (QUALICO-PC) Study [13]. QUALICO-PC is a cross-sectional survey started in 2010 to assess quality, costs and equity in PHC across 35 countries. Each participating Canadian province is being considered a separate jurisdiction in the QUALICO-PC design, with its own sampling but similar questionnaires [14]. The Quebec QUALICO-PC survey was conducted between 2013 and 2014. The complete methodology of QUALICO-PC study has been described elsewhere [13].

Study population and sample

Two groups of participants were recruited: family practitioners in PHC organizations and patients receiving care within this PHC organization by the family practitioners. Family practitioners were identified through stratified random sampling of all Quebec family practitioners, with a maximum of one participating family physician per PHC organization. The sampling of the family practitioners was obtained from a random list of 2000 family practitioners stratified by four types of regions: 1) academic (having an established faculty of medicine with high density population), 2) peripheral (being close to the academic region with high density population), 3) intermediate (having regional health care centers with moderate density population), and 4) remote (being large territories with low density population). Inclusion criteria for the family practitioners were to provide PHC services and to have a valid e-mail address. The exclusion criteria were to practice in the isolated region of Northern Quebec, or to be disengaged from the public healthcare system (representing fewer than 3.2% of all family physicians in the province [15]).

Family practitioner participants were recruited by the QUALICO-PC study team in Quebec hosted at the Quebec National Institute of Public Health. They received two consecutive invitation e-mails to participate; if they had not responded, they received later a phone call by a member of the research team.

Following the family practitioner's recruitment, the research package was sent to his clinic: the family practitioner survey, the patient experience surveys as well as the consent forms for the participants.

Patients receiving usual care in participating PHC organizations were targeted for the experience of care survey. The inclusion criteria for the patients were to be 18 years of age and over, and to speak and understand written French or English. Patients were recruited by receptionists of participating PHC clinics. The first ten patients of the participating family practitioner who presented themselves on a typical day of work were asked to participate in the study. All participants provided written informed consent.

Data source

Two types of surveys were used to collect in-depth information regarding primary care activities: providers and patients. The surveys were developed by the QUALICO-PC team and published elsewhere [16]. They were translated in French by the Quebec research team. The family practitioner survey provided data on PHC organizational characteristics. It was completed by family practitioners on paper and sent back by mail to the research team. The patient experience survey was completed on paper by the patients before and after their appointment with their family practitioner in the waiting room. The family practitioners did not know which of their patients participated. The patient experience survey were also sent back by mail to the research team.

Conceptual model

The conceptual model used in this study is shown in Fig. 1. It was adapted from Hogg and al. [4], which postulates an association between PHC organizational characteristics and its performance, including first-contact accessibility. PHC organizational characteristics are further classified according to dimensions developed by Lévesque and al. [17].

Study variables

The questions in the surveys were of different types: scaled questions, open-ended questions with numerical answers, multiple choice questions, and dichotomous questions. The independent variables are the PHC organizational characteristics (Fig. 1): number of family practitioners and physicians of all specialties in the clinic, use of specific equipment and/or electronic medical records, schedule and opening hours of the clinic, number of hours worked and the number of patients seen by the doctor on a typical day, and the presence of a nurse providing primary care services in the PHC organization. The dependent variable is first-contact accessibility, as reported by the patient participants when answering yes or no to the question: "Were you able to get the appointment with your doctor as quickly as you wanted?" This question was well validated [16, 18] and is considered to be the best question of the QUALICO-PC questionnaires to measure first-contact accessibility [19].

Participant characteristics were used as co-variates, including patients' characteristics (sex, age, income, level of fluency in French or English, education, general health status and presence of chronic conditions) and family practitioners' characteristics (sex and age).

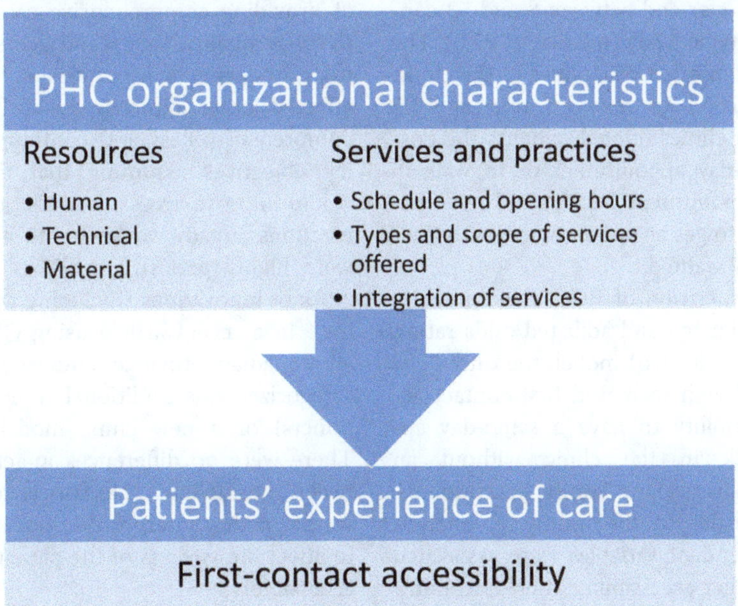

Fig. 1 Conceptual model. Legend: Adapted from Hogg et al. [4] and Lévesque et al. [14]

Analysis

Descriptive participant characteristics (patients and family practitioners) were assessed. All data were analysed in a multilevel model as the patient data was nested in the family practitioner's data. The first step was identifying associations between PHC organizations' characteristics and first-contact accessibility, using a bivariate regression analysis. Then, using a multivariate regression analysis, where all the variables were included, adjustment was made for possible confounding factors (patients' characteristics and practitioners' characteristics). Statistical significance was set at $p < 0.05$. All analyses were performed with Statistical Analysis System (SAS Institute Inc. Cary, NC, version 9.4).

Results

In total, 218 family practitioners working in 194 different PHC organizations participated in the study with 1798 of their patients. The response rate for the family practitioners was 17% with an average of 8 patient participants each. The descriptive analysis of both samples of patients and family practitioners are presented in Table 1.

The study sample for the family practitioners is representative for age and sex (FMOQ 2013). Females patients were over-represented (two thirds of respondents), but the patient sample was representative of the Quebec population for education and presence of a chronic illness [6].

In participating PHC organizations, the total number of family practitioners ranged from one to 31, the median being 4.75 family practitioners per clinic. The scope of services offered by family practitioners in the clinics varied between 3 and 80 h worked per week (median of 38.5) as a family practitioner and between 8 and 53 contacts with patients on a typical day (median of 27.5). The number of physicians from other disciplines in the clinic, ranged from none (85.6%) to between one and 25 (14.6%). The majority of clinics offered patients the possibility to have a same-day appointment or to walk in the clinic without an appointment (95.2%) and most patients (76.1%) were able to get an appointment with their doctor as quickly as they wanted.

Table 2 shows the association of PHC characteristics and access using non-adjusted and adjusted odds ratios. Using the bivariate (non-adjusted) model, the only PHC characteristic associated with increased first-contact accessibility was the possibility to have a same-day appointment or to walk in the clinic without an appointment. When adjusting for family practitioners' and patients' characteristics in the multilevel analysis model, two more independent variables were associated with increased first-contact accessibility: increased number of physicians from other disciplines in the clinic and increased number of hours worked per week by the family practitioner. Technical resources with the presence of specialized equipment in the clinic (mainly radiology and surgical equipment) was associated with decreased accessibility. The presence of nurses offering primary care services in the clinic was not associated with first-contact accessibility.

Discussion

Accessibility, especially first-contact accessibility is a fundamental issue in contemporary PHC. To our knowledge, this is the first study to examine the association between practice characteristics and better first-contact accessibility after PHC reforms in Quebec. The main finding of this study was that first-contact accessibility increased almost threefold when there was a possibility for patients to get a same-day appointment or walk-in clinic appointment in their own primary care practice. Practices where family practitioners worked longer hours per week also reported increased access.

Authors could not observe differences in access with two important targets of the PHC reforms: the use of electronic medical record and the presence of a nurse. Absence of association with nurses' role is consistent with the findings of another study in Canada [12] but different from a study conducted before the PHC reform and Family medicine group implementation in Quebec [9]. Nurses' roles in Quebec PHC during the past decade has focused mainly on increased uptake of preventive care and chronic disease management. It also has been a target of the reform to implement the goals of the patient-centered medical home into Family medicine groups [20]. The patient-centered medical home is an interprofessional model of PHC organization that aims at providing comprehensive care with particular objectives for quality, safety and access to care [20]. Accordingly, the effects of nurses in this context may have affected other dimensions of PHC performance (e.g. comprehensiveness and continuity) despite explicit policy objectives assuming that the presence of nurses would improve access. It is also possible that PHC organizations already working with nurses before the reform were highly performing clinics more opened to other types of innovations (including advanced access scheduling). In a recent article using QUALICO-PC data from all Canadian provinces, individual PHC practices were categorized as a traditional clinic model (eg. solo practitioners) or a new clinic model (eg. group practices). There were no differences in terms of accessibility between the models [21]. This is concordant with the observation that interprofessional PHC organizations tend to affect dimensions of the patient experience other than accessibility.

The number of physicians from other specialties working in the clinic was associated with better perceived

Table 1 Participant characteristics

	Frequency (n)	Proportion (%)	Khi-2 (*p*-value)
Patients			
Sex	1765[a]		0.1164
Male	593	33.6	
Female	1172	66.4	
Age	1752[a]		0.4720
18–25	100	5.7	
25–34	213	12.2	
35–44	249	14.2	
45–54	351	20.0	
55–64	393	22.4	
65 and over	446	25.5	
Income	1731[a]		0.4777
Below average	377	21.8	
About average	1011	58.4	
Above average	343	19.4	
Fluency in French or English	1752[a]		0.3931
Fluent	1520	86.8	
Sufficiently	140	8.0	
Moderately	46	2.6	
Little	35	2.0	
Not at all	11	0.6	
Education	1749[a]		0.2534
No qualifications, primary, or lower secondary	275	15.7	
Upper secondary education (grades 10–12)	622	35.6	
Post-secondary education (college, undergraduate)	852	48.7	
Employment status	1798[a]		0.0340
Working	960	53.4	
Retired	523	29.1	
Unable to work	142	7.9	
Other	192	10.7	
General health status	1778[a]		0.0044
Very good	416	23.4	
Good	881	49.6	
Fair	420	23.6	
Poor	61	3.4	
Chronic conditions	1759[a]		0.2394
Yes	918	52.2	
No	841	47.8	
Family practitioners			
Sex	215[a]		0.5886
Male	97	45.1	
Female	118	54.9	
Age	211[a]		0.6703
25–34	34	16.1	

Table 1 Participant characteristics *(Continued)*

	Frequency (n)	Proportion (%)	Khi-2 (*p*-value)
35–44	31	14.7	
45–54	64	30.3	
55 and over	82	38.9	

[a]Total n are different due to different partial non-response rate to each question

accessibility by patients. However, this variable was not distributed normally and the majority of PHC organizations had no specialists. It is possible that well performing PHC organizations offered medical services not just from family practitioners or that presence of physicians from other disciplines in the clinic was associated with other characteristics of practices influencing access that we did not measure. It is concordant with findings from the Miedema et al. study mentioned before.

A surprizing result of this study is the overall high degree of perceived access by PHC patients, with over 76% of respondents being able to get an appointment as quickly as they want. Before the reform, only 10% of patients having access to a primary care provider in Quebec were confident they could get an appointment with

Table 2 Association of organizational characteristics with patient-reported first-contact accessibility

Organizational characteristics	OR	CI 95%	*p*-value	Adjusted OR*	CI 95%*	*p*-value*
Human resources						
Number of family practitioners in the clinic[a]	1.00	(0.97–1.03)	0.89	0.96	(0.89–1.03)	0.27
Number of physicians from other disciplines in the clinic[a]	1.05	(0.996–1.10)	0.07	1.13	(1.03–1.24)	0.01
Technical and material resources						
Presence of specific equipment in the clinic[c]	0.98	(0.95–1.00)	0.08	0.89	(0.83–0.96)	0.002
Use of information technology for different tasks in the clinic[d]	0.98	(0.94–1.02)	0.37	1.02	(0.92–1.14)	0.67
Schedule and opening hours						
Typical amount of time scheduled for a regular visit with the family practitioner (in minutes)[a]	1.00	(0.98–1.02)	0.89	1.03	(0.99–1.07)	0.21
Number of opening hours per day[a]	1.01	(0.97–1.05)	0.54	1.10	(0.96–1.26)	0.18
Percentage of visits with a scheduled appointment[a]	1.00	(0.999–1.01)	0.12	1.00	(0.98–1.01)	0.66
Possibility to obtain a same-day appointment or to walk-in the clinic without an appointment[b]	1.66	(1.01–2.74)	0.04	2.94	(1.15–7.51)	0.02
Type and scope of services						
Number of hours worked per week by the family practitioner[a]	1.00	(0.99–1.01)	0.39	1.03	(1.00–1.06)	0.03
Number of hours per week worked by the family practitioner in this clinic[a]	1.00	(0.99–1.01)	0.56	0.99	(0.97–1.01)	0.26
Number of contacts with patients by the family practitioner in a typical day[a]	0.99	(0.98–1.00)	0.30	0.99	(0.97–1.01)	0.42
Integration of services						
Primary care services offered independently by a nurse in the clinic[e]	1.03	(0.90–1.18)	0.69	1.03	(0.90–1.18)	0.69

*Results are adjusted for patients and family practitioners characteristics
OR superior to 1 indicates an increase in first-contact accessibility
[a]Difference with every increase of one unit for these continuous variables (number of family practitioners, physicians, minutes)
[b]Difference between the presence or the absence of this characteristic
[c]Difference with every additional equipment present in the clinic
[d]Difference with every additional task performed with information technology
[e]Difference with every additional service provided independently by a nurse

their regular doctor if they urgently needed it [22]. This observed difference is important because in recent years, incentives for family practitioners in Quebec were to improve the ease to get a timely appointment with a family practitioner or with another healthcare professional. One should keep in mind that QUALICO-PC participants were recruited from patients who successfully obtained an appointment in primary care with their regular family practitioner, which may have overestimated our measures of patient-reported accessibility. Reported first-contact accessibility was much higher in our study than in general population surveys [6], but similar to studies surveying patients who already had access to a family practitioner [12].

Limitations

The cross-sectional nature of the family practitioner survey and the patient experience survey could not allow us to establish causality between first-contact accessibility and organizational characteristics.

Other limitations are those related to a secondary data analysis study. The surveys were not conceptualized only to measure first-contact accessibility but all dimensions of PHC and they were created in Europe [16] although validated for use in Quebec [23].

A desirability bias could also have occurred for instance if practitioners tried to give a better overall picture of their practice or if patients would embellish their ease to get an appointment. This bias could therefore have the effect of incorrectly classifying responders. We have no way to evaluate the magnitude of this effect if it is present. Work records of the clinics were not available to confirm the data collected through the family practitioners' answers.

The main limitation of this study is the low response rate of family practitioners (17%). Response rate in studies involving physicians is a common problem. The Quebec survey had the second highest response rate among Canadian provinces participating in the QUALICO-PC study [14]. Also, characteristics of participating family practitioners and practice settings were similar to those of all family practitioners in Quebec. The last data on practice profiles show 50% of family practitioners were female with a mean age of 50 years [24]. Generalizability of the results should be interpreted with caution; sampled family physicians may have worked in more highly performing practices than usual which could contribute to the overall high reported access. Information on the family practitioners and their practices that did not participate in the study was not available. Despite these limitations and overall low response rate, the data collected through the Canadian arm of QUALICO-PC represent the largest dataset on the quality and organization of primary care data in Canada. The patient sample was the same as the Quebec population for education and presence of a chronic illness. The female over-representation in the study is typical of recent cross-sectional studies in primary care in Canada [5, 25]. All the same, this gives us confidence in results of the study.

Policy implications

Our findings suggest that supporting PHC organizations to increase same-day appointment and walk-in clinics could increase first-contact access for patients. This is consistent with the goals of the recent PHC reform, most notably the implementation of Family Medicine Groups [26]. With this implementation, different financial incentives for family practitioners were provided to increase their workload, to support practice in the primary care settings outside the hospitals, and to promote wide-spread use of advanced access scheduling [27].

Conclusions

This study looked at what determines better first-contact accessibility at the organizational level in PHC organizations. First-contact accessibility increased most with the possibility for patients to have a same-day appointment or to walk-in the clinic. While patient-reported accessibility also increased with the number of hours worked per week by the family practitioner and the presence of physicians from other disciplines in the clinic, it was not associated with the use of electronic medical records or the presence of nurses. The advanced access model for practices is being implemented throughout Quebec and in the next years, it will be important to evaluate the effect of these changes on organizational characteristics and first-contact accessibility for patients.

Abbreviations

PHC: Primary health care; QUALICO-PC: Quality and Costs of Primary Care

Acknowledgments

AAPP would like to thank the Centre de recherche – Hôpital Charles-Le Moyne for statistical and bibliographical support for this research. The authors also thank Danièle Francoeur and her team at the Quebec National Institute of Public Health for the collection of the QUALICO-PC data in Quebec.

Funding

AAPP was funded by a University of Sherbrooke start-up research fund and family medicine advanced skill residency position. AB is funded by a Canada Research Chair in Patient and Public Partnership. MB is funded by Canada Research Chair in Clinical Governance in Primary Health Care. This research was completed independently and none of the funding bodies had an influence on the study design, data collection, analysis and data interpretation.

Authors' contributions

AAPP, AB, MB and MG conceptualized the manuscript and were involved in writing. AAPP and DB completed the analysis. All authors were involved in the interpretation of the results, read and approved the final manuscript.

Consent for publication
Not applicable.

Competing interests
The authors declare that they have no competing interests.

Author details
[1]Département de Médecine de Famille et de Médecine d'Urgence de l'Université de Sherbrooke, Campus de Longueuil, 150 place Charles-Le Moyne, 9e étage, Longueuil J4K 0A8, Canada. [2]Centre de recherche Charles-Le Moyne - Saguenay–Lac-Saint-Jean sur les innovations en santé, Campus de Longueuil, 150 place Charles-Le Moyne, 9e étage, Longueuil J4K 0A8, Canada. [3]Département de Médecine de Famille et Médecine d'Urgence de l'Université de Montreal, Montreal, Canada. [4]Centre de Recherche du Centre Hospitalier de l'Université de Montréal, Montreal, Canada. [5]Institut de Recherche en Santé Publique de l'Université de Montréal, Montreal, Canada. [6]Département des Sciences de la Santé Communautaire de l'Université de Sherbrooke, Sherbrooke, Canada. [7]Direction de Santé Publique, CISSS de la Montérégie-Centre, Longueuil, Canada.

References

1. World Health Organization. Declaration of Alma-Ata. In: International Conference on Primary Health Care; 1978-09-06; Alma-Ata, USSR; 1978.
2. Starfield B, Shi L, Macinko J. Contribution of primary care to health systems and health. Milbank Q. 2005;83(3):457–502.
3. Haggerty J, Burge F, Lévesque J-F, Gass D, Pineault R, Beaulieu M-D, et al. Operational definitions of attributes of primary health care: consensus among Canadian experts. Ann Fam Med. 2007;5(4):336–44.
4. Hogg W, Rowan M, Russell G, Geneau R, Muldoon L. Framework for primary care organizations: the importance of a structural domain. Int J Qual Health Care. 2008;20(5):308–13.
5. Bénigéri M. Perceptions et expériences de la population: Le Québec comparé. 2017. Accessed 3 Nov 2017.
6. Lévesque J-F, Bénigéri M. L'expérience de soins de la population: Le Québec comparé. Résultats de l'enquête internationale du Commonwealth Fund de 2010 auprès de la population de 18 ans et plus. Québec: Le Comissaire à la santé et au bien-être; 2011.
7. Breton M, Ricard J, Walter N. Connecting orphan patients with family physicians: differences among Quebec's access registries. Can Fam Physician. 2012;58(9):921.
8. Clair M, Aucoin L, Bergman H, Côté R, Ipersiel P, LeBoutillier J, et al. Commission d'étude sur les services de santé et les services sociaux: Les solutions émergentes. Rapport et recommandations. Direction des communications ed. Québec: Ministère de la Santé et des Services sociaux; 2001.
9. Haggerty JL, Pineault R, Beaulieu M-D, Brunelle Y, Gauthier J, Goulet F, et al. Practice features associated with patient-reported accessibility, continuity, and coordination of primary health care. Ann Fam Med. 2008;6(2):116–23.
10. Smithman MA, Landry G, Farah R, Breton M, Groulx A. The Multi-Level, Multi-Component Primary Healthcare Reform Underway in Québec. In: North American Primary Care Research Group Annual Meeting; 2017-11-18; Montreal; 2017.
11. Breton M, Lévesque J-F, Pineault R, Hogg W. L'implantation du modèle des groupes de médecine de famille au Québec : Potentiel et limites pour l'accroissement de la performance des soins de santé primaires. Pratiques et Organisation des soins. 2011;42(2):101–9.
12. Muggah E, Hogg W, Dahrouge S, Russell G, Kristjansson E, Muldoon L, et al. Patient-reported access to primary care in Ontario: effect of organizational characteristics. Can Fam Physician. 2014;60(1):e24–31.
13. Schäfer WLA, Boerma WGW, Kringos DS, De Maeseneer J, Gress S, Heinemann S, et al. QUALICOPC, a multi-country study evaluating quality, costs and equity in primary care. BMC Fam Pract. 2011;12:115.
14. Wong ST, Chau LW, Hogg W, Teare GF, Miedema B, Breton M, et al. An international cross-sectional survey on the quality and costs of primary care (QUALICO-PC): recruitment and data collection of places delivering primary care across Canada. BMC Fam Pract. 2015;16(20):1-10.
15. Régie de l'assurance maladie du Québec. Liste des professionnels de la santé non participants ou désengagés au régime de l'assurance maladie du Québec avec adresse de pratique au Québec. 2017.
16. Schäfer WLA, Boerma WGW, Kringos DS, De Ryck E, Greß S, Heinemann S, et al. Measures of quality, costs and equity in primary health care instruments developed to analyse and compare primary care in 35 countries. Qual Prim Care. 2013;21(2):67–79.
17. Lévesque J-F, Descôteaux S, Demers N, Bénigéri M. Measuring Organizational Attributes of Primary Care: A review and classification of measurement items used in international questionnaires. Montréal: Institut national de santé publique du Québec; 2012.
18. Shi L, Starfield B, Xu J. Validating the adult primary care assessment tool. J Fam Pract. 2001;50(2):161-75.
19. Premji K, Ryan B, Hogg W, Wodchis WP. Patients' perceptions of Access to Primary Care in Ontario: An Analysis of the QUALICO-PC Patient Experiences Survey. In: North American Primary Care Research Group Annual Meeting; 2017-11-18; Montreal; 2017.
20. Katz A, Herpai N, Smith G, Aubrey-Bassler K, Breton M, Boivin A, et al. Alignment of Canadian primary care with the patient medical home model: a QUALICO-PC study. Ann Fam Med. 2017;15(3):230–6.
21. Miedema B, Easley J, Thompson AE, Boivin A, Aubrey-Bassler K, Katz A, et al. Do new and traditional models of primary care differ with regard to access?: Canadian QUALICOPC study. Can Fam Physician. 2016;62(1):54–61.
22. Haggerty JL, Pineault R, Beaulieu M-D, Brunelle Y, Gauthier J, Goulet F, et al. Room for improvement: patients' experiences of primary care in Quebec before major reforms. Can Fam Physician. 2007;53(6):1057.
23. Francoeur D, Lévesque J-F, Boivin A, Breton M, Haggerty J. Questionnaires QUALICOPC Québec: Évaluation des services de première ligne dans la province de Québec; 2012.
24. Paré I. Profil de pratique des médecins omnipraticiens québécois: 2010–2011. 2013 [Available from: https://www.fmoq.org/pratique/enseignement-et-recherche/profil-de-pratique-des-medecins-omnipraticiens-quebecois-2010-2011/.
25. Dahrouge S, Hogg W, Russell G, Geneau R, Kristjansson E, Muldoon L, et al. The comparison of models of primary Care in Ontario (COMP-PC) study: methodology of a multifaceted cross-sectional practice-based study. Open Med. 2009;3(3):e149–64.
26. Rodríguez C, Pozzebon M. The implementation evaluation of primary care groups of practice: a focus on organizational identity. BMC Fam Pract. 2010;11:15.
27. Breton M, Maillet L, Pare I, Abou Malham S, Touati N. Perceptions of the first family physicians to adopt advanced access in the province of Quebec, Canada. Int J Health Plann Manage. 2017;32(4):e316-e332.

3

The implementation of health promotion in primary and community care: a qualitative analysis of the 'Prescribe Vida Saludable' strategy

Catalina Martinez[1], Gonzalo Bacigalupe[2], Josep M. Cortada[3], Gonzalo Grandes[1*], Alvaro Sanchez[1], Haizea Pombo[1], Paola Bully[1] and on behalf of the PVS group

Abstract

Background: The impact of lifestyle on health is undeniable and effective healthy lifestyle promotion interventions do exist. However, this is not a fundamental part of routine primary care clinical practice. We describe factors that determine changes in performance of primary health care centers involved in piloting the health promotion innovation 'Prescribe Vida Saludable' (PVS) phase II.

Methods: We engaged four primary health care centers of the Basque Healthcare Service in an action research project aimed at changing preventive health practices. Prescribe Healthy Life (PVS from the Spanish "Prescribe Vida Saludable) is focused on designing, planning, implementing and evaluating innovative programs to promote multiple healthy habits, feasible to be performed in routine primary health care conditions. After 2 years of piloting, centers were categorized as having high, medium, or low implementation effectiveness. We completed qualitative inductive and deductive analysis of five focus groups with the staff of the centers. Themes generated through consensual grounded qualitative analysis were compared between centers to identify the dimensions that explain the variation in actual implementation of PVS, and retrospectively organized and assessed against the Consolidated Framework for Implementation Research (CFIR).

Results: Of the 36 CFIR constructs, 11 were directly related to the level of implementation performance: *intervention source, evidence strength and quality, adaptability, design quality and packaging, tension for change, learning climate, self-efficacy, planning, champions, executing*, and *reflecting and evaluating*, with *—organizational tracking* added as a new sub-construct. Additionally, another seven constructs emerged in the participants' discourse but were not related to center performance: *relative advantage, complexity, patients' needs and resources, external policy and incentives, structural characteristics, available resources*, and *formally appointed internal implementation leaders*. Our findings indicate that the success of the implementation seems to be associated with the following components: the context, the implementation process, and the collaborative modelling.

Conclusions: Identifying barriers and enablers is useful for designing implementation strategies for health promotion in primary health care centers that are essential for innovation success. An implementation model is proposed to highlight the relationships between the CFIR constructs in the context of health promotion in primary care.

Keywords: Implementation Research, Program Evaluation, Qualitative Research, Organizational Innovation, Primary Health Care, Community Health Services, Health Promotion, Complex Interventions, Pilot Implementation

* Correspondence: gonzalo.grandes@osakidetza.eus
[1]Primary Care Research Unit of Bizkaia, Basque Healthcare Service – Osakidetza, BioCruces Health Research Institute, Luis Power 18 4th floor, Bilbao 48014, Spain
Full list of author information is available at the end of the article

Background

The impact of health behaviors and lifestyles on health outcomes is undisputed [1] and its individual, social, environmental and cultural determinants are well known [2]. Primary health care (PHC) professionals have many opportunities to promote healthy behaviors in patients with effective interventions [3, 4]. However, healthy lifestyle promotion is far from being integrated in routine primary care practice [5–7]. Our own research group has contributed to generate evidence on the effectiveness of clinical interventions for health promotion through several clinical trials [8, 9]. Nevertheless, the delivery of primary care interventions tends to stop after PHC professionals participate in such trials [10]. This lack of integration of evidence-based interventions may be explained by weaknesses in implementation strategies [11].

Implementation strategies can be defined as sets of methods, techniques, and interventions used to enhance the adoption and integration of evidence-based innovations into usual care [12]. In order to build strong implementation strategies, we need to identify factors that determine change in practice, namely, barriers and enablers of change [13]. This requires learning from the experiences of all innovation agents. However, when implementing a new intervention or practice most of the people that can participate in such research have little or no experience of change in practice and, instead of reporting determinants of change, they report what determines their current performance. In the 'Prescribe Vida Saludable' (PVS) innovative project for healthy promotion by PHC professionals we had the opportunity to explore the experiences of individuals who were actively involved in changing clinical practice in health promotion.

The aim of this inquiry is to identify core factors associated with success and barriers in the implementation of the PVS intervention and assess factors associated with better performance in its piloting phase. We describe the experience of the PHC professionals who have already been involved in innovation and how they assess the successes and challenges of the implementation of PVS. The analysis is based on Damschroder et al.'s Consolidated Framework for Implementation Research (CFIR) [14] which is outlined in the methods section as part of the analytical strategy. Identifying core constructs associated with implementation should strengthen future dissemination and inform the modeling process of sound and effective implementation strategies for PHC professionals practice redesign.

Methods

A qualitative comparative analysis design [15, 16] was used to comprehensively explore PVS implementation barriers and enablers. In addition to a comparative analysis of ongoing process indicators for each primary health care (PHC) center, the qualitative evaluation consisted of focus groups with PHC professionals involved. The study protocol was approved by the Primary Care Research Committee of the Basque Healthcare Services and by the Basque Country Clinical Research Ethics Committee.

Participants

The four participating PHC centers were a convenience sample, selected by the medical directors of the primary care districts of the Basque Healthcare Service on the basis of their previous involvement in health promotion programs or preventive practice optimization initiatives. The PHC professional teams initiated an action research process to design the local PVS implementation strategy for each center. In brief, a bottom-up decision making processes was initiated in the four participating centers to select actions to be included in the implementation strategy, based on discussion and consensus meetings among a multi-professional primary care team and community members. We refer to this method as collaborative modeling facilitated by the research team. A coordinator at each center was the liaison with the research team and leaded the process at the local level. The Department of Public Health supported the teams, with a district public health department representative attending the aforementioned monthly meetings.

The PVS project emerged as an initiative facilitated by the Primary Care Research Unit of Bizkaia (UIAPB) of the Basque Health Service (Osakidetza). The research team provided external facilitation for changing clinical practice. Other participants in the project were community-based organizations, including nine local municipality departments, six schools, four sports facilities, and two manufacturing companies, as well as local councils and senior management of several Osakidetza departments (information technology, primary care, and public health).

PVS innovation

The PVS first phase consisted of a collaborative modeling process to adapt evidence-based health promotion interventions to the specific contexts of the PHC centers and communities, and simultaneously change PHC professional organization (see Fig. 1). Most of the staff (80%) of the four participating PHC centers were actively involved in this process and they selected the 5 A's evidence-based clinical intervention (A1: Assess, A2: Advise, A3: Agree, A4: Assist, and A5: Arrange Follow-Up) to address three healthy lifestyles: healthy diet, physical activity, and smoking cessation [3, 4, 17]. The second phase of PVS was the pilot implementation to evaluate the feasibility of the strategy. This pilot study

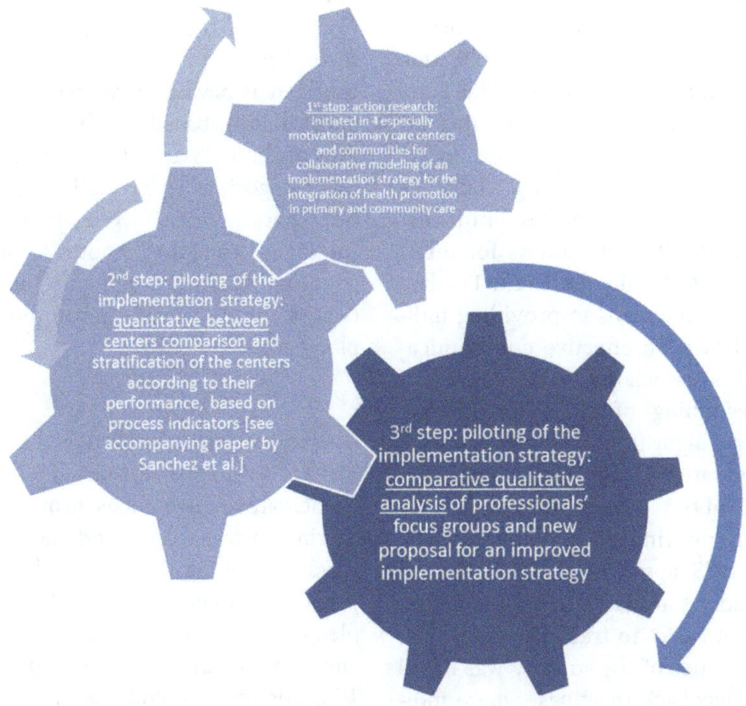

Fig. 1 PVS research steps

included all 22,459 patients 10 to 65 years old who had attended a healthcare appointment over the 2-year study period. They were assessed for physical activity, diet, and smoking in 52% of cases, 33% of them received advice at least once for changing their behavior, and 10% were prescribed lifestyle changes, with a personalized plan (see accompanying paper by Sanchez et al.).

The Primary Care Research Unit provided PHC centers with a monthly progress report outlining the results of their activities, which included indicators of assessment of habits (A1), counseling and advising (A2), and prescription of changes in behavior with tailored plans (A4). These monthly reports were a cornerstone of the audit and feedback strategy. The research team met monthly with the coordinators of the healthcare teams to evaluate the program, discuss the implementation indicators, identify ways of increasing the effectiveness of the intervention, and overall reflect on what the teams were learning about the implementation process. The coordinators organized monthly meetings in their PHC centers with the same implementation improvement objectives.

Implementation strategy

The PVS implementation strategy was focused on various levels: community involvement, top-down support from managers, bottom-up primary care organizational change, and the development of innovative e-health information and communication technologies. The study protocol has been published previously [18]. The participants adapted the 5As' strategy into a community health center's functioning plus at least one collaborative partner in the community through a collaborative modeling process. The research team facilitated a bottom-up decision making process, based on 8–10 discussion and consensus meetings among a multi-professional primary care team and community members. The intervention components did not all reside in the community health centers, A1 (Ask), for instance, could be accomplished at a school, a workplace, a PVS website link, or administrative personnel at the health center in advance of the primary care consultation. A2 (Advise) and A3 (Agree) were tasks mostly assigned to the family physicians, while the A4 (Assist) was often a role accomplished by nurses who prescribed and helped plan for health behavior modification. All the healthcare center professionals were involved in A5 (Arrange Follow Up) with client services playing an important role too.

New e-health tools were designed, tested and incorporated into the electronic health record (EHR). Screening for healthy behaviors was performed with paper-based self-report questionnaires, entered into the EHR by administrative staff, and with an electronic version publically available on the Basque Healthcare Service web portal for individual self-assessment, with online transmission of data to the EHR through a secure developed web service (see accompanying paper by Sanchez et al.). This screening provided automatic feedback to individuals and generated reminders in the EHR that prompted clinicians to implement health promotion activities guided by the PVS application integrated in the EHR information system. These reminders helped primary care staff to easily identify individuals whose lifestyles had not been assessed; to assess physical activity, diet, and smoking status of attendees; to identify those not meeting recommendations; and to select high priority populations for interventions based on data recorded in the EHR. Further, the PVS application guided clinicians in providing individually tailored advice based on effective communication of risks and benefits associated with lifestyle. It also facilitated the prescribing of plans for lifestyle modification, providing algorithms, evidence-based support, and recommendations, warnings, timetables and other information about community resources. Besides it facilitated monitoring of patients over a follow-up period. The PVS application integrated all the information, and made it available to all PHC center staff, thereby making it easier to track patients.

The fidelity and maintenance of the strategy was based on a monthly audit and feedback meetings, where indicators on patients' results were analyzed.

Implementation performance

Considering the 2-year process indicators of the PVS second phase pilot study, participating centers were categorized as having high, medium, or low implementation performance, based on their adoption and implementation of the PVS activities (see Fig. 1). One of the centers was categorized as having high and one low implementation performance, while two were assigned to the "medium" category. Another paper [see accompanying paper by Sanchez et al.] and Table 1 provide further details of the PVS intervention during the 2-year pilot implementation process.

Qualitative data collection

Staff of each of the four PHC centers were invited to participate in five focus groups (the largest center requiring two groups) and these were completed over 5 weeks (see Fig. 1). Specifically, the coordinators of the participating centers were asked to invite all the PVS implementation participants, and 75 physicians, nurses, and administrative personnel participated. An average of 15 participants attended each group (SD = 3.54). The potential pool of participants was 109 ($\overline{X} = 21.8$; SD = 4.49).

Table 1 Characteristics and implementation indicators of the primary care centers participating in this PVS pilot

		Center A	Center B	Center C	Center D
Population size		6004	5509	9915	21621
Age target in the PVS intervention, years		10–65	10–65	10–65	>10
Participation by professionals Participates/total in centre (%)	Family physicians	5/5	4/5	5/5	10/11
	Nurses	5/5	4/5	8/8	6/13
	Admission staff	5/5	3/4	5/6	5/6
	Pediatricians	1/1	0/1	2/2	0/2
	Midwives	1/1		1/1	0/2
	Others	1/1			
	Total	18/18 (100%)	11/15 (73%)	21/22 (95%)	21/34 (61%)
Community agents	Municipalities	4	2	2	1
	Schools	2	3	2	0
	Sport facilities	1	1	1	1
	Businesses	3	1	0	2
	Pharmacies	1	0	0	1
	Associations and other agencies	0	4	0	1
Two-year implementation performance indicators					
A1: % attendees assessed for physical activity, diet and smoking		3009/3635 (82.8%) (81.5–84.0%)	1640/2568 (63.7%) (62.0–65.7%)	3209/5883 (54.5%) (53.3–55.8%)	3792/10373 (36.6%) (35.6–37.5%)
A2: % of attendees advised on increasing physical activity, improving diet or smoking cessation		2136 (58.7%) (57.2–60.4%)	809 (31.5%) (29.7–33.3%)	2170 (36.9%) (35.6–38.1%)	2318 (22.3%) (21.5–23.1%)
A4: % of attendees prescribed a behavior change plan		552 (15.24%) (14.0–16.3%)	377 (14.7%) (13.3–16.1%)	406 (6.9%) (6.2–7.5%)	840 (8.1%) (7.6–8.6%)

Participants consent to their contribution to be published.

One researcher facilitated all five focus groups at the PHC centers. The research team selected this type of group interview, since one of the objectives was that all participants of each center participate jointly, in order to grasp the point of view of each individual within the group. The interviewer was selected ensuring that she had no previous direct relationship with or knowledge of participants. The discussion was guided by a set of open-ended questions to identify what factors were associated with the degree to which the PVS program had been adopted: *What are your thoughts regarding the implementation of PVS in this health center? What has been the impact of PVS on daily work? How do you interpret the indicators (participants being shown charts and graphs)? What are the factors that explain the wide variation in implementation of PVS between centers and between different members of staff within each center? What is your assessment of the way how patients are being reached? What may cause problems in the implementation and can you suggest any solutions? What are the barriers to implementation of the PVS?*

Data were shared during the interview on indicators for the sixth month of the project, from the monthly report. These data provided a clear picture of three cases depending on the degrees of success in the implementation. An observer, a representative of the public health department in the PVS efforts, accompanied the facilitator in the interviews and wrote an ethnographic report with her own analysis of the focus groups. The data analysis was ongoing, iterative, and informed by the research team's observations. The interviews were audio-recorded and transcribed for analysis.

Data analysis

A consensual qualitative research approach comprising two data analysis strategies was used to guide the systematic analysis of the barriers and enablers influencing the implementation. The two strategies included inductive and deductive data analysis to ensure not only triangulation of the data sources but also their trustworthiness.

The inductive methodology consisted of basic grounded thematic analysis. Basic themes were extracted from the transcripts analyzed separately by research team members and then consensually validated in team meetings. The ethnographic notes prepared by the observers of the group interviews also aided this thematic analysis and helped the organization of the transcribed material.

On completion of the first thematic analysis, the research team concluded that deductive analysis utilizing the CFIR model could be useful to address the wealth of data and to focus on the task of assessing implementation dimensions. This coding framework was chosen because it offers a complete taxonomy of operationally defined constructs that can influence the adoption of complex programs. CFIR constructs are organized into five major domains [15]: (1) the characteristics of the intervention, (2) the outer setting including patients' needs and resources, (3) the inner setting (i.e., how compatible the program is with existing interventions), (4) the process employed to implement the program, and (5) the characteristics of the individuals involved.

Each transcript was treated as a case and two members of the research team separately completed exhaustive within-case coding. To reach consensus, the team carried out reviews of each focus group. This within-case analysis was completed for each group and audits of the analysis were completed to ensure consistency. After completion of the within-case analysis, common themes across cases were identified and a rating value (valence) assigned to each code. These data reflect the attributes the participants associated with each of these concepts. We used the same criteria as Damschroder and Lowery [15] for assigning these ratings. Valences from +2 to −2 reflect a positive or negative influence of each construct on the organization, work processes, and/or implementation efforts [15]. The rating was completed with the same consensual data analysis as that used in the coding of the transcripts. The analysis required continuous comparison across groups, and the examination of patterns in the data. One of the researchers performed the analysis without knowing the quantitative outcomes of the health center in question to enhance the trustworthiness of the qualitative data analysis. At the end of the analysis, vignettes were selected to exemplify the CFIR dimensions and to highlight their association with the actual PVS outcomes at each center. The research team shared the analysis with the coordinators of the PHC centers to feedback the findings.

Results

What factors are associated with community health promotion and primary care innovation?

In our study, 18 of the 36 CFIR constructs proposed by Damschroder and analyzed by the research team present high levels of trustworthiness. According to the positive (+2, +1), neutral (0), or negative (−1, −2) valences assigned by participating staff, these constructs can be divided in two groups. One group includes 11 constructs associated with the actual level of success in the implementation performance; there is a trend across centers in the valences assigned by participants and this is correlated with the level of success or failure in implementation performance. The other set of seven constructs appears to be unrelated to the actual level of implementation performance (See Table 2).

For the other 18 CFIR constructs, insufficient data emerged to assess their potential association with performance. They can be considered less important for designing strategies for change in public PHC professional services. Despite the lack of data that emerged on these dimensions, they should be studied further to assess their meaning in relation to predicting implementation performance of healthy lifestyle interventions. For example, the lack of engagement of *external change agents* appeared only in one of the centers, the one which showed the highest implementation rating, and it appeared to be negatively valued (see Table 2).

Tables 3 and 4 include quotes that exemplify the dimensions that were or were not associated with the implementation performance. The valences assigned to the set of quotes are also included in each cell. The CFIR constructs not associated with the level of performance explain important barriers to and enablers of the implementation in general, but comparing the positive and negative values assigned to them by staff does not show a relation to the actual implementation observed in each center. They include: *relative advantage, complexity, patients' needs and resources, external policy and incentives, structural characteristics, available resources,* and *formally appointed internal implementation leaders.* The CFIR constructs that distinguished between health teams with low, medium, and high implementation performance included: *intervention source, evidence strength and quality, design quality and packaging, adaptability, tension for change, learning climate, self-efficacy, champions, reflecting and evaluating, planning,* and *executing.*

Our emerging conceptual implementation model for health promotion interventions synthesizes the findings. It also highlights the associations of the CFIR constructs with the implementation of innovation in community health and primary care practices (see Fig. 2). Successful implementation appears to be associated with three main components: the context, the implementation process, and the collaborative modelling. We highlight

Table 2 CFIR constructs associated with actual implementation performance

PVS Cases CFIR Constructs		Centers by level of implementation				
		High: Center A	Medium: Centers B and C		Low: Center D	
I. Intervention characteristics						
A. Intervention source		+2	+1	0	0	+ association
B. Evidence Strength & Quality		+2	+1	+1	−1	+ association
C. Relative advantage		+1	+1	+2	+1	Not associated
D. Adaptability		−2	0	−1	0	- + associated [a]
F. Complexity		−2	−1	−1	−2	Not associated
G. Design Quality & Packaging		−1	−1	+1	+1	+ association[a]
II. Outer setting						
A. Patient Needs & Resources		−1	+1	−2	−1	Not associated
D. External Policy & Incentives		−2	−1	−2	−2	Not associated
III. Inner setting						
A. Structural Characteristics		−2	−2	−2	−2	Not associated
D. Implementation climate	1. Tension for Change	+1	0	+2	−1	+ association
	6. Learning Climate	+2	0	X	−1	+ association
E. Readiness for Implementation	2. Available Resources	−2	−1	−1	−1	Not associated
IV. Characteristics of individuals						
B. Self-efficacy		+2	−1	+1	−2	+ association
V. PROCESS						
A Planning		0	0	0	−2	+ association
B Engaging	2. Formally appointed internal implementation leaders	+2	+2	+2	+1	Not associated
	3. Champions	+1	+2	X	X	+ association
C Executing		+1	0	−1	−2	+ association
D Reflecting & Evaluating		+1	+1	−1	−1	+ association
Organizational Tracking		−2	0	−2	X	- association

[a] There is a negative association with the lack of adaptability and with problems in the design and packaging of the intervention

Table 3 CFIR constructs associated with PVS performance

CFIR Constructs	Cases		
	High implementation: Center A	Medium implementation: centers B and C	Low implementation: center D
Intervention characteristics			
Intervention source	*It was a collaborative effort at all levels; everyone had internalized their commitment to health promotion.* (+2)	*We have adhered voluntarily and we have joined because we want to respond to the challenge* (of making prevention effective in increasing healthy habits). (+1)	*This is something that we initially did voluntarily but then all sorts of demands were placed on us at the same time.* (0)
Evidence strength and quality	*We are seeing how our patients are changing their habits, similar to how we have seen a change in our own.* (+2)	*This is a priority, in other words, it is so important because of the impact it has.* (+1) *Coming from pediatrics, I think other types of things could be done to make things better because this tool doesn't fit very well.* (+1)	*Everyone as much as they can (…). Haven't they told you that many folks say that five fruit or veg. portions can make you fat?* (−1)
Adaptability	*The method, in itself, is not bad. The problem is how fast. They are demanding a 95% and we are going at full speed, we can't keep up with that for a long time.* (−2)	*For this outcome data to be useful, I would have to reach 4 or 5 daily, with each consultation being half an hour, there is not enough time for me and I create a waiting list for other demands.* (0)	*The surveys are a little complicated for people, aren't they? About the portions and having to write it down every time, and all that; I think it doesn't reflect reality very well.* (−2)
Design quality & packaging	*(…) we thought, "that's fantastic, we are going to have a tool that's going to help us, and not the other way around, …" and gives us many, too many problems* (−1) *You're working with a tool that you know doesn't work; we are even having trouble printing the prescriptions* (−1) *The tools didn't work from the start, not theirs* (the nurses) *or ours* (admission)*; I'm talking about the assessment too (−1)*	*We should have better things that can help us, with this, I don't know where to fit it in* (−1) *The computer platform is amazing as a model (…) But when you want to give advice, you cannot print; it often fails completely or doesn't work properly and it could be improved. I guess… 80% of my expectations are fulfilled while 20% aren't because there are a lot of things that could be improved.* *We have to be positive, I think the tool we have is very good. In the long term, it is going to reap results (…) but it is a question of years.* (+1)	*For instance, physical exercise: I have always prescribed physical exercise; but to have the tool, the information sheets, the specifics and ways of telling individuals how much to do, in what ways, and how to orient patients about physical exercise.* (+2)
Inner setting: Implementation climate			
Tension for change	*We have committed to this and have internalized that it is not only about addressing the pathology but also about promoting health across the various levels of care.* (+1)	*We have to be positive and I think the tool is terrific. I think, in the long term, we will have good results.* (+2)	*I do tobacco prevention too (…) indeed this year, I have two or three of my patients have quit smoking; I have not managed the problem well because I don't feel comfortable with the program. I have not done the program with the patients.* (−2)
Learning climate	*All the time, we are trying to do more because everyone is saying 'let's do it, let's do it'.* (+2)	*We have to do it gradually, without stressing, and always making it better.* (0) *I haven't got as involved as him.* (0)	*I joined in December and until now I have not done anything.* (−1)
Characteristics of individuals			
Self-efficacy	*This is part of an effort on the part of the whole group and totally a personal effort, without support.* (+2)	*Going at the speed of a cruise ship, for how long do I go? Because I may not be able to.* (−1) *I am flexible with the people that really want to (…). If the patient works in the morning and wants to stop smoking, we move the appointment to the afternoon and out of the usual times; we try to do that.* (+1)	*It is very hard for me to prescribe the physical activity; it is very hard.* (−2)
Process			
Planning	*Our actions have to be organized, with everyone and directed to the patient.* (0) *I don't know where we are and where we are going; I just don't know. Sometimes we feel like we lose sight of the goal, 'listen, what do we need to do now?'.* (0)	*Our goal as professionals is to change patient lifestyle habits. If we can agree on that goal and can do it within a timeframe, that's perfect; but if not, then we will have to set other timelines.* (0) *Since during the assessment time we were getting little out of it, we told ourselves: 'let's assess here, in this other room'. That way we get to the patient in a different way and increase the rate of assessment.* (0)	*Ah, ok, later on you tell me how this is done.* (−1) *When you tell the patient, what exercise, then you write it down on a piece of paper: 'this patient is interested in doing physical exercise, please help him'. If you send them with that, the gym will pay attention and the patient will get to the appropriate person. You didn't know this?*

Table 3 CFIR constructs associated with PVS performance *(Continued)*

			No, no, I didn't know that, that you have to write it down and send the patient out with that. (−1) *At the beginning, there was talk of making more time available for PVS but I haven't done it, from the beginning I refused to do that.* (−2)
Engaging Champions	*This is a team effort, totally personal, without any support; we don't have anyone who can support it. Then, from primary care, we have been figuring out how to do it.* (+1)	*In any case, these data can be useful to check where we are, but I'm hoping it will not become a burden in our work.* (+2) *Our team coordinator is really motivated. I am with the coordinator. I don't know how to put this, but I have been surprised by the beneficial impact of PVS on our patients.* (+2)	NA
Executing	*I have the impression that we are making it better in each of our meetings and that it becomes clearer.* (+1) *You make the patient fill out the survey at the reception area, because if you don't, then he goes home and doesn't come back.* (+1)	*At the beginning, we felt a bit like: damn, it is difficult to introduce changes, and let's try to do this slowly, making changes at our own pace, bit by bit.* (0) *Me, the goals, the ones I set are not the ones defined by PVS. To me if someone eats an apple when they don't have anything to eat, I know it will not be counted by PVS but it is an achievement from my perspective.* (−1)	*We are so focused on the health problem and we are not accustomed to working through the healthy themes and how to work with them.* (−2) *In recent months, we have been doing much less assessment and this is because we show up as not doing anything. It is a failing of the computer technology; I don't know really, it is really annoying and it makes me angry that our activity is not being recognized.* (−2)
Reflecting & evaluating	*It would be interesting, even if they are very preliminary data, to have an evaluation of the first semester of the pilot and the changes that we have achieved.* (+1) *We have to look at the outcomes so that we can plan on our own, to be able to see if we are having an impact in the future.* (+1)	*I think we need to put the data in context. The data is a start of the reflection. It is to say: 'hey, how could we increase the number of patients participating?'* (+1) *Sure, but we're not sure what the "n" (the expected outcome) means, we don´t understand.* (−1)	*I realized that I was advising patients but I wasn't writing it down (…). It means that if you don't write it down, it is as if you're not doing anything.* (−2) *I don't know how the indicators are created but other information should emerge from all that, right?* (−2)
Organizational tracking	*We are running around to reach a 95% rate; if it is a pilot, why do we have to reach 95%?* (−2) *At times, we had to make decisions so that the program works and that you have been around to just bring up the statistics.* (−2)	*Man, the statistical part and all that, it is really a pain in the neck, a real drag.* (0) *It is very stressful; it doesn't, really, reflect reality.* (−2)	NA

the relationships between these dimensions and potential linkages that require further research. This includes the CFIR constructs that appeared as associated with actual implementation but also others not necessarily associated with performance [15, 19]. Even though the latter were not useful for discriminating between high and low performance, they continue to be important for the implementation model. These variables appear in lowercase in Fig. 2.

Context

The organizational conditions associated with implementation performance include *tension for change, learning climate,* and *self-efficacy* [20]. These constructs are interrelated. A positive learning climate nurtures a sense of *self-efficacy* and the development and impact of effective leaders. Similarly, higher feelings of self-efficacy made more resources available to achieve better outcomes. These organizational conditions impact, and yet are influenced by a bottom-up approach to designing and modelling the PVS intervention. The organizational climate is, therefore, the result of the characteristics of individuals, the inner setting, and the overall organizational process, dimensions that compound each other. Overall, the organizational conditions are in dialectical relationship with the context, shaping it as these conditions evolve. Several organizational constructs appear not to be associated with performance. Teams perceive, for instance, the lack of resources as a severe obstacle to change and innovation. Other constructs included in the diagram show a similar pattern. However, these constructs may not be as relevant when

Table 4 CFIR constructs not associated with PVS performance

CFIR Constructs	PVS Cases		
	A	B	C
Intervention characteristics			
Relative advantage	*It is really a great project. For a patient's own doctor, to guide their eating patterns and to encourage a healthy diet to combat their cholesterol; for my doctor, to tell me that I need to eat broccoli to prevent colon cancer, that's fantastic. It is great if a professional facilitates that conversation.* (+1)	*I am happy about this. About how to work? Obviously, it has made my clinical work better, that's clear.* (+1)	*Our profession is going in this direction and with all the chronic patients. To have expanded the work to the whole healthy population has been very important; it raises the profile of these three healthy habits.* (+1)
Complexity	*We have to attend all chronic patients, the ones we have had for a long time. We have that plus the home visits.* (−2)	*If this is a new task at work, if we have to do it and not abandon any of the other present tasks, it is just an additional task; another story is if the task can be accomplished or not, that's something else.* (−1)	*If we don't one thing, we can do another.* (−2)
Outer setting			
Patient needs & resources	*The patient's schedule, and then the patients tell you that they will do it, that they know how to eat well, or that they know how to exercise, or that they know about quitting tobacco, then they will do it when they can (…). Then you are left with the question: What do I do with this patient?* (−1)	*It is really hard, seeing the economic conditions that many of our patients are facing. If they are a homemaker and go to the grocery store and have spent a bunch of money on fruits and vegetables, to ask if they are eating their oranges* (all nod and laugh), *well, how can you say that to her, for many, there is not enough money.* (+1)	*I think people get scared, scared of being told off.* (−1)
External policy & incentives	*To be attentive to the project as well as the electronic prescription, and your own clinical work, it is exhausting.* (−2)	*The information technology depends on others and it is very slow when you want to make changes.* (−1)	*I don't know if you have the same impressions from other centers involved but the PVS is an additional task that we have compared to other centers because everything is an imposition from senior management.* (−2)
Inner setting			
Structural characteristics	*They are not short of work, nor her or any of the nurses in this center. To be able to make this program work, we need more nursing resources.* (−2)	*I doubt it; with limited resources we cannot make it all work, because there are so many other tasks that need to be accomplished.* (−2)	*The larger centers have a real difficulty in adapting to structural changes.* (−2)
Readiness for implementation: Available resources	*You bring here a scanner that doesn't work, that doesn't read correctly. Then it doesn't serve any purpose.* (−2)	*Barrier you say? For us, the time that is required.* (−1)	*We are just a physician and a nurse, so the assessment requires a tremendous effort.* (−1)
Process			
Engaging: Formally appointed internal implementation leaders	*The coordinator who runs this motivates us; she is all over us so that we achieve the goal.* (+2)	*She is really motivated. She is more involved with this and she is much more motivated.* (+2)	*A responsible peer has been helping me, many times; he has invested his own time and also mine so that I could learn in a more effective way.* (0)

making systematic decisions about which teams may be more motivated to change their practices.

Implementation process

The constructs *champions, planning, executing,* and *reflecting and evaluating,* are shaped by the aforementioned organizational conditions and generate the implementation collaborative modeling. These local leaders ensure engagement of appropriate team members and community stakeholders and the drawing of resources into the project. In centers where the figure of the local leader is highly valued, the performance was also higher. According to some of the dimensions we have analyzed, a positive set of organizational conditions and practice facilitation provided by the research team shapes successful planning and execution. The ongoing feedback provided by the researchers about the performance of the PHC professional teams plus time for learning-based discussion of these data may produce ambivalent feelings, and PHC centers with the highest implementation rating demonstrated this tension with the highest intensity. In order to avoid negative feelings associated with organizational tracking, the research team should not give feedback to the community teams without first assessing the teams' own needs and their particular decision-making process.

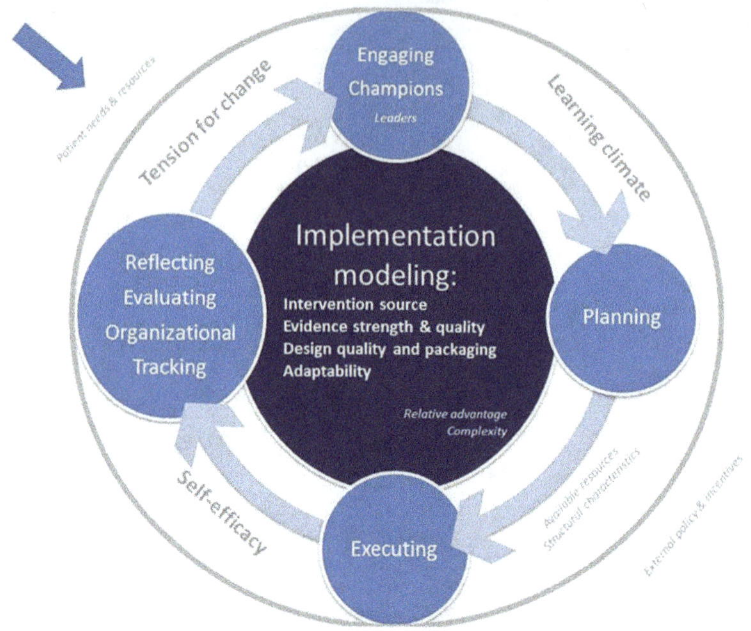

Fig. 2 Implementation model for health promotion in primary and community health care

Collaborative modeling

In the PVS first phase, the research team worked collaboratively and transparently with the PHC centers to adapt the 5 A's intervention (which includes five major steps to develop healthy habits) to the context, guided by action research principles. This engagement included discussions of epidemiological data, community demographics, evidence related to healthy behavior interventions, and the need for an ecological and community approach to prevent and ameliorate chronic illnesses. The degree to which the different teams perceived a need for change varied. However, the introduction of new information and the evolving consensus on needing to change practices may lead highly motivated teams to higher levels of implementation. Without an external research team that helps articulate this process, however, the implementation would stall. The facilitator of this process is the research team but the ownership of the intervention and its characteristics lie in the real local context [21]. The strength of the evidence, therefore, was built on this shared understanding to motivate higher performance among community health teams. The impact of the intervention, the origins of the intervention, the design of support tools and the adaptation to local context nurture the organizational conditions for successful implementation.

Discussion

Eleven of the thirty-six CFIR constructs are directly related to the level of implementation performance. From the start of the inductive qualitative analysis, we realized that the construct reflecting and evaluating is difficult to assess, since the same PHC professionals valued two distinct aspects during the focus groups. On the one hand, teams which were the most concerned about the implementation process feedback were those with higher levels of implementation effectiveness; in these cases, reflecting and evaluating was positively accepted as an appropriate reflection on action related to how the teams welcome the coaching and feedback was closely connected to the field experience. However, among teams in which the implementation had lower intensity, the impact of the evaluation process is not mentioned. On the other hand, in these cases, reflecting and evaluating generates negative feelings associated with external pressure, and a perception that the external evaluators are judging performance as well as imposing some cumbersome requirements typical of research processes. This reaction appears very strongly in the focus groups. We have reserved a section in Table 2 for this, which is called "organizational tracking". It is similar to goals and feedback, but we have not categorized it in that way because the evaluation is external to the health center.

Our findings can be compared to those of other studies that have applied the CFIR to evaluate the implementation of health promotion programs in other settings. Similarly to our results, Damschroder and Lowery [15] found that tension for change, learning climate, planning, and reflecting and evaluating clearly distinguish between centers with different effectiveness in the implementation of the MOVE! weight management program in the US Veterans Health Administration PHC centers.

These researchers did not find intervention source to be associated with different implementation performance, MOVE! being an externally developed program. In our study, the feeling of ownership of the intervention by the participants emerged as a characteristic strongly associated with implementation performance, and along with evidence strength and quality, strongly distinguished between high and low implementation performance centers. Adaptability and design quality and packaging were not useful for distinguishing between low and high implementation effectiveness of the MOVE! as materials and support tools were consistently considered helpful by all the participating centers. However, in the PVS pilot, a number of failures detected in the new information and communication technology support tools integrated into the electronic health records and delays in fixing them had a negative influence on implementation efforts of the staff of the center with the highest implementation effectiveness, while medium-to-low implementation performance centers were especially appreciative of these support tools. Unlike in the case of the MOVE!, PHC centers piloting PVS designed their own implementation strategy and agreed on well-defined milestones and standard performance measures. Specifically, process constructs were negatively associated with low implementation performance and positively associated with or unaffected by high implementation performance. See Table 4 for quotes that exemplify these constructs differentiating between centers with different levels of implementation performance.

The perception of PHC professionals of the intervention source as internal can be fostered by involving them in discussion, consensus, and a decision making process about priorities in each center according to the specific context and about workflow and the role and contributions of the different members of the PHC professional team. This bottom-up process may lead to a greater sense of ownership and commitment to adhering to the program [22, 23]. Collaborative modeling of the specific implementation strategy for each PHC center in turn favors other constructs associated with the implementation in our study, i.e., *adaptability* and *learning climate.*

In this pilot study, we identified two distinct responses to the monthly provision of clinical performance indicators. One response includes PHC professionals valuing it as a positive contribution because it encourages reflection and prompts team discussions to identify problems and look for solutions. The alternative response is related to the continuous assessment and evaluation, the provision of indicators being perceived as stressful because desired changes depend in part on factors beyond the control of the healthcare providers, i.e., excellence in the design and maintenance of the information technology support tools or requirements imposed by the research protocol associated with the implementation effort. The effectiveness of audit and feedback seems to depend on how the feedback is provided and this requires further investigation [24, 25].

Limitations

Our research design has limitations inherent to a cross-sectional study of the perception of what explains performance by healthcare professionals, the factors perceived to be associated with positive or negative implementation outcomes being based on the perceptions of the teams' post facto. The CFIR constructs and performance associations could be bidirectional, are not mutually exclusive categories, and are in continuous evolution. The focus group guide was a set of open-ended questions and was not developed using the CFIR constructs; the CFIR model oriented the analysis only after the initial stage of the grounded consensual qualitative analysis of transcripts. As a result, the lack of data about some of the constructs may be biased by the data collection process rather than a lack of significance of these constructs in the participants' experience. Our semi-structured data gathering and initial grounded data analysis, however, could have prevented a confirmation bias of the validity of the CFIR framework since the constructs were not employed in the interview design. Further research is required to establish the direction of these associations. To assess for organizational readiness for change, community health centers could be measured via surveys based on a systematic review of applications of the CFIR.

Further, the omission of some of the CFIR constructs may, in some cases, be related to the specific cultural and organizational dynamics of health service delivery in the Basque Country. Other constructs are embedded in or impacted directly by some of the dimensions not mentioned in the groups. For instance, *leadership engagement* is a core aspect of the *learning climate*, a dimension that participants found significant.

Conclusion

Strong implementation strategies are required to influence the multiple factors associated with innovation in health-promoting practices by PHC professionals. This study identifies a set of factors associated with the implementation of the PVS program (see Fig. 2). In order to develop such strategies, they should be linked to specific actions, techniques, and processes that foster change and tackle barriers [13]. Partnership between clinicians and researchers is required from the design stage. The first step is engaging the majority of the members of the PHC center in a collaborative activity led by PHC professionals appropriately informed about epidemiological and clinical evidence on health promotion interventions and evolving over time through pilot cycles within a learning organization [26].

The findings and recommendations are relevant to primary care practice as it reflects how primary care could be strengthened to highlight the relevancy of prevention measures. In many countries, primary care aims at integrating the preventive effort. Our trials intended to contribute to knowledge related to those assumptions to intentionally include a preventive dimension in family practice. We do believe the paper makes a contribution that bridges implementation and health services research in the context of primary care practice.

Abbreviations

5 A's: Ask, Advise, Agree, Assist, and Arrange follow-up; CFIR: Consolidated Framework for Implementation Research; EHR: Electronic health record; PHC: Primary Health Care; PVS: Prescribe Vida Saludable (Prescribe Healthy Life); UIAPB: The Primary Care Research Unit of Bizkaia

Acknowledgements

We gratefully acknowledge all the PVS participants who contributed to the focus groups and the representatives of the public health department who accompanied the facilitator in the interviews (see Additional file 1). The authors wish to especially thank Laura J. Damschroder, MS, MPH from Ann Arbor VA Center for Clinical Management Research for her advice in the interpretation of results and reviewing the manuscript.

Funding

The PVS project was funded by the Carlos III Health Institute of the Spanish Ministry of Economy and Competitiveness, co-financed by the European Regional Development Fund (research grant PS09/01461), the Health Department of the Basque Government (research grants 2007111009, 2009111072, 2011111145), the Basque Foundation for Social and Health Care Innovation (grant CA-2012-086), the Basque Research Center in Chronicity-Kronikgune (grant 11/056), and the Spanish Primary Care Research Network for Prevention and Health Promotion (redIAPP RD06/0018/0018 and RD12/0005/0010). The Basque Foundation for Science (Ikerbasque) funded Dr. Bacigalupe. The funding body had no role in the design of the study and collection, analysis, and interpretation of data and in writing the manuscript.

Authors' contributions

GG is the principal investigator and guarantor of the scientific quality of the PVS project and along with AS conceived the idea and designed the implementation research project. JMC, HP, CM, and PB contributed to the PVS project design, obtaining funding and coordinating the fieldwork. CM designed this qualitative evaluation, and organized and conducted the focus groups. GB, CM and JMC carried out the qualitative data analysis and triangulation. GG collaborated in and supervised quantitative and qualitative analyses. CM, GB, JMC and GG drafted the initial version and oversaw revisions of this paper. All the authors critically read and approved the final manuscript.

Competing interests

The authors declare that they have no competing interests.

Consent for publication

Not applicable.

Author details

[1]Primary Care Research Unit of Bizkaia, Basque Healthcare Service – Osakidetza, BioCruces Health Research Institute, Luis Power 18 4th floor, Bilbao 48014, Spain. [2]University of Massachusetts Boston, College of Education and Human Development, 100 Morrissey Bvld, Boston, MA 02125, USA. [3]Deusto Primary Health Care Center. Bilbao-Basurto Integrated Care Organisation. Basque Healthcare Service – Osakidetza. BioCruces Health Research Institute, Luis Power 18, Bilbao 48014, Spain.

References

1. Lim SS, Vos T, Flaxman AD, Danaei G, Shibuya K, Adair-Rohani H, et al. A comparative risk assessment of burden of disease and injury attributable to 67 risk factors and risk factor clusters in 21 regions, 1990–2010: a systematic analysis for the Global Burden of Disease Study 2010. Lancet. 2012; 380(9859):2224–60.
2. Dahlgren G, Whitehead M. Policies and strategies to promote social equity in health. Stockholm: Institute for Future Studies; 1991.
3. Whitlock EP, Orleans CT, Pender N, Allan J. Evaluating primary care behavioral counseling interventions: an evidence-based approach. Am J Prev Med. 2002;22(4):267–84.
4. Glasgow RE, Goldstein MG, Ockene JK, Pronk NP. Translating what we have learned into practice. Principles and hypotheses for interventions addressing multiple behaviors in primary care. Am J Prev Med. 2004;27(2 Suppl):88–101.
5. Grandes G, Sanchez A, Cortada JM, Balague L, Calderon C, Arrazola A, et al. Is integration of healthy lifestyle promotion into primary care feasible? Discussion and consensus sessions between clinicians and researchers. BMC Health Serv Res. 2008;8(1):213.
6. Glasgow RE, Lichtenstein E, Marcus AC. Why Don't We See more translation of health promotion research to practice? rethinking the efficacy-to-effectiveness transition. Am J Public Health. 2003;93(8):1261–7.
7. McGlynn EA, Asch SM, Adams J, Keesey J, Hicks J, DeCristofaro A, et al. The quality of health care delivered to adults in the United States. N Engl J Med. 2003;348(26):2635–45.
8. Grandes G, Sanchez A, Sanchez-Pinilla R, et al. Effectiveness of physical activity advice and prescription by physicians in routine primary care: a cluster randomized trial. Arch Intern Med. 2009;169(7):694–701.
9. Grandes G, Cortada JM, Arrazola A, Laka JP. Predictors of long-term outcome of a smoking cessation programme in primary care. Br J Gen Pract. 2003;53(487):101–7.
10. Grandes G, Sanchez G, Cortada JM, Calderon C, Balague L, Millan E. Useful strategies for promoting healthy lifestyles in primary care [Spanish]. Vitoria-Gasteiz: Eusko Jaurlaritzaren Argitalpen Zerbitzu Nagusia Servicio Central de Publicaciones del Gobierno Vasco Donostia-San Sebastián, 1–01010; 2008. p. 122.
11. Grol R, Grimshaw J. From best evidence to best practice: effective implementation of change in patients' care. Lancet. 2003;362(9391):1225–30.
12. Powell BJ, McMillen JC, Proctor EK, Carpenter CR, Griffey RT, Bunger AC, et al. A compilation of strategies for implementing clinical innovations in health and mental health. Med Care Res Rev. 2012;69(2):123–57.
13. French SD, Green SE, O'Connor DA, McKenzie JE, Francis JJ, Michie S, et al. Developing theory-informed behaviour change interventions to implement evidence into practice: a systematic approach using the Theoretical Domains Framework. Implement Sci. 2012;7(1):38.
14. Damschroder LJ, Aron DC, Keith RE, Kirsh SR, Alexander JA, Lowery JC. Fostering implementation of health services research findings into practice: a consolidated framework for advancing. Implement Sci. 2009;4(1):50.
15. Damschroder LJ, Lowery JC. Evaluation of a large-scale weight management program using the consolidated framework for implementation research (CFIR). Implement Sci. 2013;8(1):51.
16. Schneider CQ, Wagemann C. Set-Theoretic Methods for the Social Sciences: A Guide to Qualitative Comparative Analysis. Cambridge: Cambridge University Press; 2012.
17. Spring B, Ockene JK, Gidding SS, Mozaffarian D, Moore S, Rosal MC, et al. Better population health through behavior change in adults a call to action. Circulation. 2013;128(19):2169–76.
18. Sanchez A, Grandes G, Cortada JM, Pombo H, Balague L, Calderon C. Modelling innovative interventions for optimising healthy lifestyle promotion in primary health care: "Prescribe Vida Saludable" phase I research protocol. BMC Health Serv Res. 2009;9:103.
19. Emily C, Williams MLJ. Strategies to implement alcohol screening and brief intervention in primary care settings: a structured literature review. Psychol Addict Behav J Soc Psychol Addict Behav. 2011;25(2):206–14.
20. Brownson RC, Colditz GA, Proctor EK. Dissemination and Implementation Research in Health: Translating Science to Practice. Oxford: Oxford University Press; 2012.

21. Greenhalgh T, Robert G, Macfarlane F, Bate P, Kyriakidou O. Diffusion of innovations in service organizations: systematic review and recommendations. Milbank Q. 2004;82(4):581–629.
22. Lomas J. Making clinical policy explicit: legislative policy making and lessons for developing practice guidelines. Int J Technol Assess Health Care. 1993;9(01):11–25.
23. Leykum LK, Pugh JA, Lanham HJ, Harmon J, McDaniel RR. Implementation research design: integrating participatory action research into randomized controlled trials. Implement Sci. 2009;4(1):69.
24. Ivers N, Jamtvedt G, Flottorp S, Young JM, Odgaard-Jensen J, French SD, et al. Audit and feedback: effects on professional practice and healthcare outcomes. Cochrane Database Syst Rev. 2012;6:CD000259.
25. Foy R, Eccles MP, Jamtvedt G, Young J, Grimshaw JM, Baker R. What do we know about how to do audit and feedback? Pitfalls in applying evidence from a systematic review. BMC Health Serv Res. 2005;5(1):50.
26. Dixon-Woods M, Bosk CL, Aveling EL, Goeschel CA, Pronovost PJ. Explaining Michigan: developing an ex post theory of a quality improvement program. Milbank Q. 2011;89(2):167–205.

4

Implementation of cardiovascular disease prevention in primary health care: enhancing understanding using normalisation process theory

Nerida Volker[1*], Lauren T. Williams[1,2], Rachel C. Davey[1], Thomas Cochrane[1] and Tanya Clancy[1]

Abstract

Background: The reorientation of primary health care towards prevention is fundamental to addressing the rising burden of chronic disease. However, in Australia, cardiovascular disease prevention practice in primary health care is not generally consistent with existing guidelines. The Model for Prevention study was a whole-of-system cardiovascular disease prevention intervention, with one component being enhanced lifestyle modification support and addition of a health coaching service in the general practice setting. To determine the feasibility of translating intervention outcomes into real world practice, implementation work done by stakeholders was examined using Normalisation Process Theory as a framework.

Methods: Data was collected through interviews with 40 intervention participants and included general practitioners, practice nurses, practice managers, lifestyle advisors and participants. Data analysis was informed by normalisation process theory constructs.

Results: Stakeholders were in agreement that, while prevention is a key function of general practice, it was not their usual work. There were varying levels of engagement with the intervention by practice staff due to staff interest, capacity and turnover, but most staff reconfigured their work for required activities. The Lifestyle Advisors believed staff had varied levels of interest in and understanding of, their service, but most staff felt their role was useful. Patients expanded their existing relationships with their general practice, and most achieved their lifestyle modification goals.

While the study highlighted the complex nature of the change required, many of the new or enhanced processes implemented as part of the intervention could be scaled up to improve the systems approach to prevention. Overcoming the barriers to change, such as the perception of CVD prevention as a 'hard sell', is going to rely on improving the value proposition for all stakeholders.

Conclusions: The study provided a detailed understanding of the work required to implement a complex cardiovascular disease prevention intervention within general practice. The findings highlighted the need for multiple strategies that engage all stakeholders. Normalisation process theory was a useful framework for guiding change implementation.

Keywords: Practice nurse, Health coaching, Lifestyle modification, Preventative health

* Correspondence: nerida.volker@canberra.edu.au
[1]Health Research Institute, Centre for Research & Action in Public Health, University of Canberra, College Road, Bruce, Canberra, ACT 2601, Australia
Full list of author information is available at the end of the article

Background

Cardiovascular disease (CVD) was the leading cause of death in Australia in 2011 [1]. Primary health care has an important role in supporting CVD prevention, however prevention-orientated activities are not routinely undertaken in Australian general practice [2, 3]. While the need for more heath promoting health systems has long been recognised, attempts to reorientate health services towards prevention have proven highly resistant to change [4]. The need for greater expertise in how to implement CVD prevention strategies in practice has been identified as key to addressing the CVD burden worldwide [5].

The Model for Prevention study (MoFoP) is a case study exploration of a whole-of-system CVD prevention intervention framed by the Expanded Chronic Care Model (ECCM) [6].

The ECCM provides an evidence-based approach to health system redesign for prevention and management of chronic disease integrating the Chronic Care Model and the five action areas from the Ottawa Charter for Health Promotion [7]. The intervention was of 12 months duration, with strategies including improvement of clinical and community information systems, support for health practitioner decision making for CVD risk management, provision of a health coaching service to support patients to develop lifestyle modification skills and health system redesign to provide greater health behaviour change support across the general practice setting.

Patients from six general practices in the Australian Capital Territory (ACT) identified via existing clinical data as being at high risk for CVD disease were provided with enhanced risk management support, including access to a Lifestyle Advisor service (health coach) for up to 12 months (average of four sessions). The intervention also included strategies to build the capacity of community-based lifestyle modification services to support patients in the community setting.

Interventions to address chronic disease are complex and, while guidelines-based care has been shown to be effective in very controlled situations, translating these outcomes into real world practice has proven difficult to sustain. In their review of Chronic Care Model-framed interventions which aim to improve chronic disease outcomes, Kadu and Stolee found the need for more research focused on understanding the inner settings of organisations, including the characteristics of the work of individual practitioners, in order to better understand how to achieve and sustain positive outcomes [8]. One of the main aims of the MoFoP study was to focus on the feasibility of embedding the intervention approach into real world practice, both in the general practice and community setting. The community setting aspects of the study have been reported elsewhere [9].

This paper focuses on the aspects of the intervention that occurred within general practice involving general practitioners (GP), practice nurses (PN), practice management (PM), lifestyle advisors (LA) and patients who participated in the intervention (P). To make sense of the social and organisational aspects of the intervention Normalisation Process Theory (NPT) was chosen as a tool to frame the analysis. NPT is a mid-level theory developed to understand and evaluate the processes by which complex interventions are embedded into routine practice [10]. The theory takes a whole-of-system perspective, which aligned well with the intervention design. NPT has also been used as a tool for assessing the suitability of trial approaches or providing information to optimise trials [11].

Methods

Data collection

The study used a qualitative design employing semi-structure interviews. The interviews were conducted with staff of all the six practices, who delivered the CVD prevention intervention. All staff members were sent individual invitations by the research team to participate in the interviews. Additionally, all patients who participated in the intervention ($n = 30$) and both Lifestyle Advisors were sent invitations to be interviewed. Semi-structured interviews were used instead of focus groups due to the nature of the general practice environment, which makes it difficult for groups to get together at one time. Interviews also provide a degree of anonymity for staff members who were often employees or junior staff of other interviewees. Topic guides for practice staff and LAs were informed by NPT constructs. These constructs help to explain the work involved in embedding interventions into routine practice. This includes making meaning and sense of the intervention (coherence), committing to and engaging with the intervention (cognitive participation), delivering the intervention (collective action) and reflecting and appraising the intervention approach (reflective monitoring).

Topic guides for the interviews with patients were developed in very early stages of the research and contained evaluation questions not directly informed by NPT. The decision was made to include patient data in this analysis given the identified need to include service user evaluation in the NPT literature [12]. All topic guides were pilot tested before data collection commenced. Interview questions for all stakeholders are provided in Additional file 1.

Purposive sampling was used to ensure representation from a range of practice staff across all of the intervention general practices. Practice staff were invited to participate via a letter from the researcher, which was distributed by practice management. Patients and LAs were also invited by letter to participate after the completion of the intervention. Interviews with general practice staff were conducted mostly on site at practices and lasted between 20 and 60 min. Interviews were conducted individually rather than in a group due to sensitivity to employee/employer relationships which may have impacted on the ability of some staff to answer questions honestly. Patients were interviewed face to face at their general practice or by phone (for their convenience) and lasted between 30 and 60 min. LAs were interviewed face to face at the office of the interviewer and these interviews lasted around 60 min. Interviews were conducted between December 2013 and July 2014. All interviews were conducted by the first author, audio taped and transcribed. Ethical approval for the study was obtained from University of Canberra Human Research Ethics Committee (Project number 11–141).

A description of each of the stakeholder groups is outlined in Table 1.

Data analysis

The study used NPT constructs to frame the data analysis. May and colleagues proposed that NPT could structure the way that qualitative data is coded, analysed and understood [13]. In this instance, the four constructs (and components) were used to code the data in line with Strauss and Corbin's single coding approach [14]. Drawing on the work of Murray, Blakeman, and Gallacher, a NPT informed coding framework was developed and interview transcripts were coded against the framework [15, 16]. The framework is described at Table 2.

A subset (20%) of transcripts were coded independently by a second researcher and then compared and discussed to ensure consistent coding against NPT constructs. The data generally aligned with the constructs and, where data did not fit, it was coded as "other". Data handling was facilitated using NVivo 10 software. After coding, narratives were developed under each of the constructs.

Results

There were 40 face to face interviews conducted with participants in all six general practices involved in the MoFoP study. Interviews were held with 11 General Practitioners (GPs) (26% of GP participants), 12 Practice Nurses (PNs) (75% of PN participants), six Practice Managers (PMs) (100% of PM participants), two LAs (100% of LA participants) and nine patients (30% of patient participants). Characteristics of interview participants are detailed in Table 3.

While male and female practice staff members were interviewed, gender is not reported for each category to maintain confidentiality of individuals. All patients interviewed were male, consistent with the total MoFoP intervention population, where all but one participating patient was male.

The stakeholder interviews provided a rich description of the processes of implementation of the MoFoP intervention. After the data were analysed using the NPT coding framework, narratives were developed for each of the four NPT constructs. These narratives were summarised and are presented below with illustrative quotes. While not all elements within each construct had the same density of coded information, overall most stakeholders could comment across most of the NPT constructs. The quotes are attributed to participants by professional grouping, years working in that role, and age for patients.

Making sense of the intervention

For the general practices and their patients, the intervention was the first time they had taken a systematic approach to identification and management of CVD risk.

The prevention-orientated service was considered by practice staff to be important for the health of their patients and an important function of general practice, as one GP stated:

> *I feel this is what general practice is about. We are here to prevent health problems and manage patients.* (GP11, 25 years as a GP).

While practice staff saw the intervention approach to be consistent with the goals of general practice, most

Table 1 Description of key stakeholder groups

Title	Description of key stakeholder groups
General Practitioner	GPs are medical practitioners who provide primary, comprehensive and continuing care to patients and their families within the community. General practice is a medical speciality. Entry to the speciality may be achieved by admission to Fellowship of the Royal Australian College of General Practice [22].
Practice Manager	PMs perform all or some of the practice management tasks in a healthcare setting [23].
Practice Nurse	PNs are registered or enrolled nurses who are employed by, or whose services are otherwise retained, by a general practice [24].
Lifestyle Advisor	LAs (health coaches) perform a relatively new care extender role helping patients gain the knowledge, skills, tools and confidence to become active participants in their own care so that they can reach their self-identified health goals [25]. LAs were fitness professionals provided with additional training in the Health Change Australia approach [26].
Intervention Participant (patient)	Ps were those patients who responded to the recall and participated in the intervention.

Table 2 Coding framework for analysis

Coherence (sense making work)	Cognitive participation (Relationship work)	Collective action (Enacting work)	Reflexive monitoring (Appraising work)
Differentiation	Enrolment	Interactional workability	Reconfiguration
Were staff and patients clear on their roles regarding the intervention? Were staff and patients clear on other's roles regarding the intervention?	Did staff engage with other staff around the intervention? Did patients engage with the practice for the intervention? Who initiated the engagement? Who did and who didn't 'buy-in' to the intervention?	How was the intervention enacted by staff, Lifestyle Advisors and patients? How did the intervention fit with existing work of all stakeholders? How did patients, staff and lifestyle advisors adapt to the introduction of the intervention? What effect did the intervention have on usual practice?	Has the approach to CVD prevention in the practices been adapted based on the intervention experience? If so, how? Has the patients approach to their CVD risk changed based on the intervention experience? If so, how?
Individual specification	Initiation	Relational integration	Individual appraisal
Did the staff and patients know what the intervention was? Was the intervention easy for the staff and patients to describe? What benefits did the intervention bring, and to whom?	Who was engaged in the intervention? What organisational skills did staff use to contribute to the intervention? Were staff prepared to invest time, energy and work to the intervention? If so, what did they do? Were patients prepared to invest time, energy and work into the intervention? If so what did they do? What organisation skills did they use?	How did the intervention affect trust and confidence between all parties (i.e. patients, staff, lifestyle advisors)? How did the intervention affect the relationships between all stakeholders? How did all stakeholders work to maintain relationships?	Was it clear to staff and patients what effects the intervention has had? Did patients and staff make efforts to reflect on and appraise the intervention? If so, how? Has appraisal work informed whether the intervention was advantageous for patients and staff?
Communal specification	Activation	Skill set workability	Communal appraisal
Did the staff have a shared sense of purpose around the intervention? Did staff and patients have a shared sense of purpose around the intervention? Who thought the intervention was a good idea? Who did not? Were the benefits of the intervention valued by all patients and all staff? Did the intervention fit with the overall goals and activity of the general practice?	Did the patients and staff undertake work to arrange a shared contribution to the implementing the intervention? If so, what is this work? How did the intervention feature in practice meetings? How did the practice communicate with patients about the intervention?	How was the intervention work distributed within the patients and staff? What impact did the introduction of the intervention have on the distribution/division of labour, resources, power and responsibility? Was the work for the intervention devolved to others not usually doing the work? If so, how and for what reason? Was there alignment in the intervention approach throughout the patients and staff? Did the introduction of the intervention alter the awareness of the work done by other members within a practice team?	How did patients and staff know that the intervention approach is being carried out? Did staff and patients contribute/share feedback about the intervention with others? If so, what was discussed? Has appraisal work informed whether the intervention approach is advantageous for patients and staff?
Internalisation	Legitimation	Contextual integration	Systematisation
Was there an understanding by staff of how to learn to implement the intervention approach? Did the patients relate their CVD risk and their need to seek support to the intervention? Did staff have the time to learn to understand and carry out the intervention approach?	Was there work undertaken to ensure that participating in the intervention was viewed by patients and staff as the right thing to do? If so, what was this work? Did staff have the permission to use the intervention approach?	How was the intervention resourced? Did patients bring their own resources to the intervention? Could they integrate lifestyle changes into their everyday life? Are tasks compatible with existing work practices? Was the intervention linked to, and resourced through, organisational structures (e.g. clinical information systems, decision support tools)? How did the intervention affect the relationship with existing structures?	Has the practice developed ways of keeping patients and staff up to date with best practice approaches to CVD prevention?

Table 3 Characteristics of stakeholders interviewed

PNs	Years as PN	PMs	Years as PM	GPs	Years as GP	LAs	Years in lifestyle modification	Patients (P)	Age in years
PN1	3	PM1	19	GP1	N/A	LA1	27	P1	69
PN2	6	PM2	4	GP2	<1	LA2	27	P2	72
PN3	6	PM3	16	GP3	25			P3	66
PN4	10	PM4	8	GP4	1			P4	66
PN5	1	PM5	1.5	GP5	25			P5	69
PN6	7.5	PM6	18	GP6	1			P6	73
PN7	1.5			GP7	8			P7	65
PN8	1			GP8	1			P8	70
PN9	1			GP9	2			P9	75
PN10	0.5			GP10	20				
PN11	3			GP11	25				
PN12	5								

agreed it was different from their everyday experience, which focused on responding to acute illness. As one PN put it, *"Normally it is about treating; this was about prevention"* (PN7, 1 year as a PN).

The patients who participated in the intervention also agreed that preventing CVD was important and they expected their general practice to have a role in supporting them to reduce their risk. Most reported that they had existing risk factors for CVD and felt the intervention was therefore relevant to them. However, not all participants were convinced that they were at high risk and for one patient the recall letter was totally unexpected.

He said, *"I think the word I would use is bemused. I didn't know, or didn't really suspect, that I might have been at high risk"* (P4, 66 years old).

Stakeholder investments in the intervention

While the six general practices volunteered to be involved in the intervention, the degree of commitment and engagement varied across the practices, between practice staff groups and for patients in each of the different practices.

One PN noted that in their practice *"there was great support from management, but I think the clinicians (GPs) had varying levels of commitment to the project."* (PN 2, 6 years as a PN).

In another practice a strong interest in CVD prevention by one particular staff member led to a high level of engagement with the intervention. A GP from this practice noted, *"Having a nurse with a background in cardiovascular disease meant that we weren't going to let anything cardiovascular pass us by"* (GP 1, 20 years as a GP). While many practice staff reported that they participated in the intervention in the interests of their patients, others undertook activities because they were expected to as part of their employment. As one GP said *"I did what I was told"* (GP3, 25 years as a GP). Both LAs also felt that there were varying levels of support for the intervention across practices with one LA stating that, *"I would probably say one of the four (GPs) was committed"* (LA2, 27 years in lifestyle modification).

Communication with practice staff regarding the delivery of the intervention was generally good. However, staff turnover in all practices meant that as the intervention progressed some practitioners were not informed of their required activities. One GP noted that *"I think the doctors who came along after the intervention had started did not know what was involved...they did not go to the talks"* (GP1, 20 years as a GP).

The patients interviewed had all made the effort to participate in the intervention by reading the provided information on CVD risk, making an appointment to see their GP, and in some cases, having a blood test to update lipid levels. Most patients considered the intervention to be a normal extension of care from their general practice. They had established relationships with the practice and its staff and assumed that participation would be beneficial. As one patient said *"It seemed ordinary, in a sense that this practice does look after me"* (P5, 69 years old).

Stakeholders work to enact the intervention

While all practices reported following the intervention protocol, the size of the practice, skills and preferences of the workforce, and the business model led to the work of the intervention being configured in a range of ways. These ranged from a nurse led approach to the intervention, with limited input by the GP, to non-participation where individual GPs in a practice would not allow their patients to be recalled because they did not receive a direct incentive payment. One GP explained:

> *It depends on how the practice is set up and what your nursing staff are like. I suppose also how you like to do things as a GP as well. If you like to maintain*

> *that relationship and do the education yourself rather than pass the buck to whoever it may be.* (GP9, 2 years as a GP)

Successful implementation of the intervention relied on administration staff undertaking a wide range of tasks, including many considered central to achieving a systems approach. While clinicians were responsible for recording most of the clinical and demographic data, administration staff took the lead in most practices in educating and reminding staff about the need to enter the key demographic and CVD risk factor data and how to enter this data correctly. They used their usual practice communication strategies such as staff meetings and some novel approaches, for example, messages on the back of staff toilet doors. One PM recounted her approach, *"We were sticking little stickers* [Post It notes] *all over the GP's computers saying, "please do this or please do that".* (PM4, 8 years as a PM).

Other tasks that were central to successful implementation were related to navigating patients through the intervention processes, such as responding appropriately to phone calls about the recall visits. When administration staff failed to perform these tasks the practice experienced difficulties communicating with eligible patients. One patient recalled his experience of contacting his practice and the receptionist not being fully aware of her role in the intervention.

> *I had to ring up the practice and tell them that I wanted an appointment for this program. So I did that and they made me feel that I was stupid...why did I need this appointment she said.* (P8, 70 years old).

All GPs reported that the intervention did not add a significant workload and they were happy to refer patients to the LA service. They frequently commented that it was beneficial to give patients access to a broader range of team members who could spend more time with them on lifestyle modification issues. As one GP said:

> *I can only do so much for this patient because I have 15 minutes ... so that team-based model... I think the program got that team approach.* (GP1, 20 years as a GP).

For the PNs the intervention activities led to a greater consultation role, which most of them enjoyed. This work differed from their usual task-orientation and provided opportunities to build deeper relationships with patients.

One practice nurse said, *"There is not a lot of relationship building (usually). When talking about prevention, we need to build relationships, and be in it for the long haul"* (PN2, 6 years as a PN).

The LAs were highly motivated to develop good working relationships with the GPs from the beginning of the intervention. While they reported to be disappointed that the contact was generally restricted to written communication, they did feel that being present at the practice made their service more credible with the clinical staff.

One LA said *"they had more confidence in what we do because we were actually in the medical centre."* (LA1, 27 years working in lifestyle modification).

While the intervention introduced an LA as a new health care provider to the usual practice based care team, the patients did not feel that their relationship with their GP or other practice staff was diminished. As one participant stated, *"I don't think he thought I was being poached away."* (P 3, 66 years).

Most found that the health coaching approach used by the LAs was non-judgemental, allowing them to be honest about areas they were willing to change and supported in achieving the goals they set for themselves. One patient outlined how the process worked for them:

> *Basically what happened is I told her what I wanted to do, she listened and I took over. She steered me in another direction sometimes or pointed something out I might need.* (P7, 65 years old).

Stakeholder appraisal of the intervention

All those interviewed considered the intervention to be worthwhile at some level. Most patients made positive changes to their lifestyle as a result of the intervention. One patient had good outcomes for issues that had previously been resistant to change. He said:

> *I have certainly reduced smoking and alcohol. I have been able to put alcohol free days into my program which I found difficult before* (P1, 69 years old).

Practice staff and LAs recalled positive health and wellbeing outcomes for patients and the practice and systems level changes achieved. These changes included both practice and opportunistic risk factor data captured for enhanced CVD risk assessment and management. As explained by one of the PNs interviewed:

> *Since the program was introduced I think it improved our collection of data, when patients come now all patients who come through the treatment room get height, weight, blood pressure, allergies and smoking assessment* (PN12, 5 years as a PN).

The key role of administrative staff improving the systems response to CVD prevention was also recognised during the study. One experienced PM noted that *"Since my involvement with this project I train my staff that are sending out the recall letter... so when a patient calls and makes an appointment they know exactly what to tell them*" (PM6, 18 years as a PM).

Some staff believed the intervention resulted in a greater awareness by GPs of the importance of managing CVD risk and an increased number of CVD risk assessments being conducted. One PN reported that in her practice, CVD risk assessment had increased, stating that "*Doctors are doing a lot more cardiovascular assessments...they are actually doing them!*" (PN2, 6 years as a PN). There were staff in every practice that identified barriers to them reorganising practice to align with the intervention approach. While practice nurses were interested in an expanded role, many felt underprepared to address lifestyle modification and felt they needed more training in the area. This was highlighted by one nurse who said, "*I haven't been trained for any of this, it has all been a learning curve for me*" (PN6, 7 years as a PN). Current financing models, time pressures and practical issues such as poorly integrated clinical software were also considered issues to be addressed if they were to become a more prevention-orientated practice. One GP was very clear about this, stating that:

> *Anything that puts more work on the staff or the doctors is unrealistic... If there's no incentive for us, at least make it that simple that I don't have to invest extra work into it.* (GP10, 20 years as a GP).

When reflecting back on the intervention, almost all practice staff identified the difficulty of achieving sustained lifestyle modification itself as a major impediment to providing prevention-orientated services. They also considered these challenges would be exacerbated if there were out of pocket costs for patients.

> *It's a hard sell and that is why it should be free.* (PN7, 1 year as a PN).

Discussion

The study examined the work required by general practice staff, Lifestyle Advisers and patients to implement CVD prevention in primary care consistent with existing evidence-based practice guidelines [17]. The findings provide insight into the feasibility of intervention approach being embedded into real world practice. There were many aspects of the existing general practice system that could be supported, some with very small investment, to achieve and sustain more health promoting general practice setting. However, significant barriers to system change did exist, such as the design of current funding and the challenging nature of lifestyle modification, making it difficult for practitioners, and their patients, to move away from their usual practice.

While usual practice did not normally include prevention-orientated activities, practice staff felt that prevention-orientated care was part of their role and that of general practice. Patients agreed that CVD prevention was important, important to their own health and they expected their General Practice to support them to reduce their risk of CVD. To enhance the likelihood of the intervention approach being adopted, the study outcomes highlight the need for an increased focus on strategies that build relationships across general practice. Mazza and colleagues found that for patients, having trust and a good rapport with a GP encouraged them to participate in prevention-orientated care [18]. Consistent with this finding, most patients in the intervention identified strongly with the General Practice or their particular GP. The study outcomes also emphasised the value of nurturing relationships between patients and other members of the practice team. Practice Nurses were open to building these relationships and developing more comprehensive clinical roles. The administration staff also had an important role in engaging patients into the intervention particularly in areas related to coherence, supporting patients to see their general practice as interested in prevention and cognitive participation, getting the multiple internal and external relationships to work for the intervention and making it easy for patients to engage in the new activities. Greater recognition of the importance of this workforce and the development more specific strategies to support their role, should be a feature of future interventions.

Redistribution of the work undertaken by general practice staff to support patients in health behaviour change was an important element of the intervention approach. This included the adoption of new or enhanced tasks related to health information quality, CVD risk assessment and behaviour change support for the practice staff. There was also the integration of a new primary health care workforce in the Lifestyle Advisors. The GPs were generally happy to undertake small additions to practice to deliver the intervention and to transfer more lengthy discussions on lifestyle modification to the LA. Most PNs welcomed the opportunity to expand their role, but found lifestyle modification a challenging area of practice because they had had little previous training or experience in the area. Limitations in health behaviour change skills of nurses working in primary health care and has been previously identified as a barrier to PN's more active engagement in chronic disease prevention [19]. Ongoing professional development, particularly using an academic detailing approach that offers tailored on-site support for the different needs of individual staff and practices, is needed to build the competence and confidence of this workforce in this new role.

The positioning of a health coaching service in a primary care practice is a relatively new innovation. While most patients and practice staff reported positive outcomes from the LAs service, the LAs themselves perceived varying levels of interest, or as they put it "curiosity" about their service, particularly by practice staff. Liddy and colleagues found that it does take time for practices to adjust to having this new role in place and that a poor understanding of health coaching by other practice staff can limit its effectiveness [20]. Therefore the addition of this new workforce has potential to make prevention-orientated services easier to deliver in the general practice setting, but it will need to be supported over an extended period to allow the potential benefits to be fully recognised. To continue this role would be an area requiring a new source of recurrent funding, as in the current intervention these positions were fully supported with short term project funds.

The need for more recurrent funding for prevention activities and the challenging nature of lifestyle modification were identified as fundamental barriers to the intervention approach being adopted as usual practice. The lack of adequate funding, funding along with limited time and other competing priorities have been found by other researchers to be barriers to lifestyle modification in general practice [21]. This ambivalence remains a fundamental barrier to prevention-orientated general practice, with the benefits of moving to delivery of more prevention services over remaining with the status quo, not yet compelling for the practices involved in the study. However, if positive patient health and practice system outcomes could be maintained, even at some level, over time the experience of CVD prevention could improve and help to build the value proposition for prevention-orientated services. The need to build the value proposition for prevention was also emphasised by the community-based lifestyle modification providers in their attempt to operate viable businesses [9]. Until prevention-orientated services hold greater value for everyone and attract the collective action and subsequent advocacy for policy and funding reform, it is unlikely there will be the community and political will required to achieve change.

The study demonstrated the utility of exploring implementation processes and the work required at an individual and organisational level to see translation of evidence-based CVD prevention practice into everyday general practice. It also showed the benefit of using NPT as a tool for examining implementation of a prevention-orientated activity. It allowed the researchers to 'think through' the data in a structured way and highlighted the work required by all stakeholders to implement such a complex intervention. Much of this information was unlikely to have been captured systematically in other ways. In particular, it helped to expose the 'hidden work' that needs to occur to create health promoting systems.

The limitations of the study relate to the sample and the timing of the interviews. The study took place in a single city with a generally high standard of living. The sample of practice staff included only those willing to be interviewed, who may have been more interested in the intervention outcomes. Not all staff interviewed worked at one of the six practices over the entire period of the intervention, which limited their capacity to comment on the earlier stages of implementation. Data was collected at the completion of the pilot study, those interviewed may have forgotten aspects relevant to the early stages of the intervention.

While consideration was given to collecting baseline information from stakeholders about what they expected from enhanced CVD prevention, given the novel nature of the intervention for many of the staff and patients, it was decided that this step would provide little additional information to justify the increased burden on participants. However, the study team did use the NPT constructs in the development of the strategies for the intervention.

The study was strengthened by inclusion of all key workforce groups in general practice, and in particular, by including the patients who were the users of the service. The practices in the study operated using a range of business models and serviced a range of demographic groups. While some of the issues raised were directly related to the predominately fee-for-service funding model of general practice in Australia, many of the findings are relevant to the challenges faced by health systems globally in attempts to improve prevention-orientated primary health care. Finally, use of the NPT provided a rich and detailed framework for analysis and a strong theoretical grounding to the study.

Conclusion

Despite widespread agreement that increasing CVD prevention activities in primary care is important, progress in reorientating health systems towards prevention-orientated practice has been limited. This study highlights the value of examining the implementation processes at a detailed level, including the experience of all stakeholders, in understanding of the feasibility of a complex intervention being embedded into usual practice. While many barriers will continue to impede the translation of the intervention approach, the study was able to highlight parts of the system that are highly influential to improving CVD prevention and are ready to change. Over time, supporting these areas will increase the capacity of general practice to become

a health promoting setting and a true primary health care setting, which is a goal definitely worth pursuing.

Abbreviations
CVD: Cardiovascular disease; ECCM: Expanded Chronic Care Model; GP: General Practitioner; LA: Lifestyle Advisor; NPT: Normalisation Process Theory; P: Patient; PM: Practice Manager; PN: Practice Nurse

Acknowledgements
The authors thank all interview participants for their time and their thoughtful insights around the intervention.

Funding
NV was supported for PhD studies through a scholarship from Australian Capital Territory (ACT) Health. The intervention that was the focus of this study was funded by ACT Health. The organisation was not involved in the development of this publication.

Authors' contributions
NV designed the study, carried out the interviews, drafted and finalised the manuscript. TC, TCI, RD and LTW contributed to the study design and drafts of the manuscript. TCI also helped to organise interviews. All authors conributed to, read and approved the final manuscript.

Competing interests
The authors declare that they have no competing interests.

Consent for publication
Not applicable.

Author details
[1]Health Research Institute, Centre for Research & Action in Public Health, University of Canberra, College Road, Bruce, Canberra, ACT 2601, Australia. [2]Menzies Health Institute of Queensland, Griffith University, Parklands Drive, Southport, QLD 4222, Australia.

References
1. Australian Bureau of Statistics. Causes of Death Australia, ABS cat. no. 3303.0. Canberra: Australian Bureau of Statistics; 2013.
2. Heeley EL, Peiris DP, Patel AA, Cass A, Weekes A, Morgan C, et al. Cardiovascular risk perception and evidence-practice gaps in Australian general practice (the AusHEART study). MJA. 2010;192(5):254–9.
3. Denney-Wilson E, Fanaian M, Wan Q, Vagholkar S, Schütze H, Mark M. Lifestyle risk factors in general practice–routine assessment and management. Aust Fam Physician. 2010;39(12):950–3.
4. Ziglio E, Simpson S, Tsouros A. Health promotion and health systems: some unfinished business. Health Promot Int. 2011;26 suppl 2:ii216–25.
5. Yusuf S, Wood D, Ralston J, Reddy KS. The World Heart Federation's vision for worldwide cardiovascular disease prevention. Lancet. 2015;386(9991):399–402.
6. Volker N, Davey RC, Cochrane T, Williams LT, Clancy T. Improving the Prevention of Cardiovascular Disease in Primary Health Care. The Model for Prevention Study Protocol. JMIR Res Prots. 2014;3(3):e33.
7. Barr VJ, Robinson S, Marin-Link B, Underhill L, Dotts A, Ravensdale D, Salivaras S. The Expanded Chronic Care Model: an integration of concepts and strategies from population health promotion and the Chronic Care Model. Hosp Q. 2003;7(1):73–82.
8. Kudu MK, Stolee R. Facilitators and barriers of implementing the chronic care model in primary care: a systematic review. BMC Fam Pract. 2015;16:12.
9. Volker N, Williams LT, Davey RC, Cochrane T. Community-based lifestyle modification workforce: an underutilised asset for cardiovascular disease prevention. Aust J Prim Health. http://dx.doi.org/10.1071/PY14178. Accessed 18 Jan 2017.
10. May C, Finch T. Implementing, embedding, and integrating practices: an outline of normalization process theory. Sociology. 2009;43:535–54.
11. Murray E, Treweek S, Pope C, MacFarlane A, Ballini L, Dowrick C, et al. Normalisation process theory, a framework for developing, evaluation and implementing complex interventions. BMC Med. 2010;8:63.
12. McEvoy R, Ballini L, Maltoni SC, O'Donnell A, Mair FS, MacFarlance A. A qualitative systematic review of studies using the normalisation process theory to research implementation processes. Implement Sci. 2014;9:2.
13. May C, Murray E, Finch T, Mair F, Treweek S, Ballini L, et al. Normalization Process Theory On-line Users' Manual and Toolkit. 2010. http://www.normalizationprocess.org. Accessed 18 Jan 2017.
14. Strauss A, Corbin JM. Basics of qualitative research: Grounded theory procedures and techniques. Thousand Oaks, CA: Sage; 1990.
15. Blakeman T, Protheroe J, Chew-Graham C, Rogers A, Kennedy A. Understanding the management of early-stage chronic kidney disease in primary care: a qualitative study. Br J Gen Pract. 2012;62(597):e233–42.
16. Gallacher K, May CR, Montori VM, Mair FS. Understanding patients' experiences of treatment burden in chronic heart failure using normalization process theory. Ann Fam Med. 2011;9(3):235–43.
17. National Vascular Disease Prevention Alliance. Guidelines for the management of absolute cardiovascular disease risk. 2012. https://strokefoundation.org.au/What-we-do/Treatment-programs/Clinical-guidelines/Guidelines-for-the-assessment-and-management-of-absolute-CVD-risk. Accessed 18 Jan 2017.
18. Mazza D, Shand LK, Warren N, Keleher H, Browning CJ, Bruce EJ. General practice and preventive health care: a view through the eyes of community members. MJA. 2011;195(4):180–3.
19. McIlfatrick S, Keeney S, McKenna H, McCarley N, McIlwee G. Exploring the actual and potential role of the primary care nurse in the prevention of cancer: a mixed methods study. Eur J Cancer Care. 2014;23(3):288–99.
20. Liddy C, Johnston S, Nash K, Ward N, Irving H. Health coaching in primary care: a feasibility model for diabetes care. BMC Fam Pract. 2014;15:60.
21. Laws RA, Kemp LA, Harris MF, Davies GP, Williams AM, Eames-Brown R. An exploration of how clinician attitudes and beliefs influence the implementation of lifestyle risk factor management in primary healthcare: a grounded theory study. Implement Sci. 2009;4:66.
22. Royal College of General Practice. http://www.racgp.org.au/becomingagp/what-is-a-gp. Accessed 18 Jan 2017.
23. Australian Association of Practice Management. http://www.aapm.org.au/About-AAPM/Definition-of-a-Practice-Manager. Accessed 18 Jan 2017.
24. Australian Practice Nurse Association. http://www.apna.asn.au/scripts/cgiip.exe/WService=APNA/ccms.r?PageId=11012. Accessed 18 Jan 2017.
25. Wolever R, Simmons L, Sforzo G, Dill D, Kaye M, Bechard E, et al. A Systematic Review of the Literature on Health and Wellness Coaching: Defining a Key Behavioral intervention in Healthcare. Glob Adv Health Med. 2013;2(4):38–57.
26. Gale J. The HCA Model of Health Change: An integrated model of health behaviour change for chronic disease prevention and chronic condition self-management. Health Change Australia. 2010. http://www.healthchange.com/resource-library.htm.

5

Exploring why a complex intervention piloted in general practices did not result in an increase in chlamydia screening and diagnosis: a qualitative evaluation using the fidelity of implementation model

R. Allison[1*], D. M. Lecky[1], K. Town[2], C. Rugman[3], E. J. Ricketts[4], N. Ockendon-Powell[5], K. A. Folkard[2], J. K. Dunbar[2] and C. A. M. McNulty[1]

Abstract

Background: *Chlamydia trachomatis* (chlamydia) is the most commonly diagnosed sexually transmitted infection (STI) in England; approximately 70% of diagnoses are in sexually active young adults aged under 25. To facilitate opportunistic chlamydia screening in general practice, a complex intervention, based on a previously successful Chlamydia Intervention Randomised Trial (CIRT), was piloted in England. The modified intervention (3Cs and HIV) aimed to encourage general practice staff to routinely offer chlamydia testing to all 15–24 year olds regardless of the type of consultation. However, when the 3Cs (**c**hlamydia screening, signposting to **c**ontraceptive services, free **c**ondoms) and HIV was offered to a large number of general practitioner (GP) surgeries across England, chlamydia screening was not significantly increased. This qualitative evaluation addresses the following aims:

a) Explore why the modified intervention did not increase screening across all general practices.
b) Suggest recommendations for future intervention implementation.

Methods: Phone interviews were carried out with 26 practice staff, at least 5 months after their initial educational workshop, exploring their opinions on the workshop and intervention implementation in the real world setting. Interview transcripts were thematically analysed and further examined using the fidelity of implementation model.

Results: Participants who attended had a positive attitude towards the workshops, but attendee numbers were low. Often, the intervention content, as detailed in the educational workshops, was not adhered to: practice staff were unaware of any on-going trainer support; computer prompts were only added to the female contraception template; patients were not encouraged to complete the test immediately; complete chlamydia kits were not always readily available to the clinicians; and videos and posters were not utilised. Staff reported that financial incentives, themselves, were not a motivator; competing priorities and time were identified as major barriers.
(Continued on next page)

* Correspondence: Rosie.Allison@phe.gov.uk
[1]Primary Care Unit, National Infection Service, Public Health England, Microbiology Dept, Gloucestershire Royal Hospital, Great Western Road, Gloucester GL1 3NN, UK
Full list of author information is available at the end of the article

(Continued from previous page)

Conclusion: Not adhering to the exact intervention model may explain the lack of significant increases in chlamydia screening. To increase fidelity of implementation outside of Randomised Controlled Trial (RCT) conditions, and consequently, improve likelihood of increased screening, future public health interventions in general practices need to have: more specific action planning within the educational workshop; computer prompts added to systems and used; all staff attending the workshop; and on-going practice staff support with feedback of progress on screening and diagnosis rates fed back to all staff.

Keywords: Chlamydia, Testing, Training, Educational intervention, General practice, Implementation, Adherence, Fidelity, Qualitative, Evaluation

Background

Chlamydia trachomatis (chlamydia) is the most commonly diagnosed STI in England, with 206,774 diagnoses made in 2014 [1]. Sexually active young adults aged under 25 years old continue to be at the highest risk of contracting an STI [1]. Chlamydia infection can cause significant short and long-term morbidity with complications including: pelvic inflammatory disease (PID), tubal infertility and ectopic pregnancy in females; and epididymo-orchitis and possible infertility in males [2–4].

The National Chlamydia Screening Programme (NCSP), established in 2003, aims to control chlamydia through early detection and treatment of asymptomatic infection, so reducing onward transmission and the consequences of untreated infection [5, 6]. A means of achieving this is through opportunistic screening [7–9]. As the majority of young people visit their GP surgery at least once annually, young people see it as an accessible and acceptable setting to receive sexual health services [10–12].

To facilitate opportunistic screening, Public Health England (PHE), in consultation with a primary care led advisory group comprising of general practitioners and practice nurses, developed a more complex intervention, based on a previously successful Chlamydia Intervention Randomised Trial (CIRT) [13, 14]. Whereas the only aim of CIRT was to increase chlamydia screening, the modified intervention, 3Cs and HIV [15], incorporated updated national policy change, such as the integration of chlamydia testing with other sexual health and reproductive services. It aimed to encourage general practice staff to routinely offer chlamydia testing, and provide information about the provision of contraceptive services and free condoms (the '3C's) to all 15–24 year olds, regardless of their reason for consultation. Additionally, practice staff were encouraged to offer HIV screening in line with national guidelines [16].

The 3Cs and HIV intervention, based on the Theory of Planned Behaviour [17], consisted of two educational workshops, delivered by trained local sexual health staff, and an optional follow up with the trainer (see Fig. 1 for details). The first workshop focussed on the routine offer of 3Cs (chlamydia, contraception and condoms); and the second on facilitating HIV screening. The workshops, delivered between August 2013 and July 2015, were supported by a range of materials to engage practice staff and patients (posters, invitation cards and/or leaflets) [18], such as: advertising the availability and confidentiality of the service, in waiting areas; as a prompt for clinicians, in consultations. These resources were developed based on the Theory of Planned Behaviour [17], with engagement in mind. The intervention encouraged a 'whole practice' approach to screening, encouraging all staff members (clinical and non-clinical) to attend the educational workshops; and suggested a 3Cs champion be appointed to motivate, encourage and facilitate discussions and feedback within team meetings.

Following the protocol for the 3Cs & HIV programme [15], both quantitative and qualitative methods were planned to evaluate the effectiveness of the intervention in relation to increasing chlamydia screening (see Fig. 2 for more details on how the intervention was designed to increase chlamydia screening, specifically).

Although immediately after the workshop, practice staff who attended the educational workshops fed back that they intended to increase their chlamydia screening as a result of the training, the quantitative evaluation shows that there was no overall significant increase in chlamydia testing or diagnosis across all of the practices offered the workshops [19]. However, chlamydia testing and diagnosis significantly increased in practices that received specific payments for testing before the intervention began. These practices were reminded about these incentives during the educational workshop.

This qualitative arm of the service evaluation aimed to: a) explore why an intervention based on a successful trial [13, 14] did not achieve the same sustained results in the wider pilot, b) make recommendations for future interventions, and their implementation, within the general practice setting in an effort to improve outcomes.

The fidelity of implementation model (Fig. 3) has been used to facilitate this research. The theory provides a conceptual framework referring to the degree to which an intervention or programme is delivered as intended

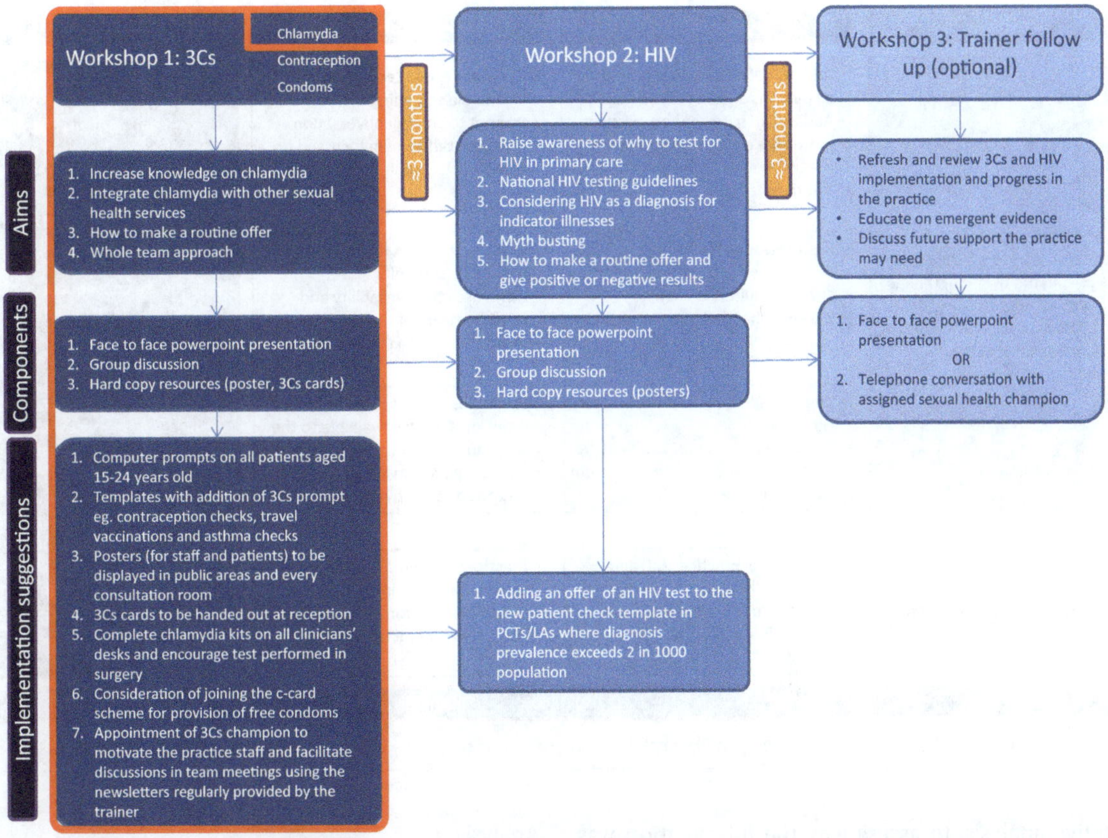

Fig. 1 The 3Cs and HIV intervention with the components that aim to increase chlamydia screening and diagnosis rate highlighted in red

[20]. Unless such an assessment is made, it cannot be determined whether a lack of impact is due to poor implementation or inadequacies inherent in the programme itself, so called Type III error [21, 22]. The concept of implementation fidelity can be described in terms of five elements: adherence to an intervention; exposure or dose; quality of delivery; participant responsiveness; and programme differentiation [23]. This paper will explore each of the first four elements, the relationship between them and suggest essential components of the intervention (programme differentiation, the fifth element) based on the qualitative and quantitative findings.

Methods

Recruitment and sampling

Practices that had participated in the 3Cs and HIV intervention were stratified by chlamydia screening rate per 100 registered 15–24 year old patients, from January 2013 until September 2014 [19]. Practices were then contacted in a random order from this list via the practice managers. Interviews were arranged with practice staff that had previously attended the educational workshops. Data saturation was achieved after 18 interviews [24]. However, as the quantitative analysis showed locally enhanced service (LES) payments to be a relevant factor [19], purposive sampling [25] was used recruit a further 8 participants from areas with an existing LES, at the time of the intervention. At this stage, male practice staff were prioritised, where there was an option, to reduce the gender imbalance.

Interview schedule

The interview schedule explored staff's opinions on the 3Cs and HIV educational workshop as a whole; which components of the intervention they had implemented and their opinion on these (ie. posters, cards, prompts, champion, further discussion); and the impact the intervention had had on their chlamydia testing, HIV testing and sexual health provision. Participants were specifically asked about any barriers to offering basic sexual health services in their practice and ideas on how these could be alleviated. In the initial stages of qualitative data collection, the interviewers were not aware of the quantitative findings. The semi structured interview schedule [26] was modified and developed throughout the data collection process, based on the findings from previous interviews and, following the results of the

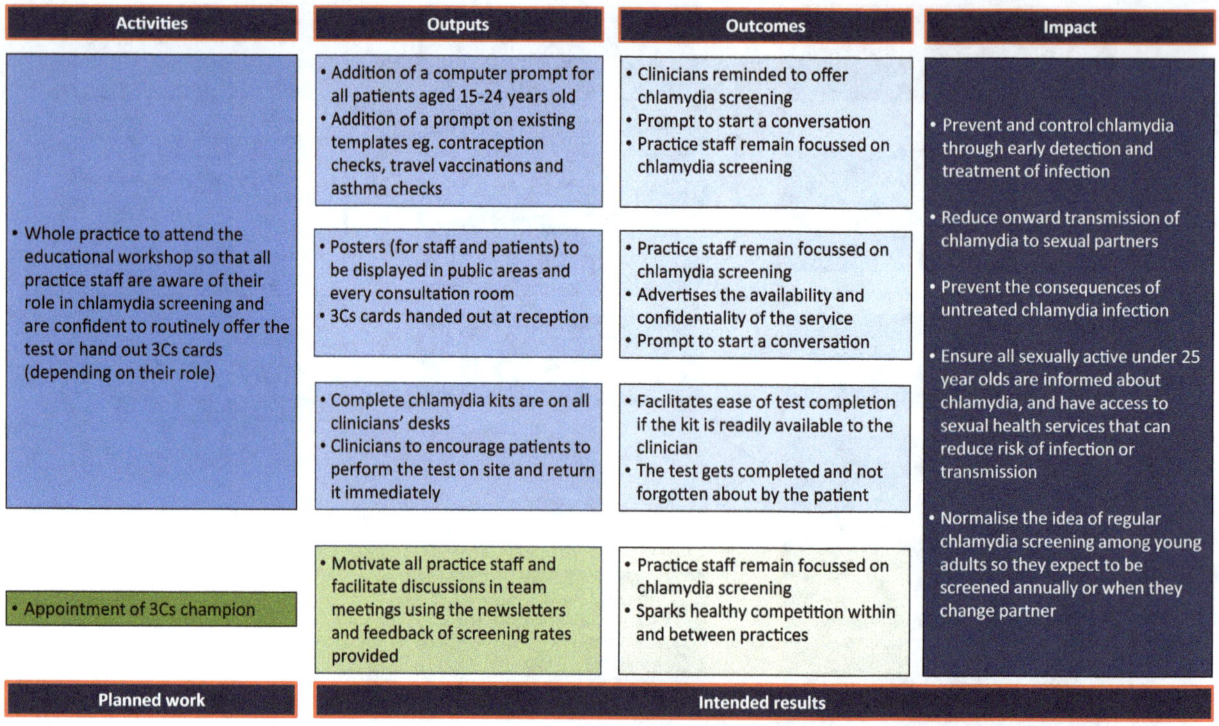

Fig. 2 Modified logic model of how the suggested components of the intervention could have been implemented to increase chlamydia screening

quantitative analysis, to assess why the intervention was not successful, overall (Additional file 1: Appendix 1 and Additional file 2: Appendix 2). Interviewers were practiced in the skill of interviewing, using probing as opposed to leading questions. Length of interviews ranged from 12.8 to 50.6 min, with an average length of 31.6 min.

Interview sessions

Interviews were conducted by telephone, as practice staff reported that they had insufficient time for face-to-face interviews. Although visual cues cannot be obtained during telephone interviews [27, 28], results compared between telephone and face-to-face interviews are very similar [29]. In order for the interviewee to feel they could speak openly and not be influenced by a pre-existing relationship with the interviewer, the interviewer had not facilitated the training or had any previous contact with the participants. Therefore, in order for the interviewer to build rapport with the practice staff, emails and phone calls were exchanged, in order to: set up a time for the interview; discuss the purpose of the research; and ensure the participant was fully informed before written consent was provided. Interviewees were explicitly encouraged to discuss all positive and negative features of the intervention, in order to understand facilitators and barriers to implementation.

Analysis

Interviews were recorded and transcribed verbatim. Transcripts were analysed using a modified framework analysis [30]. Transcripts were initially read through for accuracy and data familiarisation. Two researchers independently coded categories and themes: the lead researcher coded all transcripts and a second researcher coded 10% of the transcripts, to ensure coding consistency; minor discrepancies over specific terminology of themes were resolved through discussion and referral to the original transcripts until agreement was reached. Use of NVivo software (version 10) facilitated the organisation of the data. The one sheet of paper (OSOP) method [31] was used to clarify findings within, and between, themes. As the quantitative evaluation found that the intervention was not successful in increasing chlamydia screening and diagnosis rates in all general practices [19], deductive analysis [32] was used, whereby the principles of the fidelity of implementation model (Fig. 2) were applied to further analyse the themes.

Results

From July 2014 to May 2016, at least 5 months post intervention, 26 members of practice staff were interviewed to see whether there had been a sustained behaviour change. Both clinical and non-clinical staff were interviewed, as everyone had been encouraged to attend the educational workshops. More women participated in

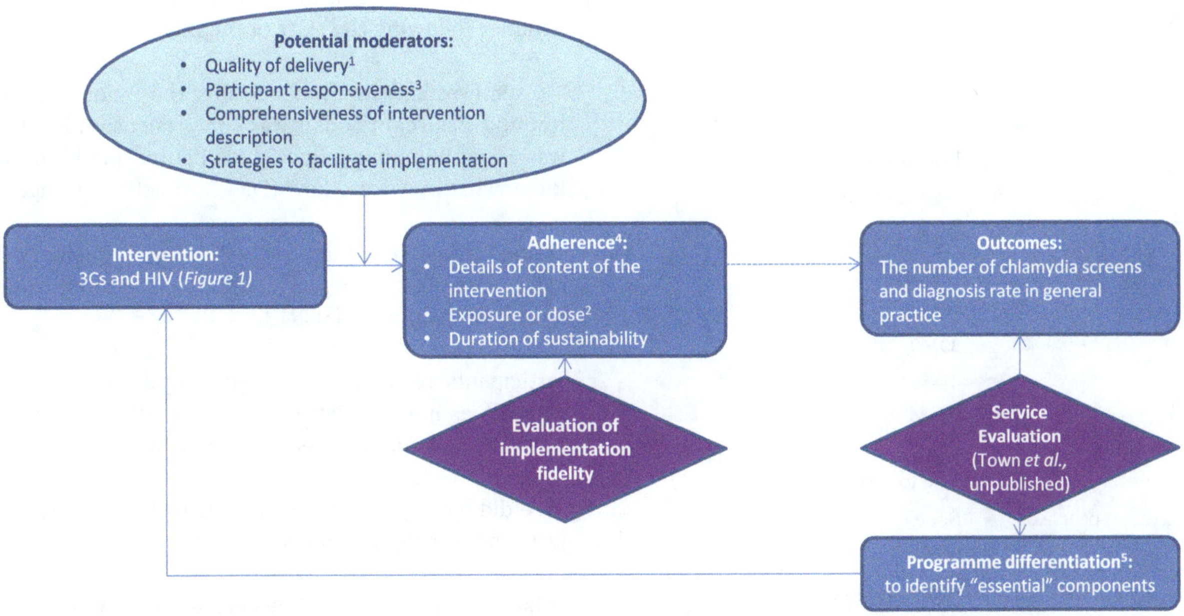

Definition of Terms

[1]**Quality of delivery:** the manner in which the trainer delivered the educational workshops

[2]**Exposure or dose:** the amount of an intervention received by participants (both practice staff and 15-24year olds)

1. Frequency and duration of the intervention: whether all elements of the intervention were delivered as often as specified
2. Coverage: whether all of the people who should be participating in or receiving the benefits of the intervention did so

[3]**Participant responsiveness:** measures how far participants responded to, or were engaged by, an intervention. It involves judgments by participants or recipients about the outcomes and relevance of an intervention.

[4]**Adherence:** whether the 3Cs intervention was being implemented in general practice as it was intended

[5]**Programme differentiation:** identifying which elements of the intervention are essential without which the programme will not have its intended effect

Fig. 3 Modified conceptual framework for fidelity of implementation [20]

the interviews than men, which is also reflected in attendance of the educational workshops. See Table 1 for more details.

The themes that emerged from the interviews were further examined using the fidelity of implementation model as outlined below.

Quality of delivery

Opinion on the trainer/training

Practice staff were very positive about the trainer, quality and format of the training received.

> "actually quite interested to hear all the statistics because she did say a lot about the (*geographical location*) area and what was relevant to us rather than just about the whole country" (KIKT122- receptionist)

> "The advantages of training like the 3C are that staff can talk to each other at in group sessions, and any sort of group training is good because, people, not from what you learn particularly from the lecturers, but from what you learn from the colleagues" (YNYCR126- nurse)

Participants felt that it was relevant to all staff, regardless of their previous sexual health training or their current role within the practice.

> "I found it very useful, and it was... delivered at the right level... we had admin staff with varying knowledge and years of experience working in the NHS as well as two clinical staff attend. So she pitched it at the right level, made it interesting, made it informative and yeah, she's a very pleasant lady and I think she did very well... Yes, no complaints whatsoever. It was easy to understand. There wasn't any massive medical jargon. It gave a bit of background history as to each point and yeah, she delivered it well." (DRA2- practice manager)

The training raised staff awareness of chlamydia and was facilitated by the fact that the trainer came to the practice and held the training over lunch, so it was not an added burden to staff's workload. In a couple of practices, the 3Cs and HIV educational workshop prompted individuals within the practice with an interest in sexual health to provide further training sessions for staff.

Table 1 Characteristics of participants ($n = 26$) and practices ($n = 19$)

Participant characteristic	Variable	Number of participants
Job Role	GP	9
	Practice Nurse	13
	Practice Manager	3
	Receptionist	1
Gender	Male	5
	Female	23
Age	30–40	3
	41–50	6
	51–60	6
	Unknown or did not wish to declare	11
Treating young people or providing sexual health services	None	7
	Some	6
	Heavily involved	13
Practice characteristic	Variable	Number of participants
Local Authority	Devon	3
	Kingston	4
	Luton	2
	North Somerset	5
	York and North Yorkshire	10
	Lincolnshire	2
Phase of implementation (stepped wedge design) [15]	1	4
	2	19
	3	3
Enhanced service	Yes	14
	No	8
	Unknown	4
Chlamydia testing rate higher than England median (pre-intervention)	Yes	19
	No	7
Number of GPs employed	2–5	8
	6–10	5
	11–15	4
	16+	9

> "I think it's made people more aware, because what we did was, we also expanded on the contraceptive side of things and we actually gave a very short training session to the staff as to the types of contraceptive that we actually offer..." (DRA2- practice manager)

Suggestions for the future

Most staff said that they did not: receive the 3Cs and HIV newsletter provided by the trainer to the practice for dissemination; or any other feedback on their progress; and were not aware of any further contact with the trainer following the start of the intervention.

> "Never, ever had any feedback after the training...The training was very good, it was comprehensive, but I was asked then, to produce these figures and I'll never know what they were for." (DRA2- practice manager)

> "I don't think we got any support from my memory, I can't remember having anything...which I think would have been helpful" (NSCR122- GP)

Participants recommended regular updates circulated to all staff, as initially staff were motivated and focussed, but as time passed, this was not sustained.

> "We did have quite a big drive originally, and things just tend to drop off sometimes...
>
> What do you think could be changed so that it doesn't drop off?
>
> I think just keeping up with this kind of training, really, and keeping us on our toes, I suppose.... we just need to do the reminders, I think, more than anything else." (LIRA2- nurse)

Suggested formats included: the trainer coming back to train new staff; shorter but more regular training slots; making the training mandatory; training for a group of GP surgeries rather than individual surgeries; more regular updates on STIs.

> "...you do a big screening event, for the few weeks after the event, it's foremost in everyone's mind because they've just had the training. A year later, they've forgotten all about it... If the same person that delivered the first training turned up 6 months later and said I'm only here for 10 minutes, do you remember we did the screening, the training, how are you getting on? Have any anything you want to discuss about difficulties?... You know if you just had a 10 minute refresher every 6 months that would, that would keep the plant watered" (NSCR121- GP)

> "I think probably tiny amounts of training on a on a frequent basis...may be better than a big training session which nobody has got time for... I think small but regular training inputs are more effective" (NSCR121- GP)

"Following the training, were you clear on what your role was in taking the 3Cs forward and offering a routine chlamydia test?

At the time I was. I think I was crystal clear. Yeah. I'd like, I wouldn't say I am now.

And why do you think it is?

...I need things repeating to me every so often and I think that's what's missing. I think if we had something like the 3Cs training yearly, that would keep it fresh in my mind... Yeah we do a lot of things yearly. It's mandatory for a lot of things and that's how we remember it. Because we're all rubbish at remembering... So it would fit with something like that." (YORA4- GP)

"The GPs have training every month... and that is the best way to get to GPs, because they're all there at the same time... there's nurse training as well, that we have every month." (YORA1- nurse)

Exposure or dose

Who attended the training vs. who the training would be most useful for

Data from the quantitative analysis showed that 58% (268/460) of practices that agreed to participate in the intervention received at least one educational workshop [19]. When discussing reasons for their colleagues non-attendance at the educational workshops, participants reported reasons, such as: lack of time (especially GPs); staff feeling that it is not their field, role, or area of expertise (especially male, older GPs); and the perception that chlamydia tests are offered in contraception consultations, which are generally for female patients, who prefer to see female staff.

"We didn't complete it... only did the chlamydia and it's not because she didn't try, she kept trying to get in, but we had a massive, massive staff change round and then we've had a lot of sickness so I couldn't, I just cannot get the meetings together for the rest of them." (YNYER121- nurse)

"you're going to find that female staff will go... it's also in your area of speciality and it's going to be interesting whereas, yeah, someone who's just not got that in their kind of bag is not, unless it's a learning need for them, they're probably not going to rush to be there... are going to miss training" (DCR120- GP)

"[male GP talking about patient's preference]...see the female doctors for, for consultations... I think it's less of an issue less of something I've had to deal with than some of my colleagues but that of course puts me at risk of being less good at it" (NSKT124- GP)

Some participants felt that the training would be most beneficial for the staff that do not deal with sexual health or young people on a regular basis, but it was felt that these were often the members of staff that did not attend the training.

"If we didn't already have the experience of talking to young people because we are a university eh campus site then I think that those for those clinicians then it would be hugely beneficial" (YNYKT125- nurse)

Staff's perception of young people's beliefs

It was felt that 15–24 years olds are overall more aware and responsive to the offer of a chlamydia screen than previously, due to campaigns related to screening, and education in personal, social, health and economic education (PSHE) and sex and relationship education (SRE) in schools. As such, participants reported that chlamydia screening has become more routine.

"Yeah, they are more aware and a lot of them have had, yeah a, well a lot of them say that they have had chlamydia screening in the last 3 months, when I've asked them, and they're aware to do it every year if they've got a regular partner or when they change their partner" (NSCR122- GP)

"It's part of their, you know, obligatory PHSE training in school now, they all have a lot of time erm being taught that, so I think, perhaps, patients don't feel the need to come in and be taught that in the surgery, because they've already had it" (NSCR120- GP)

Practice staff reported that the 3Cs were mainly offered to young women in contraception consultations, as there was a reminder on the contraception template. It was the opinion of some practice staff that if a patient wanted to be tested for chlamydia, they would just pick up a self-screening kit, and therefore, did not need to be offered a test.

"I haven't had the personal experience that that many people are coming in asking for screening. I think, if they want screening, they know they can pick up the self-testing kits" (NSCR120- GP)

It was the opinion of many practice staff that young people have a preference for receiving sexual health advice from services other than general practices. Reasons included: lack of GP appointments at appropriate times; preference to be in an environment with people of similar age to them; and the worry about the lack of confidentiality in general practice, especially if practice staff know the patient's family members. Several sources gave their opinion that young people would rather attend sexual health or GUM clinics to get advice on sexual health or pick up a chlamydia screening kit.

> "But for the young, with the time, they might talk about after school, before school, and general practice is quite restricted in time." (LUCR120- nurse)

> "They like that so and I think they feel more comfortable about accessing that service if there is people of a similar age to them" (KICR123- nurse)

> "Young people that, they like to go somewhere where they think no one knows them and they're worried maybe if they know the receptionist, or someone's going to tell their parents, and they don't realise how confidential the service is really, so that's why I think they like anonymity of going maybe to a CASH service or an integrated contraception and sexual health service" (KICR123- nurse)

Participant responsiveness

Practice staff's responsiveness

Whose role is sexual health?

There were differing perceptions from participants on whose role sexual health was and whose responsibility it was to implement the suggested changes of the intervention.

> "[talking about their colleagues' perceptions] Not their field not their problem. Those sorts of patients go to family planning or women's health or the nurses" (DCR120- GP)

This lack of clarity often resulted in components of the intervention not being completed, as individuals expected someone else to be doing it.

> **"Do you know whether, following the training, you had a sexual health champion or someone that reminded, kept prodding you to**

> Do you know what? We didn't. That would have been a good idea. We didn't. I think we rely on Dr ** in the practice and Dr ** [female GPs], an awful lot with this. But I think we haven't actually got a champion.

> **Do you know whether that was something that was discussed or within the training?**

> Do you know, I think it was. I think actually in the meeting afterwards I think it was, and for my knowledge I don't know if we've got one. But there could be, well be one in place and I'm just not aware of it." (YORA4- GP)

> "Doctors will be aware of it but they just I suppose haven't got the time and they just think that nurse, the nurses are doing it [laughs] they just think the nurses are doing it" (KICR123- nurse)

Participants also reported a lack of discussion amongst staff members about chlamydia testing, especially between clinical and non-clinical staff.

> "Probably if we had a meeting with the GPs and had a discussion about it and as to what the policy should be, that would probably be more useful, then we'd know where we stand really, If the GPs were on board with offering it then we would if, we'd probably do it ourselves more often as well" (YNYCR122- nurse)

There was a mixed response from non-clinical staff on their willingness to participate in the implementation, for example, some reception staff felt uncomfortable handing out the 3Cs invitation cards to patients.

> "Because I kind of did all the spiel and left all the kits at reception and various information, only to discover when I checked a little while later if they'd been offering it, they said, 'oh, well no one's asked'" (KICR123- nurse)

> "It's not considered our role to ask patients if they want to have chlamydia screening done or anything like that...if someone wants a chlamydia test we'd book them in with Nurse C*" (KIKT122- receptionist)

Patient responsiveness

The majority of staff felt that young people are receptive to a discussion about 3Cs.

> "Where we work, there's decent awareness of chlamydia amongst young people as an issue, so provided its phrased sensitively, I don't think there's a particular issue with making that offer" (NSKT124- GP)

Some participants stated that young people expect to be offered 3Cs as they are in the target age range. It was highlighted that the best approach was to phrase the offer of 3Cs correctly; emphasising the routine, non-judgemental nature of the offer. Gender difference in response to the offer was not identified, but it was highlighted that young men are especially hard to target as they did not attend as frequently.

> "I mean men of that age, boys don't, if they're not coming for contraception they don't consult... and when they do consult they're not consulting about anything to do with sexual health... so for men, you've got somebody coming in about their asthma, and then you're saying to them, as the doctor, 'while you're here, do you want a chlamydia check?' Its, they're going to look at you, thinking, 'I've come about my asthma, why are you suggesting I need sexual, you know, why are you suggesting I've got a sexually transmitted disease?'" (NSCR121- GP)

In contrast, young women were often offered sexual health advice and chlamydia testing at contraception check-ups, as there was usually a tick box for this on the contraception computer template. Some sources said that it was more difficult to offer the 3Cs if the young person was accompanied. Despite the educational workshops, some sources still perceived that patients responded negatively to an offer of a chlamydia test, citing reasons, such as: the perception that patients are offended and feel judged if offered in a non- sexual health consultation; and that there is an excess of chlamydia testing offers to this age group, which causes frustration.

> "And there are, some youngsters are constantly being offered chlamydia tests. They get offered them at college, they get offered them every time they go into the toilet there's a poster about it and if you're just unlucky enough to be the seventh person that week that's offered them a test...they can actually be slightly irritated that it's being overdone" (NSCR121- GP)

The difference between wanting to implement change and making that behaviour change

A locally enhanced service, including financial incentives was mentioned as a facilitator that could make a small difference, but targets set to gain these payments were often reported by participants as unrealistically high. One interviewee highlighted that offering the 3Cs becomes easier, more routine and more comfortable with practice.

Adherence to an intervention

Practice adherence: prompts and templates

Most staff said that they now had a reminder to offer a chlamydia test on the contraception template, which was useful, but no practices had added it to any other consultation template.

> "The contraception template, there's, you know, a tick box for condom supplied, tick box for chlamydia discussed or offered, and tick box for contraception counselling. So, you know, it does kind of, if you use the template, it does trigger you to go through those three things." (DCR120- GP)

> "...prompts on our, just for contraception about screening for chlamydia. We don't have any other prompts" (NSCR122- GP)

Very few had added a computer prompt based solely on the age of the patient, which would encourage offering a chlamydia test to anyone in the age range, not just females presenting for their contraception consultations.

> "I don't think we could manage to make it toggle into our template, so I think then, it's a separate thing we have to search for, and I think that is probably something that gets missed" (DCR120- GP)

Practice adherence: hard copy resources

All of the practices interviewed had made use of the posters and 3Cs cards provided in the 3Cs and HIV intervention. Many had positive views on the resources, reporting that they acted as good marketing tools to advertise the chlamydia screening service and highlight its confidential nature.

> "We've got notices up saying that it's about confidentiality... And I think, actually, it's really useful having the posters because you can say, 'this is a national screening programme.'" (NSCR120- GP)

The majority displayed the posters in the waiting rooms or a prominent place in corridors.

> "We actually set up a campaign in the waiting rooms... to say that we were going to ask about chlamydia" (YNYER121- nurse)

Very few displayed the posters in clinical rooms, but those that did said that it was a useful prompt to open the conversation, as suggested in the intervention training videos used in some educational workshops. 3Cs cards were mainly left on reception or in the waiting area for patients to pick up, however, interviewees often did not know whether the receptionists had handed these out, as follow up discussions between practice staff about how the intervention had been implemented had not occurred.

Practice adherence: sexual health champion

Although it was suggested in the educational workshops, some practices were unaware of whether they had a sexual health champion; and when appointed, a couple of sexual health champions were unclear of the requirements of their role.

> "I think we just need an update, and a reminder that we need to be thinking, that involves more of our staff. I'm sure, if somebody came, they wouldn't tell us anything more than we already know, but sometimes you need that prompt every now and again.
>
> **Was there anyone within the practice that was giving those prompts?**
>
> No, I probably should do it as lead, but again, you just, it just gets absorbed into everything else that you've got to do." (YORA1- nurse)

Barriers to adherence

Competing priorities; lack of time as patients often come in with more than one issue to discuss; or forgetting to offer the 3Cs, especially in a non-sexual health consultation, appeared to be the main barriers for practice staff.

> "If a young person has come to talk about something else, it's not always appropriate to then start talking about 3Cs...sometimes they kind of come with a shopping list of things that they want to come and get dealt with in 10 min, which is all, all medical, and then you are then going to add in well let's talk about 3Cs, and if you do that properly, that really... can be a 10 min consultation itself, because it opens can often open up a whole can of worms and a whole other consultation and discussion with the patient, just, just to talk about the 3Cs" (YNYKT125- nurse)

> "If a young man presents with back pain or shoulder pain then I wouldn't really, I'm not very good at remembering" (NSCR122- GP)

However, a couple of participants pointed out that, although offering the 3Cs may mean a little extra work, it is something they are meant to, or should routinely be doing.

> **"So has working in a way, offering the 3Cs, meant that you've got any more work to do?**
>
> No... It's just made me do the work that I was meant to do." (YORA4- GP)

Lack of complete chlamydia kits or condoms in clinicians' rooms were also limiting factors.

> "Our support staff don't have the kits made up... and that has hindered it... you know, if each time, I've got to go and find it, sort it out myself... and you look a plonker, you look a right wally. You know, if you say, 'oh there's a kit in the waiting room go' and there isn't... it's down to couple of key individuals that just they perhaps see their role as that." (NSKT123- GP)

> "It's all very well for me to sit here running 20 min late and think and four people in the waiting room waiting for me, and to think, 'oh, I should offer this person chlamydia screening'. But, unless that's at my fingertips, in terms of information for the patient all the testing materials... it makes me think, 'oh I just can't I just can't do that now.'" (NSKT124- GP)

Lack of privacy in the reception area and lack of opportunity proved the main barriers for receptionists handing out the 3Cs cards.

> "Because, if you're a receptionist who's not, not a clinician, it's difficult to ask. You can't. How can you ask someone, in the reception area, with a queue of people?" (NSCR120- GP)

Due to time pressures or lack of facilities, not all practices viewed the video clips as part of their educational workshop. These videos suggested "scripts" that could be used in different consultations to facilitate the offer of 3Cs.

Discussion

Summary

Although participants were very positive about the educational workshops, they reported that not all staff attended and, therefore, a whole practice approach was not attained. Some practices did not plan who was going to take the intervention components forward and how this would be done. For example, patients often did not complete the test immediately and the main reason given was that kits often were not made up and in the clinicians' rooms.

Additionally, although the educational workshops specifically encouraged the use of computer prompts and templates, practices generally only added a 3Cs prompt to the female contraception template. Many practices did not develop automatic computer prompts for all patients aged 15–24 years old; therefore, men were excluded [4, 33]. Nevertheless, if all patients attending their GPs for a contraception consultation had completed a chlamydia screen, the intervention effect would have been greater than observed [34], suggesting that this did not happen.

Furthermore, although the educational workshop explicitly addressed some misconceptions of patients' preferences, practice staff's opinions and beliefs had not always changed. This is highlighted in the opinion of a few practice staff that patients would just pick up a self-testing kit if they wanted to be screened; although the point of the intervention was to routinely offer a chlamydia screen to all 15–24 years olds, even if unsymptomatic and in un-related consultations. Although screening may be available through other services, the evidence provided at the educational workshops showed that young people see the GP setting as a non-threatening place for them and therefore an appropriate setting to be offered chlamydia screening [10]. Many participants stated that, as chlamydia screening is becoming more routine, many patients had already completed a test recently and therefore refused the offer. It should be acknowledged that the number of times practice staff offered the test was not reported in the quantitative results; only the number of complete chlamydia screens. It may be that, as chlamydia screening kits are more readily available, young people are getting screened through other means, but as data shows that 60–70% of young people in the target age group visit the GP surgery at least annually [6], practice staff should still be encouraged to offer chlamydia screening to 15–24 year olds, routinely.

Practice staff were not aware of any on-going support with the trainer, which is a key difference from the successful CIRT trial; and, although trainers provided regular newsletters, these were not always circulated around the whole practice [13, 14]. Furthermore, in CIRT, the trainer was funded from a research grant; whereas the 3Cs & HIV intervention used existing staff resources to see whether the intervention was achievable and sustainable in a real world setting. The results suggest there are many challenges with moving from an RCT to real world setting.

Competing priorities, and time were the main barriers for implementation [35]. These competing priorities were: within the general practice, overall; within a consultation, when the patient came in with many symptoms to discuss. Staff reported that financial incentives themselves were not a motivator as targets were too hard to achieve, however the quantitative results show that the practices with financial incentives had a significant increase in chlamydia screening and diagnosis [19]. It is possible that the presence of LES agreements is an indicator of a pre-existing interest in the topic.

Strengths and limitations

Complimenting a quantitative service evaluation with a qualitative evaluation can achieve various aims, including: corroborating findings; generating more complete data; and using results from one method to enhance insights attained with the complementary method [36, 37]. This paper utilised a qualitative approach to attempt to explain and provide insights into the quantitative results. The qualitative findings reflect real issues with any intervention implementation in primary care [38, 39] and the approach enables understanding of ways to improve interventions to facilitate better implementation of already proven effective complex intervention strategies on larger scales outside of trial conditions, with existing local authority funded staff [40, 41].

An additional strength of the study is the range of staff, and characteristics of practices, interviewed. For example, a mixture of male and female: GPs, nurses, practice managers and receptionists; from a range of sized practices with or without a LES, were interviewed. Furthermore, data saturation was reached and no new themes emerged, confirming rich data and a rigorous methodology.

A further strength includes the consideration of the role of the interviewers. The interviewers had not delivered the workshop to the participants and therefore had not developed a relationship with the participants around the intervention delivery. However, the interviewers had been involved in intervention development and/or analysis and therefore had a good understanding of how the intervention was intended to be delivered and the reasoning behind this. This allowed for informed probing by the interviewer, but the participant was not affected by social desirability bias [42] as they did not link the intervention and the interviewer. The primary analyst had not been involved in the intervention development, and therefore was not biased in their analysis.

As this was a service evaluation across England, it was not possible to video the educational workshops to ascertain whether they were delivered as intended. Trainers were encouraged to adapt the presentation to suit their own presentation style and add statistics to make it applicable to the local authority. Therefore, it cannot be confirmed whether the presentation was delivered exactly as intended and whether the key messages were relayed in their entirety. This highlights the difficulty in ensuring a high fidelity of delivery when working with a wide range of people in differing contexts. For example, trainers reported that, sometimes, there were not the facilities to play the video clips role-playing typical situations, and occasionally there was no training room, so the educational workshop was delivered in the waiting room with staff huddled around the trainer (data not shown).

Comparison to other literature and recommendations

Complex interventions have greater scope for variation in their delivery, and so are more vulnerable to one or more components not being implemented as they should; both in delivery and actions following this [20, 41]. The fidelity of implementation model (Fig. 2) details that various moderators should be taken into consideration when implementing an intervention:

Facilitation

Participants in this study were familiar with and positive about the use of prompts and templates. A study by Walker et al., [33] suggest that alerts alone may not be sufficient to significantly increase chlamydia screening, but that they could be included as part of a more complex intervention, such as the 3Cs and HIV. This complex intervention uses prompts in combination with hard copy resources, such as posters and leaflets. Therefore, strategies such as: providing a manual on how to set up a computer prompt based on age; or training the trainer on how to add this prompt to the system, and have the trainer set up the prompt at the first educational workshop, could facilitate implementation, which could have improved the outcomes [33].

Provision of chlamydia kits was not part of the 3Cs and HIV intervention, which relied on the use of existing kits, provided by the Clinical Commissioning Group (CCG). The chlamydia kits' supplier was not recorded as part of the intervention, but future work may be necessary to liaise with the commissioners of primary care resources, to highlight the importance of providing the complete kits in GP surgeries, as this would resolve the problem of incomplete kits, identified by some participants. This further highlights the differences between an RCT and sustainably implementing change in real-life conditions, using existing resources and procedures.

Intervention complexity

Research on guidelines intended for GPs found that detailed and clear recommendations were almost twice as likely to be followed as vague and non-specific recommendations [20, 43]. It could have facilitated implementation if trainers had been explicit about the need for chlamydia kits to be available in every consultation room, to facilitate staff making the offer and facilitate patients completing the tests immediately.

Additionally, more specificity was necessary in regards to where the posters should have been displayed, as the educational workshops suggested that posters displayed in consultation rooms could be used as a prompt or conversation starter, but this was not always adhered to. Furthermore, as the 3Cs and HIV is a complex intervention with multifaceted components and outcomes, a specific action plan detailing staff's roles and responsibilities to implement the intervention should have been agreed at the end of the training session and re-visited at practice meetings [44, 45].

The lack of fidelity of implementation of the intervention may also have been a result of not everyone attending the educational workshops. The workshop highlighted that if everyone within a practice understands what the 3Cs offer is and how it works in their practice, it makes a huge difference in increasing successful outcomes [46]. Francis and Young [47] define a team as "an energetic group of people who are committed to achieving common objectives". However, as not everyone attended the training sessions, there was rarely a whole team approach, which may have resulted in an inconsistent approach to testing, reported by participants, and thus, an overall reduction in fidelity of implementation. By: accessing existing protected learning time and networks; making attendance mandatory; or providing more regular training opportunities, the educational workshop would be attended by a higher percentage of staff, and therefore a whole team approach would be more likely.

Robbins and Finley [48] argue that team failure is often due to: mismatched needs; confused goals; unresolved roles; insufficient feedback and/or information; ill-conceived reward systems, some of which are consistent with the findings of this study.

Conclusions

The findings of this qualitative study indicate that the overall lack of significant increases in chlamydia testing across all general practices involved in the intervention could be due to lack of adherence to the intervention as it was intended, and how it was suggested in the educational workshops. CIRT [49] highlighted key components of the chlamydia intervention that resulted in a successful and sustained increase in chlamydia screening. However, this study highlights that, although in theory these components are known, it is not always possible to implement them outside of a research setting. Further research is required to explore the differences between research and real-life settings; however, this qualitative evaluation suggests minor modifications to the presentation, and support provided within the intervention, which could greatly facilitate implementation and may increase chlamydia screening (Table 2).

The majority of practices were initially very motivated by the educational workshop, but were not able to sustain this focus, which resulted in drop off in fidelity of implementation. To counter this, it is essential that contact is sustained between the trainer and the sexual health champion identified within the educational workshop, so that any questions are answered and ensure that the suggested changes have been implemented. Although the third educational workshop was optional, the majority of practices opted for this to be carried out by phone or felt that they did not need or have time for it

Table 2 Programme differentiation: "key" components identified, without which, the intervention may not have its intended effect

Components of the intervention that were not implemented as intended	Importance of the component	Recommendations for improvements
Whole practice attendance at the educational workshops	If everyone understands what the 3Cs offer is and how it works in their practice, it makes a huge difference in increasing successful outcomes	Make the 3Cs and HIV training mandatory and offer more frequent educational workshops. In the meantime, continue working with the practice manager to find an appropriate time when as many people as possible can attend.
Age-based prompt as well as addition to templates	A prompt solely on the contraception template will not target young men [4] and therefore a prompt is needed for all patients aged 15–24 years old to ensure that clinicians are reminded to offer the 3Cs to everyone in this age group [33].	Be more specific in the educational workshop and facilitate by providing a manual on how to add the prompt; or train the trainer on how to add this prompt to the system, and have the trainer set up the prompt at the first educational workshop.
Complete screening kits in all clinicians' rooms	Screening kits at the clinician's fingertips act as a reminder and facilitates ease of testing, which saves time and will facilitate completion of the tests on-site	Be more specific in the educational workshop and ensure a detailed action plan including who makes up kits is completed in the workshop. Liaise with the commissioners to suggest provision of complete kits as this would facilitate chlamydia testing. Encourage all staff to attend the training so that the whole team: is committed; are clear on their roles; and understand the testing process in their practice.
Reminders and feedback on progress of testing and diagnosis rates	Regular feedback ensures that: 3Cs is not forgotten; staff remain focussed on any targets; and 3Cs are kept as a high priority.	Identify a sexual health champion during the educational workshop ensures that the champion is clear on their role of feeding back and discussing staff's progress of 3Cs in team meetings. A locally enhanced service (LES) should increase the priority of 3Cs in the CCG and the GP surgery. LES financial incentives, in themselves, may not be a driver, but CCG reminders that coincide may improve chlamydia screening rates [50, 51].

[19]. In an attempt to build relations, it could be advised that the trainer return to the practice to be able to see in person whether the intervention is being implemented as intended, give suggestions for improvements, and their presence would act as a reminder for staff to re-focus on their role. Although trainers attempted to find a suitable time to return to the practice, this was not always possible due to lack of time, both for the trainer who was not given additional funding or time to complete the role; and the practice who highlighted lack of time as their main barrier for implementation. It is a suggestion that practices without a locally enhanced service should be targeted first for extra support as there was not a significant increase in chlamydia testing within this group [19].

It is possible that the additional complexity of the 3Cs and HIV intervention in contrast to CIRT was not fully appreciated, and the additional support and facilitators required for implementation was not foreseen. Therefore, in an attempt to increase fidelity of implementation and consequently improve likelihood of increased screening, the intervention needs to have: more specific action planning; computer prompts added to systems and used; all staff attend the workshop in dedicated learning time; and on-going practice staff support.

Abbreviations

3Cs and HIV: Chlamydia, Contraception, Condoms, HIV; CCG: Clinical Commissioning Group; CIRT: Chlamydia Intervention Randomised Trial; GP: General Practitioner; ITT: Intention to treat; LA: Local authority; LES: Local enhanced service; NCSP: National chlamydia screening programme; OSOP: One sheet of paper; PHE: Public Health England; PID: Pelvic inflammatory disease; PSHE: Personal, social, health and economic education; RCT: Randomised controlled trial; SRE: Sex and relationship education; STI: Sexually transmitted infection

Acknowledgements

We wish to thank the National Chlamydia Screening Programme (NCSP) and wider project group in England, especially John Saunders, Anthony Nardone, and Thomas Hartney, and all members of the 3Cs & HIV Project Group (Deborah Shaw, Sharron Ainslie). Also, the 3Cs & HIV Advisory Group in England (Sebastian Kalwij, Farah Paruk, Farhana Lockhart, Jane Wilkinson, Jason Warriner, Richard Ma, Suzie Clements, and Vicki Courage). We also wish to express our thanks to the CATTE Project Audit Committee (Karin Haar, Chris Foy, Ruth Lowbury, Olga Rostowska, and Torsten Berglund). We thank all of the practice staff who were involved.

Funding

This study was supported by a Leonardo Da Vinci Lifelong Learning programme project ChlamydiA Testing Training in Europe (number 2012-1-GB2-LEO05.08044) and Public Health England.

Authors' contributions

CAM and EJR wrote the grant application and designed the study/project, and wrote the draft interview schedules and protocols for discussion. CR, KT, DML, CAM and RA discussed and agreed the protocols and interview schedule and were involved in adapting interview schedules. CAM, CR, KT, NO-P and RA conducted the interviews, and RA and KT analysed the transcripts. RA, DML, KT, CR, EJR, NO-P, KAF, JKD, and CAM contributed to the resource adaptation process. RA wrote the manuscript with contributions from all authors. RA, DML, KT, CR, EJR, NO-P, KAF, JKD, and CAM have reviewed and approved the final manuscript.

Competing interests
CAM leads on the development of PHE quick reference infection diagnostic guides for GPs; KF is the National Chlamydia Screening Programme (NCSP) Manager; and KD is the Director of the National Chlamydia Screening Programme (NCSP). No other staff declare competing interests.

Consent for publication
Not applicable as no personal information is provided in the manuscript.

Ethics approval and consent to participate
The 3Cs & HIV project is a service development programme that aims to support sexual health teams in Local Authorities (LA) improve general practice engagement using existing sexual health services and resources. After review, the Research Governance Coordinator for PHE confirmed that no ethical approvals were needed. Local research and development approvals were obtained for the qualitative interviews from West Midlands (Ref: COV210514), Devon and Exeter (Ref: VL/MC/R&D/CG), South London (Ref: 121512PC), Lincolnshire, Luton, Avon (Ref: 2014–027), York, North Yorkshire and Humber (Ref: 227). Informed verbal and written consent was obtained from the participants and they were given the opportunity to receive a transcript of the interview. A short code was allocated to each participant, so as to uphold anonymity of quotes used.

Author details
[1]Primary Care Unit, National Infection Service, Public Health England, Microbiology Dept, Gloucestershire Royal Hospital, Great Western Road, Gloucester GL1 3NN, UK. [2]HIV/STI Department, Centre for Infectious Disease Control and Surveillance, Public Health England, London, UK. [3]Formerly Public Health England, Primary Care Unit, Microbiology Dept., Gloucester GL1 3NN, UK. [4]Formerly Public Health England, Primary Care Unit, Microbiology Dept., Gloucester, now Derriford Hospital, Derriford Road, Plymouth, UK. [5]Formerly Public Health England, Primary Care Unit, Microbiology Dept., Gloucester, now Biotechnology and Biological Sciences Research Council (BBSRC), Polaris House, North Star Avenue, Swindon, UK.

References
1. Public Health England. Sexually transmitted infections and chlamydia screening in England, 2014, vol. 9. 2015.
2. Akande V, Turner C, Horner P, Horne A, Pacey A. Impact of Chlamydia trachomatis in the reproductive setting: British Fertility Society Guidelines for practice. Hum Fertil. 2010;13(3):115–25.
3. Nwokolo NC, Dragovic B, Patel S, Tong CW, Barker G, Radcliffe K. 2015 UK national guideline for the management of infection with Chlamydia trachomatis. Int J STD AIDS. 2015;27:251–67. doi:10.1177/0956462415615443.
4. Tebb KP, Pantell RH, Wibbelsman CJ, Neuhaus JM, Tipton AC, Pecson SC, Pai-Dhungat M, Ko TH, Shafer MB. Screening sexually active adolescents for Chlamydia trachomatis: what about the boys? Am J Public Health. 2005;95(10):1806–11.
5. LaMontagne D, Fenton K, Randall S, Anderson S, Carter P. Establishing the National Chlamydia Screening Programme in England: results from the first full year of screening. Sex Transm Infect. 2004;80(5):335–41.
6. Salisbury C, Macleod J, Egger M, McCarthy A, Patel R, Holloway A, Ibrahim F, Sterne AC, Horner P, Low N. Opportunistic and systematic screening for chlamydia: a study of consultations by young adults in general practice. Br J Gen Pract. 2006;56(523):99.
7. Adams J, Turner ME, Edmunds WJ. The cost effectiveness of opportunistic chlamydia screening in England. Sex Transm Infect. 2007;83(4):267.
8. Robinson S, Roberts T, Barton P, Bryan S, Macleod J, McCarthy A, Egger M, Sanford E, Low N, Chlamydia SG. Healthcare and patient costs of a proactive chlamydia screening programme: the Chlamydia Screening Studies project. Sex Transm Infect. 2007;83(4):276.
9. Turner KME, Adams EJ, Lamontagne DS, Emmett L, Baster K, Edmunds WJ. Modelling the effectiveness of chlamydia screening in England. Sex Transm Infect. 2006;82(6):496.
10. Hogan AH, Howell-Jones RS, Pottinger E, Wallace LM, McNulty CA. "...they should be offering it": a qualitative study to investigate young peoples' attitudes towards chlamydia screening in GP surgeries. BMC Public Health. 2010;10:616.
11. Ginige S, Fairley CK, Hocking JS, Bowden FJ, Chen MY. Interventions for increasing chlamydia screening in primary care: a review. BMC Public Health. 2007;7:95.
12. Guy RJ, Ali H, Liu B, Poznanski S, Ward J, Donovan B, Kaldor J, Hocking J. Efficacy of interventions to increase the uptake of chlamydia screening in primary care: a systematic review. BMC Infect Dis. 2011;11:211.
13. McNulty CA, Hogan AH, Ricketts EJ, Wallace L, Oliver I, Campbell R, Kalwij S, O'Connell E, Charlett A. Increasing chlamydia screening tests in general practice: a modified Zelen prospective Cluster Randomised Controlled Trial evaluating a complex intervention based on the Theory of Planned Behaviour. Sex Transm Infect. 2014;90(3):188–94.
14. McNulty CA, Thomas M, Bowen J, Buckley C, Charlett A, Gelb D, Foy C, Sloss J, Smellie S. Interactive workshops increase chlamydia testing in primary care–a controlled study. Fam Pract. 2008;25(4):279.
15. Town K, Ricketts E, Hartney T, Dunbar J, Nardone A, Folkard K, Charlett A, McNulty C. Supporting general practices to provide sexual and reproductive health services: protocol for the 3Cs & HIV programme. Public Health. 2015;129(9):1244–50.
16. National Institute for Health and Care Excellence (NICE), Public Health England (PHE). HIV testing: increasing uptake among people who may have undiagnosed HIV (Joint NICE and Public Health England guideline). 2016;1–62.
17. Ajzen I. Perceived behavioral control self-efficiacy locus of control and theory of planned behavior. J Appl Soc Psychol. 2002;32(4):665–83.
18. Freeman E, Howell-Jones R, Oliver I, Randall S, Ford-Young W, Beckwith P, McNulty C. Promoting chlamydia screening with posters and leaflets in general practice–a qualitative study. BMC Public Health. 2009;9:383.
19. Town K, McNulty CA, Ricketts EJ, Hartney T, Nardone A, Folkard KA, Charlett A, Dunbar JK. Service evaluation of an educational intervention to improve sexual health services in primary care implemented using a step-wedge design: analysis of chlamydia testing and diagnosis rate changes. BMC Public Health. 2016;16(1):1.
20. Carroll C, Patterson M, Wood S, Booth A, Rick J, Balain S. A conceptual framework for implementation fidelity. Implement Sci. 2007;2:40.
21. Dobson D, Cook TJ. Avoiding type III error in program evaluation: Results from a field experiment. Eval Program Plann. 1980;3(4):269–76.
22. Craig P, Dieppe P, Macintyre S, Michie S, Nazareth I, Petticrew M. Developing and evaluating complex interventions: the new Medical Research Council guidance. BMJ. 2008;337:a1655.
23. Mihalic S. The importance of implementation fidelity. Emotional and Behavioral Disorders in Youth. 2004;4(4):83–105.
24. Fusch PI, Ness LR. Are we there yet? Data saturation in qualitative research. Qual Rep. 2015;20(9):1408.
25. Patton MQ. Qualitative research. In: Wiley Online Library. 2005.
26. Newton N. The use of semi-structured interviews in qualitative research: strengths and weaknesses. Exploring qualitative methods. 2010;1(1):1–11.
27. Novick G. Is there a bias against telephone interviews in qualitative research? Res Nurs Health. 2008;31(4):391–8.
28. Garbett R, Mccormack B. The experience of practice development: an exploratory telephone interview study. J Clin Nurs. 2001;10(1):94–102.
29. Vogl S. Telephone Versus Face-to-Face Interviews Mode Effect on Semistructured Interviews with Children. Sociol Methodol. 2013;43(1):133–77.
30. Braun V, Clarke V. Using thematic analysis in psychology. Qual Res Psychol. 2006;3(2):77–101.
31. Ziebland S, McPherson A. Making sense of qualitative data analysis: an introduction with illustrations from DIPEx (personal experiences of health and illness). Med Educ. 2006;40(5):405–14.
32. Pope C, Ziebland S, Mays N. Analysing qualitative data. BMJ. 2000;320(7227):114–6.
33. Walker J, Fairley K, Walker M, Gurrin C, Gunn M, Pirotta V, Carter R, Hocking S. Computer reminders for Chlamydia screening in general

practice: a randomized controlled trial. Sex Transm Dis. 2010;37(7):445.
34. Bowden J, Currie J, Toyne H, McGuiness C, Lim L, Butler R, Glasgow J. Screening for Chlamydia trachomatis at the time of routine Pap smear in general practice: a cluster randomised controlled trial. Med J Aust. 2008;188(2):76.
35. Wallace L, McNulty C, Hogan A, Bayley J. Exploring attitudes and practices of General Practice staff towards offers of opportunistic screening for chlamydia: a UK survey. Prim Health Care Res Dev. 2012;13(3):255.
36. Curry LA, Nembhard IM, Bradley EH. Qualitative and mixed methods provide unique contributions to outcomes research. Circulation. 2009;119(10):1442–52.
37. Creswell JW, Clark VLP. Designing and conducting mixed methods research. 2007.
38. Smeets HM, Kuyvenhoven MM, Akkerman AE, Welschen I, Schouten GP, Van Essen GA, Verheij TJ. Intervention with educational outreach at large scale to reduce antibiotics for respiratory tract infections: a controlled before and after study. Fam Pract. 2009;26(3):183–7.
39. Cabana MD, Rand CS, Powe NR, Wu AW, Wilson MH, Abboud P-AC, Rubin HR. Why don't physicians follow clinical practice guidelines?: A framework for improvement. JAMA. 1999;282(15):1458–65.
40. Pope C, Mays N, Popay J. Synthesising Qualitative and Quantitative Health Evidence: A Guide to Methods: A Guide to Methods. UK: McGraw-Hill Education; 2007.
41. Greenhalgh T, Annandale E, Ashcroft R, Barlow J, Black N, Bleakley A, Boaden R, Braithwaite J, Britten N, Carnevale F, et al. An open letter to The BMJ editors on qualitative research. BMJ. 2016;352:i563.
42. Fisher RJ. Social desirability bias and the validity of indirect questioning. J Consum Res. 1993;20(2):303–15.
43. Grol R, Dalhuijsen J, Thomas S, Rutten G, Mokkink H. Attributes of clinical guidelines that influence use of guidelines in general practice: observational study. BMJ. 1998;317(7162):858–61.
44. Lorch R, Hocking J, Guy R, Vaisey A, Wood A, Donovan B, Fairley C, Gunn J, Kaldor J, Temple-Smith M, et al. Do Australian general practitioners believe practice nurses can take a role in chlamydia testing? A qualitative study of attitudes and opinions. BMC Infect Dis. 2015;15:31.
45. Lorch R, Hocking J, Temple-Smith J, Law M, Yeung A, Wood A, Vaisey A, Donovan B, Fairley CK, Kaldor J, et al. The chlamydia knowlegde awreness and testing practices of Australian General practitioners and practice nurses: survey findings from the Australian Chlamydia Control Effectiveness Pilot (ACCEPt). BMC Fam Pract. 2013;14(169):1471–2296.
46. Castka P, Bamber CJ, Sharp JM, Belohoubek P. Factors affecting successful implementation of high performance teams. Team Performance Management: An International Journal. 2001;7(7/8):123–34.
47. Francis D, Young D. Improving work groups, a practical manual for team building. La Jolla: University Associates; 1979.
48. Robbins H, Finley M. The new why teams don't work: What goes wrong and how to make it right. San Francisco: Berrett-Koehler Publishers; 2000.
49. Ricketts EJ, Francischetto EOC, Wallace LM, Hogan A, McNulty CA. Tools to overcome potential barriers to chlamydia screening in general practice: Qualitative evaluation of the implementation of a complex intervention. BMC Fam Pract. 2016;17(1):1.
50. Bilardi E, Fairley K, Temple-Smith J, Pirotta V, McNamee M, Bourke S, Gurrin C, Hellard M, Sanci A, Wills J, et al. Incentive payments to general practitioners aimed at increasing opportunistic testing of young women for chlamydia: a pilot cluster randomised controlled trial. BMC Public Health. 2010;10:70.
51. Kalwij S, French S, Mugezi R, Baraitser P. Using educational outreach and a financial incentive to increase general practices' contribution to chlamydia screening in South-East London 2003–2011. BMC Public Health. 2012;12:802.

6

Health care resource use by patients before and after a diagnosis of chronic fatigue syndrome (CFS/ME): a clinical practice research datalink study

Simon M. Collin[1*], Inger J. Bakken[2], Irwin Nazareth[3], Esther Crawley[1] and Peter D. White[4]

Abstract

Background: Our aim was to investigate patterns of health care resource use by patients before and after a diagnosis of CFS/ME, as recorded by Clinical Practice Research Datalink (CPRD) GP practices in the UK.

Methods: We used a case–control study design in which patients who had a first recorded diagnosis of CFS/ME during the period 01/01/2001 to 31/12/2013 were matched 1:1 with controls by age, sex, and GP practice. We compared rates of GP consultations, diagnostic tests, prescriptions, referrals, and symptoms between the two groups from 15 years (in adults) or 10 years (in children) before diagnosis to 10 years after diagnosis.

Results: Data were available for 6710 adult and 916 child (age <18 years) matched case–control pairs. Rates of GP consultations, diagnostic tests, prescriptions, referrals, and symptoms spiked dramatically in the year when a CFS/ME diagnosis was recorded. GP consultation rates were 50% higher in adult cases compared to controls 11–15 years before diagnosis (rate ratio (RR) 1.49 (95% CI 1.46, 1.52)) and 56% higher 6–10 years after diagnosis (RR 1.56 (1.54, 1.57)). In children, consultation rates in cases were 45% higher 6–10 years before diagnosis (RR 1.45 (1.40, 1.51)) and 62% higher 6–10 years after diagnosis (RR 1.62 (1.54, 1.70)). For adults and children, rates of tests, prescriptions, referrals, and symptoms were higher in cases compared to controls for up to 10 years before and after diagnosis.

Conclusions: Adults and children with CFS/ME have greater health care needs than the rest of the population for at least ten years before their diagnosis, and these higher levels of health care resource use continue for at least ten years after diagnosis.

Keywords: Chronic fatigue syndrome, CFS/ME, fibromyalgia, Diagnosis, Adults, Children, Primary care, CPRD, Health care resource use

Background

Chronic fatigue syndrome (CFS, also known as 'ME') is a debilitating illness of unknown aetiology and pathophysiology [1]. Characterizing patients' long-term health status before and after the onset and diagnosis of CFS/ME is important if we are to quantify the health economic and societal costs of CFS/ME, and the effects of diagnosis on health care use. Productivity losses due to CFS/ME in the UK have been estimated to be more than £100 M per annum [2]. These estimates of indirect costs were based on self-reported duration of illness (median 3 years) among patients who were able to access specialist CFS/ME services and who do not include all patients with CFS/ME. Direct costs of CFS/ME have been estimated from health care resource use by patients presenting to GPs in England, but only for short periods (3–6 months) prior to diagnosis [3, 4].

The aim of our study was to investigate long-term patterns in health care resource use before and after a diagnosis of CFS/ME using data from the Clinical Practice Research Datalink (CPRD). The CPRD provides data from approximately 7% of primary care (GP) practices in

* Correspondence: simon.collin@bristol.ac.uk
[1]School of Social and Community Medicine, University of Bristol, Oakfield House, Oakfield Grove, Bristol BS8 2BN, UK
Full list of author information is available at the end of the article

the UK [5]. We hypothesised that health care resource use would increase from around the time of patient-reported onset of illness (median self-reported duration of illness among patients who attend NHS specialist services is 3 years (adults), 16 months (children age 12–18 years) and 12 months (children <12 years old)) [1] until diagnosis. We did not have a prior hypothesis about post-diagnosis health care resource use, although this might be expected to fall if diagnosis led to referral and effective treatment. We also investigated whether health care resource use varied by sex and by socioeconomic status, given earlier evidence of a social gradient in access to CFS/ME specialist services in England [6] and in incidence of CFS/ME diagnoses [7], and we investigated adult and paediatric patients, given differences in presentation and prognosis [1].

Methods

Data source

The Clinical Practice Research Datalink (CPRD), formerly known as the General Practice Research Database (GPRD), is an anonymised research database aggregating medical records data from participating general practices across the UK (approximately 7% of 10,000 practices in 2012) [5]. Practices contributing to CPRD are broadly representative of general practices in the UK in terms of practice size and geographical distribution, and the source population (approximately four million 'active' patients, i.e. alive and registered with a GP) is broadly representative of the population of the UK in terms of age, sex, and ethnicity. GPs enter medical diagnoses and symptoms as Read codes, a hierarchical coding system used to record clinical information. Procedures, prescriptions, and referrals to secondary care are also recorded. CPRD provides two sets of data quality criteria: 'up-to-standard' (UTS) date for practices and 'acceptability' for patients [5]. These criteria do not ensure data quality, but they are used to delineate periods of quality data recording. UTS date is the date from which data in the practice are considered to be of sufficiently high quality by checking that events are being recorded continually and that recording of deaths matches projections for the practice (allowing for geographical and seasonal variation). For this study, data recorded since the practice UTS date were obtained from 660 general practices in the UK from 01/01/2001 to 31/12/2013. The acceptable patient metric is based on registration status, consistency and completeness of recording of events in the patient record, and valid information on age and sex [5]. Patients with non-contiguous records or poor data recording, which thereby raises suspicion about the validity of that patient's record, are excluded. This study used the medical record data of patients who had acceptable data from a period beginning with the latest of the patient's current registration period and the practice UTS date, and ending with the earliest of the patient's transfer out date, the practice last collection date and the study end date.

Cases

Cases were patients who had a new diagnosis of CFS/ME during the study period (01/01/2001 to 31/12/2013), as indicated by an index event with a Read code for diagnosis of CFS/ME (nine possible Read codes [8]) or referral to a CFS/ME specialist service (Additional file 1: Table S1). We considered new CFS/ME diagnoses to be those index events for which there was no preceding diagnosis of CFS/ME, FM, PVFS or asthenia/debility in the patient's CPRD medical record as indicated by prior events with the corresponding Read codes (Additional file 1: Table S1). Read codes for referral to specialist services were introduced in 2010. Diagnoses which were made after a referral (and for which there was no prior diagnosis) were treated as new diagnoses.

Controls

For each case, one control was matched on index event date, practice, year of birth, and sex. Controls were selected at random from patients who had no recorded diagnosis of CFS/ME, post-viral fatigue syndrome, asthenia/debility or fibromyalgia. Matching on index event date meant that the index event of the case must have occurred within the control's registration period.

Health care resource use

GP consultations, tests, prescriptions, and referrals were counted if they had been recorded in the patient's medical record at any time during the patient's current registration period with the primary care practice. Multiple GP consultations on one day were counted as a single consultation. Multiple tests per day were counted in order to reflect the total number of tests ordered. Multiple prescriptions per day were counted, but only new prescriptions were included, i.e. repeat (recurring) prescriptions were not counted. Cases and controls were required to have at least 12 months of UTS and acceptable data prior to the index event date, in order to avoid the excess events which tend to occur shortly after a patient has registered with a practice [9].

Symptoms

Symptoms were flagged as 'all' symptoms, i.e. a symptom of any type, and 'fatigue' symptoms (if the symptom had a Read code as listed in Additional file 1: Table S1).

Practice-level socioeconomic status

Index of Multiple Deprivation (IMD) score was used as a measure of socioeconomic status for the practice, based on its postcode. The IMD is the UK government's official measure of deprivation.[10] It is a composite score derived from seven domains: income, employment, health and disability, education skills and training, barriers to housing and services, crime and disorder, and living environment. We grouped the top three (least deprived) quintiles and bottom two (most deprived) quintiles into two IMD strata to simplify our analysis and because our study of trends in CFS/ME diagnoses using CPRD data had shown a difference in incidence rates across these groupings [7].

Statistical analyses

Annual rates (and 95% confidence intervals (CIs)) per patient of health care resource use events and symptoms were calculated by summing the number of events during each calendar year (for up to 15 years before and up to 10 years after the year of first recorded diagnosis of CFS/ME), and dividing by the number of patients whose medical data extended up until that time. We calculated rate ratios for cases compared with controls by fitting negative binomial regression models including a term for interaction between case status and time period, coded as three 5-year periods pre-diagnosis (11–15, 6–10 and 1–5 years before diagnosis), year of diagnosis (year 0), and two 5-year periods post-diagnosis (1–5 and 6–10 years). This allowed us to estimate the mean ratio between rates for cases compared with controls during each time period. Models were fitted using Stata (StataCorp. 2015. Stata Statistical Software: Release 14. College Station, TX: StataCorp LP).

Results

Study population

7901 patients had a new CFS/ME diagnosis recorded during the study period. Matched controls were available for 7626 (96.5%) of these patients. The population comprised 916 child (age <18 years) and 6710 adult patients. At the time of the index event, the median (interquartile range (IQR)) age of child patients was 15 (13–16) years, and 63.9% (585/916) were female; the median (IQR) age of adult patients was 43 (33–53) years, and 72.6% (4874/6710) were female.

The durations of pre-diagnosis data were the same in cases and controls, with a median (IQR) of 6 (3–11) years for both adult cases and controls, 8 (4–12) years for child cases, and 8 (4–11) years for child controls. Post-diagnosis data were available for 5 (3–9) years for adult cases, 5 (2–8) years for adult controls, and 4 (2–7) years for both child cases and controls. Up to 10 years of pre-diagnosis data were available for 25.9% (1737/6710) and 26.0% (1744/6710) of adult cases and controls, respectively (Additional file 1: Table S2), and 10 years of post-diagnosis data were available for 19.8% (1328/6710) and 18.4% (1232/6710) of adult cases and controls. Ten years of pre-diagnosis data were available for 32.3% (296/916) and 31.0% (284/916) of child cases and controls (Additional file 1: Table S3), and post-diagnosis data up to 10 years were available for 11.7% (107/916) and 12.1% (111/916). Fifteen years of pre-diagnosis data were available for 7.6% (509/6710) and 7.9% (529/6710) of adult cases and controls, respectively.

Health care resource use

Adults

At 11–15 years before their first recorded CFS/ME diagnosis, GP consultations per patient per year were 49% higher in cases compared with controls (rate ratio (RR) 1.49 (95% CI 1.46, 1.52)) (Table 1, Fig. 1). During the 5 years before diagnosis, the rate of GP consultations was 76% higher (RR 1.76 (1.75, 1.77)) and, in the year when the diagnosis was recorded, the rate was 2.5 times higher (RR 2.48 (2.44, 2.51)). The rate ratio fell steeply after diagnosis, and was 56% higher (RR 1.56 (1.54, 1.57)) over the period 6–10 years post-diagnosis. Rates of tests, new prescriptions and referrals were, respectively, 64% (RR 1.64 (1.59, 1.68)), 56% (RR 1.56 (1.53, 1.58)) and 53% (RR 1.53 (1.46, 1.60)) higher in cases compared with controls at 11–15 years pre-diagnosis (Table 1, Fig. 1). Rate ratios for tests, prescriptions and referrals peaked at 3.0, 2.4 and 3.5, respectively, in the year when a CFS/ME diagnosis was first recorded. At 6–10 years post-diagnosis, rates of tests, prescriptions and referrals were, respectively, 50% (RR 1.50 (1.49, 1.51)), 85% (RR 1.85 (1.82, 1.87)) and 78% (RR 1.78 (1.72, 1.85)) higher in cases compared with controls.

Children

At 6–10 years before their first recorded CFS/ME diagnosis, GP consultations per patient per year were 45% higher in cases compared with controls (RR 1.45 (1.40, 1.51)) (Table 2, Fig. 2). During the 5 years before diagnosis the rate of GP consultations in cases was more than double the rate in controls (RR 2.34 (2.28, 2.41)), peaking at a 4-fold higher rate (RR 4.10 (3.90, 4.31)) in the year when the diagnosis was recorded. The rate ratio fell steeply after diagnosis, and was 62% higher (RR 1.62 (1.54, 1.70)) over the period 6–10 years post-diagnosis. Test rates in cases began almost 3-fold higher than in controls at 6–10 years pre-diagnosis (RR 2.70 (2.51, 2.89)), peaked at a 13-fold higher rate (RR 12.9 (12.3, 13.5)) and fell back to >2 times higher 6–10 years later (RR 2.37 (2.29, 2.44)) (Table 2, Fig. 2). Relative rates of new prescriptions were 44% higher 6–10 years pre-diagnosis (RR 1.44 (1.39, 1.50)), peaking at 3.3 times higher in the year of diagnosis, and falling back to 84% higher 6–10 years later (RR 1.84 (1.74, 1.93)). Referral rates were 40% higher at 6–10 years pre-diagnosis (RR 1.40

Table 1 Rates per patient year (95% CI) and rate ratios (95% CI) of GP consultations, tests, prescriptions and referrals from 15 years before until 10 years after a first recorded diagnosis of CFS/ME in adult cases compared with controls

	Year −15 to −11	Year −10 to −6	Year −5 to −1	Year 0	Year 1 to 5	Year 6 to 10
Total person years						
Cases	4579	12,183	24,478	6710	25,447	10,815
Controls	4649	12,258	24,564	6710	25,038	10, 508
GP consultations						
Cases (rate)	6.42 (6.35, 6.49)	6.77 (6.72, 6.81)	8.06 (8.02, 8.09)	10.6 (10.6, 10.7)	7.11 (7.08, 7.14)	6.59 (6.54, 6.64)
Controls (rate)	4.31 (4.25, 4.37)	4.53 (4.49, 4.56)	4.58 (4.56, 4.61)	4.29 (4.24, 4.34)	4.10 (4.07, 4.12)	4.24 (4.20, 4.28)
Rate ratio	1.49 (1.46, 1.52)	1.50 (1.48, 1.51)	1.76 (1.75, 1.77)	2.48 (2.44, 2.51)	1.73 (1.72, 1.75)	1.56 (1.54, 1.57)
Diagnostic tests						
Cases (rate)	2.50 (2.46, 2.55)	8.01 (7.96, 8.06)	20.4 (20.3, 20.4)	37.0 (36.9, 37.2)	23.1 (23.0, 23.1)	26.4 (26.3, 26.5)
Controls (rate)	1.53 (1.49, 1.57)	4.98 (4.94, 5.02)	9.75 (9.71, 9.79)	12.3 (12.2, 12.3)	14.2 (14.1, 14.2)	17.6 (17.5, 17.7)
Rate ratio	1.64 (1.59, 1.68)	1.61 (1.59, 1.62)	2.09 (2.08, 2.10)	3.02 (3.00, 3.05)	1.63 (1.62, 1.64)	1.50 (1.49, 1.51)
Prescriptions						
Cases (rate)	6.83 (6.76, 6.91)	6.26 (6.21, 6.30)	6.63 (6.60, 6.67)	7.84 (7.78, 7.91)	6.48 (6.45, 6.51)	6.63 (6.58, 6.68)
Controls (rate)	4.39 (4.33, 4.45)	3.84 (3.81, 3.88)	3.47 (3.45, 3.50)	3.34 (3.29, 3.38)	3.31 (3.29, 3.33)	3.59 (3.56, 3.63)
Rate ratio	1.56 (1.53, 1.58)	1.63 (1.61, 1.65)	1.91 (1.89, 1.93)	2.35 (2.31, 2.39)	1.96 (1.94, 1.98)	1.85 (1.82, 1.87)
Referrals						
Cases (rate)	0.99 (0.96, 1.02)	0.86 (0.84, 0.87)	0.86 (0.85, 0.87)	1.38 (1.35, 1.41)	0.76 (0.75, 0.77)	0.71 (0.70, 0.73)
Controls (rate)	0.65 (0.63, 0.67)	0.55 (0.54, 0.57)	0.43 (0.42, 0.43)	0.39 (0.37, 0.40)	0.38 (0.37, 0.39)	0.40 (0.39, 0.41)
Rate ratio	1.53 (1.46, 1.60)	1.55 (1.50, 1.60)	2.02 (1.98, 2.07)	3.54 (3.39, 3.70)	2.00 (1.95, 2.05)	1.78 (1.72, 1.85)

(1.22, 1.60)), peaked at a 9-fold higher rate (RR 8.83 (7.38, 10.6)) and were 2.5-fold higher 6–10 years post-diagnosis (RR 2.53 (2.12, 3.03)).

Symptoms

Adults

Relative rates of all (any) recorded symptoms were 55-69% higher in cases compared with controls from 6–15 years pre-diagnosis and 1–10 years post-diagnosis, peaking at a >2-fold higher rate in the year of diagnosis (RR 2.34 (2.28, 2.39)) (Table 3, Fig. 3, Additional file 1: Table S4). Relative rates of fatigue symptoms were much higher in cases compared with controls, rising from an 8-fold higher rate 11–15 years pre-diagnosis (RR 8.12 (4.83, 13.7)) to a 22-fold higher rate in the year of diagnosis (RR 21.9 (18.8, 25.5)), then falling to a 4-fold higher rate 6–10 years post-diagnosis (RR 3.75 (3.26, 4.32)).

Children

Symptoms of any kind were recorded at a 68% higher rate (RR 1.68 (1.57, 1.79)) in child cases compared with controls 6–10 years before diagnosis, peaking at a >4-fold higher rate in the year of diagnosis (RR 4.40 (4.04, 4.79)), and falling back to a 79% higher rate (RR 1.79 (1.65, 1.94)) 6–10 years after diagnosis (Table 3, Fig. 3, Additional file 1: Table S4). Fatigue symptoms were recorded at a 7-fold higher rate (RR 6.93 (2.44, 19.7)) in cases compared with controls 6–10 years pre-diagnosis, peaking at a 52-fold higher rate (RR 51.6 (27.6, 96.5)), and falling back to an almost 5-fold higher rate 6–10 years post-diagnosis (RR 4.73 (2.47, 9.07)).

Variation in health care resource use by sex and socioeconomic status

Women had higher rates of health care resource use than men (Fig. 4). Case *vs.* control rate ratios tended to be lower in female than in male patients (Table 4, Additional file 1: Tables S5a, b), but the overall patterns of relative health care resource use were similar (Fig. 4). Practice-level IMD data were available for 78.5% (5266/6710) and 85.8% (786/916) of adult and child patients, respectively. Rates of health care resource use in the upper three (least deprived) IMD quintiles were similar to rates in the lower two quintiles, although rates of prescriptions were higher in the bottom two quintiles (Fig. 5). There was little discernible difference in relative rates of health care resource use comparing cases *vs.* controls between the two socioeconomic strata (Table 5, Additional file 1: Tables S6a, b), although rate ratios for tests and prescriptions were lower in the bottom two than in the top three IMD quintiles in the pre-diagnosis periods and in the year of diagnosis.

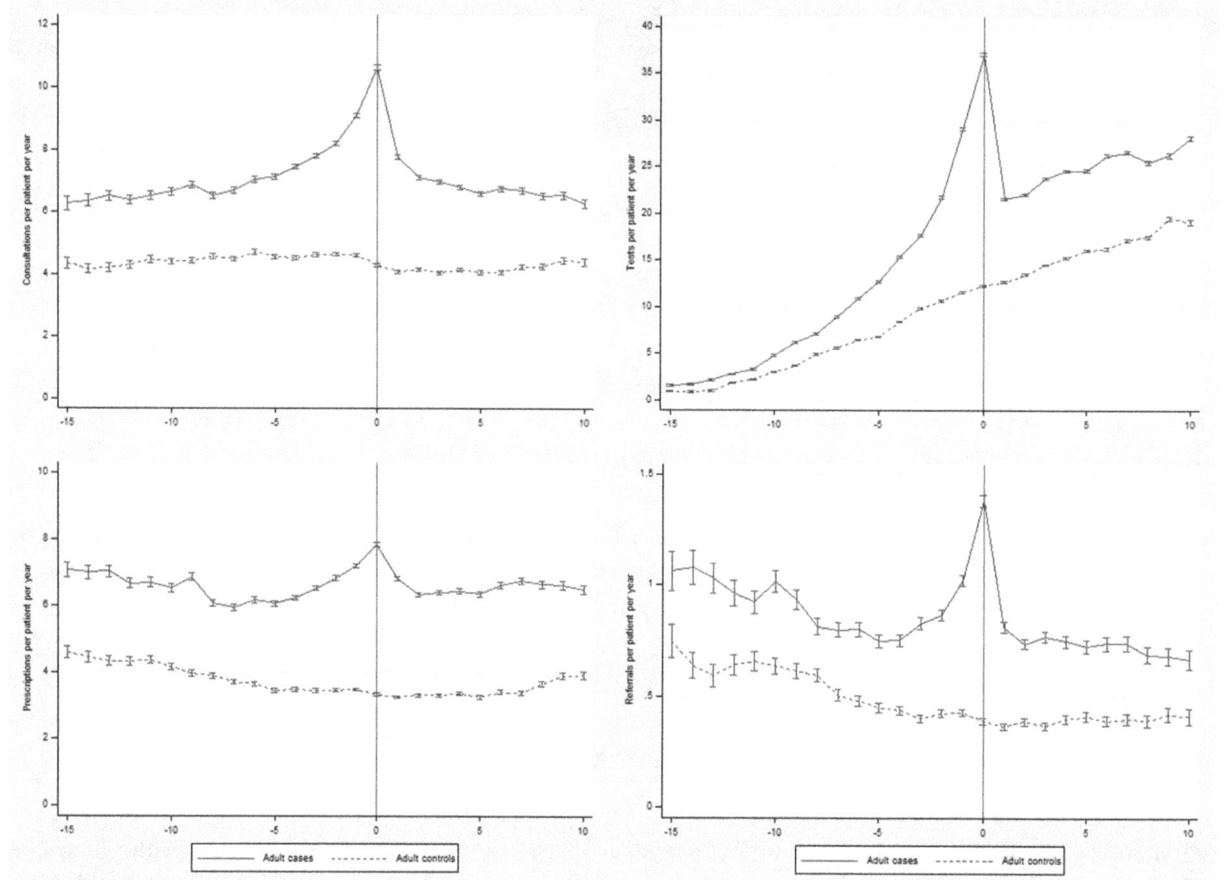

Fig. 1 Rates of GP consultations, tests, prescriptions and referrals from 15 years before until 10 years after a first recorded diagnosis of CFS/ME in adult cases compared with controls

Discussion

Statement of principal findings

Our study has revealed three main features of long-term patterns in health care resource use before and after a diagnosis of CFS/ME: 1) adults and children diagnosed with CFS/ME have greater health care needs than the rest of the population for at least ten years before the diagnosis; 2) from this higher baseline, there were steep increases in use of health care resources 2–4 years before diagnosis in adults and 1–2 years before diagnosis in children; and 3) a steep drop in resource use immediately after diagnosis was followed by sustained higher levels of health care resource use for at least ten years after diagnosis. These patterns were broadly similar in women and men, and in social strata defined by IMD quintiles, and were also seen in rates of symptoms generally and fatigue symptoms specifically.

The second of these three features was not unexpected. We had hypothesised that health care resource use would increase from around the time of patient-reported onset of illness, and the dramatic peaks in health care resource use and symptoms are consistent with CFS/ME being defined clinically as a disease of new or distinct onset. However, the higher levels of health needs and symptoms predating diagnosis by up to 15 years is a somewhat unexpected finding. It conflicts with patients reporting that they were fit and well prior to the onset of their illness [11, 12] (albeit in small qualitative studies), and it raises interesting questions about the natural history of CFS/ME.

Our study in relation to other studies

In relation to onset of illness, seven case definitions for CFS/ME have been used in clinical practice and research since the first was published in 1988, and these definitions have differed mainly in the minimum duration of fatigue and the type and number of additional symptoms [13]. That the fatigue must be of new or distinct onset was a feature of the original CDC case definition [14], and was also part of the Fukuda [15], Oxford [16], and the (original) Canadian [17] case definition. The Canadian criteria and its subsequent revision allowed for a gradual onset, but recognised that onset was typically distinct [18]. The recently-introduced US Institute of

Table 2 Rates per patient year (95% CI) and rate ratios (95% CI) of GP consultations, tests, prescriptions and referrals from 10 years before until 10 years after a first recorded diagnosis of CFS/ME in paediatric cases compared with controls

	Year −10 to −6	Year −5 to −1	Year 0	Year 1 to 5	Year 6 to 10
Total person years					
Cases	2088	3715	916	3290	1076
Controls	1996	3591	916	3257	1077
GP consultations					
Cases (rate)	3.77 (3.69, 3.85)	4.43 (4.36, 4.49)	8.22 (8.04, 8.41)	4.42 (4.35, 4.49)	4.01 (3.89, 4.13)
Controls (rate)	2.59 (2.52, 2.66)	1.89 (1.84, 1.93)	2.01 (1.91, 2.10)	2.36 (2.31, 2.42)	2.47 (2.38, 2.57)
Rate ratio	1.45 (1.40, 1.51)	2.34 (2.28, 2.41)	4.10 (3.90, 4.31)	1.87 (1.82, 1.92)	1.62 (1.54, 1.70)
Diagnostic tests					
Cases (rate)	1.42 (1.37, 1.47)	8.44 (8.35, 8.54)	29.4 (29.1, 29.8)	10.3 (10.2, 10.4)	11.8 (11.6, 12.0)
Controls (rate)	0.53 (0.49, 0.56)	1.21 (1.17, 1.24)	2.28 (2.19, 2.38)	3.90 (3.83, 3.97)	5.00 (4.87, 5.14)
Rate ratio	2.70 (2.51, 2.89)	7.01 (6.79, 7.23)	12.9 (12.3, 13.5)	2.64 (2.59, 2.70)	2.37 (2.29, 2.44)
Prescriptions					
Cases (rate)	3.00 (2.93, 3.08)	3.37 (3.31, 3.43)	5.67 (5.52, 5.83)	3.83 (3.77, 3.90)	3.65 (3.54, 3.77)
Controls (rate)	2.08 (2.02, 2.14)	1.46 (1.42, 1.50)	1.71 (1.62, 1.79)	1.92 (1.88, 1.97)	1.99 (1.91, 2.07)
Rate ratio	1.44 (1.39, 1.50)	2.31 (2.23, 2.38)	3.33 (3.14, 3.52)	1.99 (1.93, 2.05)	1.84 (1.74, 1.93)
Referrals					
Cases (rate)	0.25 (0.23, 0.27)	0.43 (0.41, 0.45)	1.28 (1.21, 1.35)	0.42 (0.40, 0.44)	0.39 (0.36, 0.43)
Controls (rate)	0.18 (0.16, 0.20)	0.14 (0.13, 0.15)	0.15 (0.12, 0.17)	0.16 (0.15, 0.17)	0.16 (0.13, 0.18)
Rate ratio	1.40 (1.22, 1.60)	3.08 (2.79, 3.41)	8.83 (7.38, 10.6)	2.61 (2.36, 2.89)	2.53 (2.12, 3.03)

Medicine criteria for Systemic Exercise Intolerance Disease (SEID) require that the fatigue be "of new or definite onset (not lifelong)" [19], as do current UK National Institute of Health and Care Excellence (NICE) clinical guidelines [20].

The distinct peak in health care resource use that we observed matches the duration of illness reported to clinicians by patients when first assessed by specialist CFS/ME services in England. For patients assessed during the period 2004–2014, the median (IQR) duration of illness for adult patients was 3 (1–8) years, and for adolescent patients (who comprise the majority of child patients) it was 1.5 (1 to 2) years [1]. The upper and lower bounds of these IQR encompass the steep upward slope in health care resource use in each patient group, i.e. the rapid increase in health care needs is consistent with patients' (or parents') self-report of the time since onset.

However, the sustained higher use of health care resources and numbers of symptoms predating this onset is inconsistent with patients' (or parents') recollections that they (or their child) had been healthy prior to the onset of CFS/ME [11, 12], and conflicts somewhat with case definitions worded to exclude fatigue that is lifelong or not of new onset. There are several possible explanations for this discrepancy.

Firstly, people may simply have had CFS/ME for a very long time. The previously quoted durations of illness (3 years for adults, 18 months for children) were self-reported, and people with CFS/ME may be underestimating the length of time for which they have been ill. Also, these are patients who access specialist services, who will not include all patients with CFS/ME. CFS/ME may begin as a mild form which develops quite suddenly into more severe CFS/ME, thereby setting the patient on a pathway to diagnosis. Patients' (and parents') recall of their health status prior to the onset of more severe symptoms could be distorted by the debilitating nature of moderate to severe CFS/ME, leading them to report having been healthy. This is particularly plausible if the milder form of CFS/ME had not prevented them from being in full-time employment or had not led to notable absences from school or college. We know that adults often persevere in employment whilst coping with the symptoms of CFS/ME for years before obtaining a diagnosis [2], and an active case finding study in three secondary schools in England led to 5% (23/461) of children whose attendance was below 80% being diagnosed with CFS/ME, giving a CFS/ME prevalence of 1% (28/2855) in the three schools in the study [21]. Also, CFS/ME is accompanied by comorbidities including depression, anxiety, chronic pain, migraine and irritable bowel disease [1], which can mask CFS/ME as the primary disorder.

Secondly, it is possible that people who develop CFS/ME have pre-existing risk factors which lead to higher

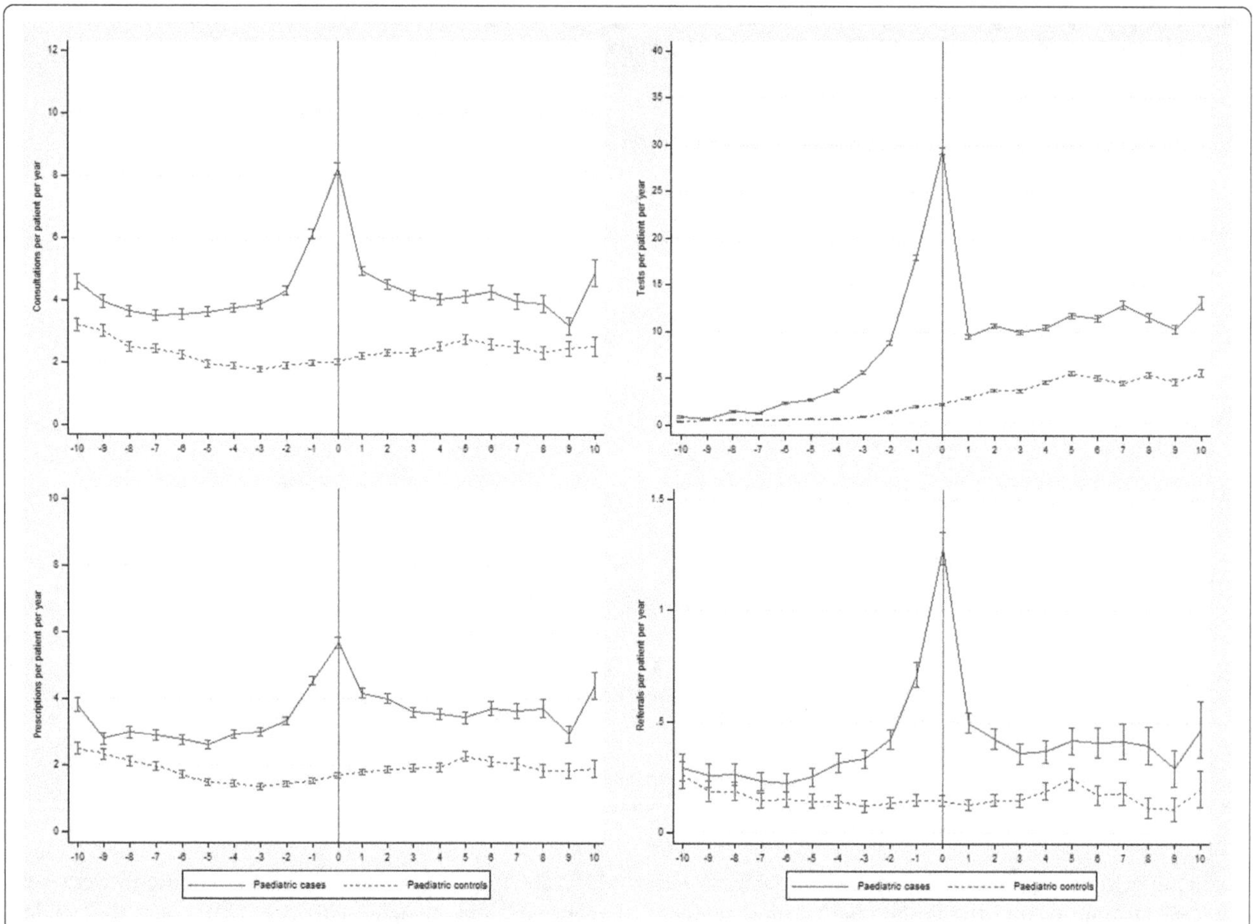

Fig. 2 Rates of GP consultations, tests, prescriptions and referrals from 10 years before until 10 years after a first recorded diagnosis of CFS/ME in paediatric cases compared with controls

rates of health care resource use. Presentation for other illnesses would be consistent with a subsequent diagnosis of CFS/ME if patients were generally more susceptible to illness, e.g. immunologically or if patients with CFS/ME have different health care seeking behaviour. A small case–control study in England reported higher GP consultation rates over three 5-year periods before a diagnosis of CFS/ME, as we observed in our study [22]. The consultations were for a wide range of symptoms, and the authors concluded that behaviour traits such as disease conviction and somatic concern could not be discounted as aetiological factors. Finally, it is possible that patients who present repeatedly and regularly to primary care are more likely to be given a diagnosis of CFS/ME by their GP.

Relative rates of health care resource use and symptoms 6–10 years after diagnosis were not substantially different from rate ratios 6–10 years before diagnosis, except perhaps for lower relative rates of diagnostic tests and (in child patients) fatigue symptoms, and higher relative rates of prescriptions and referrals post-diagnosis. The overall patterns in our study were similar to those observed in a study of fibromyalgia using data from the General Practice Research Database (GPRD, the precursor to CPRD) [23]. We are unable to determine from our data whether the type of health care resource use by patients changes following diagnosis, and we do not know how many patients in our study received specialist treatment. Receiving a diagnosis may change health care resource use, because patients have an identifiable illness which explains the fatigue and symptoms that they have been experiencing and GPs may be able to provide specific advice. Adult patients in England have access to approximately 50 NHS specialist services, many of which were established under the CFS/ME Service Investment Programme (2004–2006) [24]. These services follow NICE guidance, including specific guidelines for diagnosis, specialist care, and ongoing management, with an overall patient-centred approach to treatment [20]. Although outcomes up to 20 months after treatment are favourable for some patients [25], long-term treatment outcomes for these services have not been reported. Children have better prognosis than adults [26], but specialist service

Table 3 Rates (95% CI) of all symptoms and of fatigue symptoms and rate ratios (95% CI) from 15 years before (adults) or 10 years before (paediatric) until 10 years after a first recorded diagnosis of CFS/ME

	Year −15 to −11	Year −10 to −6	Year −5 to −1	Year 0	Year 1 to 5	Year 6 to 10
Total adult person years						
Cases	4579	12,183	24,478	6710	25,447	10,815
Controls	4649	12,258	24,564	6710	25,038	10, 508
Adults (all symptoms)						
Cases (rate per patient year)	1.14 (1.11, 1.17)	1.53 (1.51, 1.55)	2.46 (2.44, 2.48)	3.19 (3.15, 3.23)	2.35 (2.33, 2.37)	2.40 (2.37, 2.43)
Controls (rate per patient year)	0.67 (0.65, 0.70)	0.98 (0.96, 1.00)	1.30 (1.29, 1.32)	1.36 (1.34, 1.39)	1.41 (1.40, 1.43)	1.55 (1.53, 1.57)
Rate ratio	1.69 (1.62, 1.77)	1.57 (1.53, 1.60)	1.89 (1.87, 1.92)	2.34 (2.28, 2.39)	1.67 (1.65, 1.69)	1.55 (1.52, 1.58)
Adults (fatigue symptoms)						
Cases (rate per patient year)	2.80 (2.31, 3.28)	6.15 (5.71, 6.59)	19.4 (18.9, 20.0)	57.5 (55.7, 59.3)	10.9 (10.5, 11.3)	8.61 (8.06, 9.16)
Controls (rate per patient year)	0.34 (0.18, 0.51)	1.61 (1.38, 1.83)	2.31 (2.12, 2.50)	2.62 (2.24, 3.01)	2.66 (2.45, 2.86)	2.29 (2.00, 2.58)
Rate ratio	8.12 (4.83, 13.7)	3.83 (3.27, 4.48)	8.40 (7.70, 9.16)	21.9 (18.8, 25.5)	4.10 (3.77, 4.46)	3.75 (3.26, 4.32)
Total paediatric person years						
Cases		2088	3715	916	3290	1076
Controls		1996	3591	916	3257	1077
Paediatric (all symptoms)						
Cases (rate per 100 patient years)		1.14 (1.10, 1.19)	1.74 (1.70, 1.78)	3.12 (3.01, 3.24)	1.62 (1.58, 1.66)	1.53 (1.46, 1.61)
Controls (rate per 100 patient years)		0.68 (0.64, 0.72)	0.67 (0.64, 0.69)	0.71 (0.66, 0.76)	0.81 (0.78, 0.84)	0.86 (0.80, 0.91)
Rate ratio		1.68 (1.57, 1.79)	2.60 (2.48, 2.73)	4.40 (4.04, 4.79)	2.00 (1.91, 2.10)	1.79 (1.65, 1.94)
Paediatric (fatigue symptoms)						
Cases (rate per 100 patient years)		1.39 (0.88, 1.89)	11.6 (10.5, 12.7)	56.3 (51.5, 61.2)	7.36 (6.43, 8.28)	4.83 (3.52, 6.15)
Controls (rate per 100 patient years)		0.20 (0.00, 0.40)	0.56 (0.31, 0.80)	1.09 (0.42, 1.77)	1.81 (1.35, 2.27)	1.02 (0.42, 1.62)
Rate ratio		6.93 (2.44, 19.7)	20.8 (13.3, 32.6)	51.6 (27.6, 96.5)	4.06 (3.05, 5.40)	4.73 (2.47, 9.07)

provision for is much less comprehensive, with one large paediatric service in the south west of England, and patchy or non-existent provision elsewhere in the UK.

Strengths and limitations

The main strength of our study is that it is based on a large sample from a cohort of approximately four million patients registered with a GP, representing approximately 7% of the population in the UK [5]. Patients have a median of 9.4 years (IQR 3.4-13.9) of data [5], which gives us some (but not absolute) confidence in classifying diagnoses as 'new' if the patient's medical record has no previously recorded diagnoses. Two limitations of our study are that we do not know how many cases of CFS/ME in the population are undiagnosed or misdiagnosed, or what proportion of CFS/ME cases in our study were correctly diagnosed. Although knowledge and awareness of CFS/ME in primary care has improved over the past decade [27], some GPs still lack confidence in diagnosing CFS/ME [28]. This is consistent with a relatively high rate of misdiagnosis by GPs when referring to specialist services [29, 30]. The estimated incidence of adult CFS/ME diagnoses in CPRD data in the period 2008–2010 was broadly consistent with incidence estimated from data obtained directly from NHS specialist CFS/ME services in 2009, which gives some reassurance that CFS/ME diagnoses recorded by GPs towards the end of the period covered by our study were made or confirmed by a specialist CFS/ME service [7]. However, CFS/ME diagnoses in CPRD data have yet to be validated through linkage or other means.

Two other potential limitations of our study were that people who contributed the longest durations of pre- and post-diagnosis data may not have been representative of CFS/ME patients and healthy controls, and that biases in rate ratios could be introduced at the extremes of follow-up if there were differential losses between the case–control pairs. However, there were no differential losses by age, sex and IMD quintile, and sensitivity analyses restricted to patients who had either 10 years of pre-diagnosis or 10 years of post-diagnosis data yielded rate ratios which were similar to those in our main analysis.

Unanswered questions and future research

The extent to which the elevated health care needs of adults and children who were subsequently

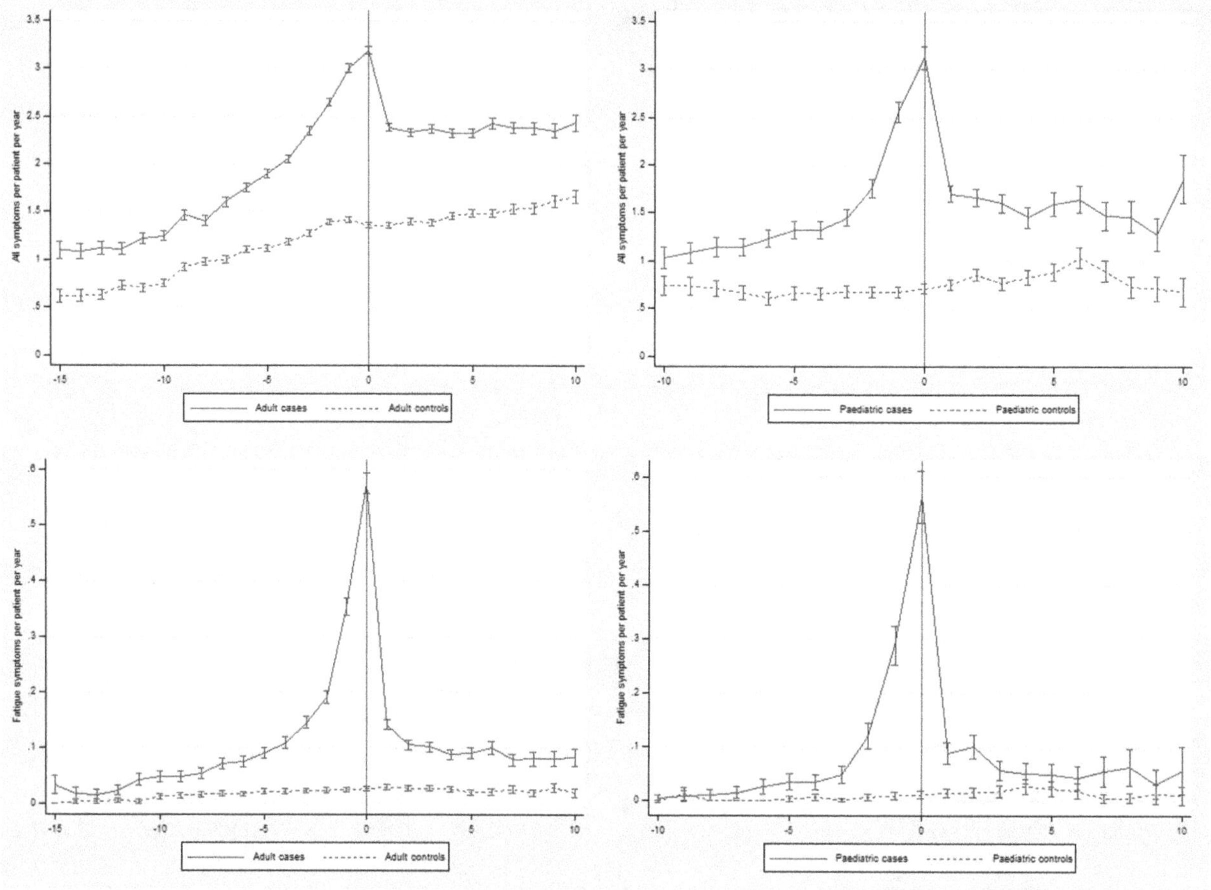

Fig. 3 Rates of all symptoms and fatigue symptoms from 15 years before (adults) or 10 years before (paediatric) until 10 years after a first recorded diagnosis of CFS/ME in cases compared with controls

diagnosed with CFS/ME reflect long-term undiagnosed illness requires further investigation. Ideally this would be accomplished by means of a large long-term prospective cohort study with deep phenotyping of participants, including repeated measurements of symptoms, biological markers, psychological states, and objective measures of health and function. The sample size for such studies could be reduced by following patients who have an acute infectious illness, given that CFS/ME will be triggered in a fairly constant proportion of patients [31]. However, these patients will not represent all patients who develop CFS/ME if the illness is triggered by other events. Electronic primary care records can be used to investigate whether specific illnesses occur more frequently in patients who are subsequently diagnosed with CFS/ME [32], and to investigate what the overall higher rates of health care resource use actually represent, in terms of specific tests, prescriptions, and referrals. With regard to post-diagnosis health care resource use, cohort studies are needed to quantify long-term treatment outcomes among patients who are treated by specialist CFS/ME services after diagnosis. Qualitative methods could be used to investigate how health care needs before and after diagnosis relate to patients' health status and quality of life.

Conclusions

We cannot discount the possibility that patients in our study have presented over a period of 10 or more years with symptoms related to CFS/ME, even if a very long prodromal period before the onset of CFS/ME appears to be inconsistent with patients' own reports of when their illness began and with patients describing themselves as being fit and healthy prior to onset. We are also mindful of the known heterogeneity within CFS/ME, and that patterns of health care resource use could vary substantially across different CFS/ME phenotypes. Diagnosis of CFS/ME coincided with a dramatic peak in health care resource use, and had little or no impact on health resource use in the longer term.

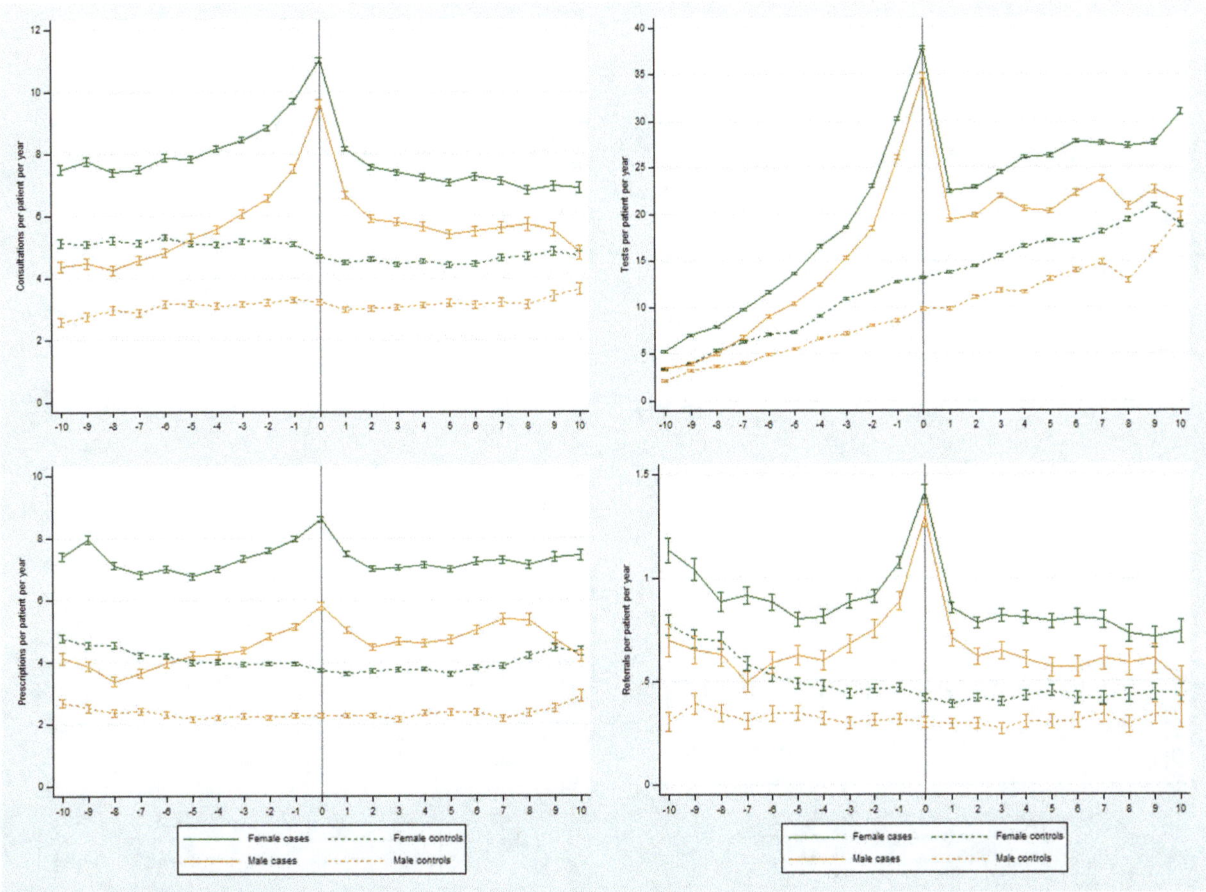

Fig. 4 Rates of GP consultations, tests, prescriptions and referrals from 10 years before until 10 years after a first recorded diagnosis of CFS/ME in adult cases compared with controls by sex

Table 4 Rate ratios (95% CI) of GP consultations, tests, prescriptions and referrals from 10 years before until 10 years after a first recorded diagnosis of CFS/ME in adult cases compared with controls by sex

	Year −10 to −6	Year −5 to −1	Year 0	Year 1 to 5	Year 6 to 10
	Year −10 to −6	Year −5 to −1	Year 0	Year 1 to 5	Year 6 to 10
GP consultations					
Female	1.47 (1.45, 1.49)	1.70 (1.69, 1.71)	2.35 (2.31, 2.38)	1.68 (1.66, 1.69)	1.52 (1.50, 1.54)
Male	1.56 (1.53, 1.60)	1.99 (1.96, 2.02)	2.98 (2.90, 3.07)	1.95 (1.92, 1.99)	1.69 (1.65, 1.74)
Diagnostic tests					
Female	1.60 (1.58, 1.62)	2.01 (2.00, 2.02)	2.87 (2.85, 2.90)	1.58 (1.57, 1.59)	1.51 (1.50, 1.52)
Male	1.61 (1.58, 1.65)	2.39 (2.37, 2.42)	3.56 (3.50, 3.61)	1.80 (1.79, 1.82)	1.49 (1.47, 1.51)
Prescriptions					
Female	1.63 (1.61, 1.65)	1.87 (1.85, 1.89)	2.30 (2.26, 2.34)	1.93 (1.91, 1.95)	1.79 (1.77, 1.82)
Male	1.55 (1.51, 1.60)	2.07 (2.03, 2.11)	2.56 (2.47, 2.65)	2.07 (2.03, 2.11)	2.08 (2.03, 2.14)
Referrals					
Female	1.49 (1.44, 1.54)	1.95 (1.90, 2.00)	3.34 (3.18, 3.50)	1.95 (1.89, 2.00)	1.78 (1.71, 1.86)
Male	1.77 (1.65, 1.90)	2.30 (2.18, 2.41)	4.32 (3.93, 4.73)	2.18 (2.07, 2.30)	1.80 (1.67, 1.95)

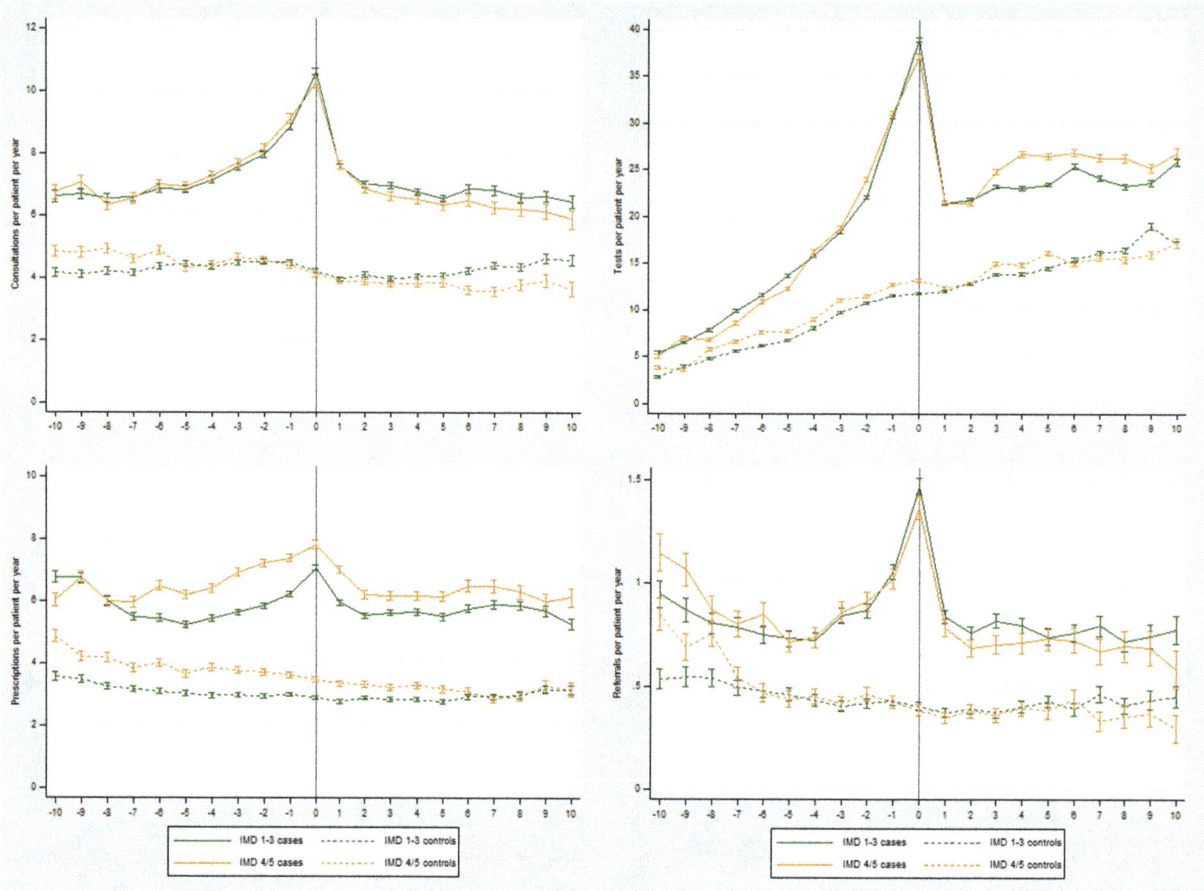

Fig. 5 Rates of GP consultations, tests, prescriptions and referrals from 10 years before until 10 years after a first recorded diagnosis of CFS/ME in adult cases compared with controls by Index of Multiple Deprivation (IMD) quintiles

Table 5 Rate ratios (95% CI) of GP consultations, tests, prescriptions and referrals from 10 years before until 10 years after a first recorded diagnosis of CFS/ME in adult cases compared with controls by Index of Multiple Deprivation (IMD) quintiles

	Year −10 to −6	Year −5 to −1	Year 0	Year 1 to 5	Year 6 to 10
GP consultations					
Top 3 quintiles	1.58 (1.55, 1.60)	1.75 (1.73, 1.77)	2.52 (2.47, 2.57)	1.75 (1.73, 1.76)	1.52 (1.50, 1.55)
Bottom 2 quintiles	1.40 (1.37, 1.43)	1.77 (1.75, 1.80)	2.49 (2.42, 2.56)	1.78 (1.76, 1.81)	1.70 (1.66, 1.75)
Diagnostic tests					
Top 3 quintiles	1.78 (1.76, 1.81)	2.20 (2.19, 2.22)	3.30 (3.27, 3.34)	1.69 (1.68, 1.70)	1.48 (1.46, 1.49)
Bottom 2 quintiles	1.39 (1.37, 1.42)	2.02 (2.00, 2.03)	2.80 (2.76, 2.84)	1.69 (1.68, 1.71)	1.68 (1.66, 1.71)
Prescriptions					
Top 3 quintiles	1.81 (1.78, 1.85)	1.92 (1.89, 1.94)	2.43 (2.38, 2.49)	2.00 (1.97, 2.02)	1.90 (1.86, 1.93)
Bottom 2 quintiles	1.50 (1.47, 1.53)	1.85 (1.82, 1.88)	2.23 (2.16, 2.30)	1.93 (1.90, 1.96)	2.07 (2.01, 2.13)
Referrals					
Top 3 quintiles	1.59 (1.52, 1.66)	2.02 (1.95, 2.09)	3.64 (3.43, 3.86)	2.03 (1.97, 2.10)	1.78 (1.69, 1.87)
Bottom 2 quintiles	1.45 (1.38, 1.53)	1.97 (1.88, 2.05)	3.53 (3.25, 3.84)	1.95 (1.86, 2.05)	1.84 (1.69, 1.99)

Additional file

Additional file 1: Table S1. READ codes defining diagnoses, referrals and fatigue symptoms. **Table S2.** GP consultations, tests, prescriptions and referrals from 15 years before until 10 years after a first recorded diagnosis of CFS/ME in adult cases and controls. **Table S3.** GP consultations, tests, prescriptions and referrals from 10 years before until 10 years after a first recorded diagnosis of CFS/ME in paediatric cases and controls. **Table S4.** Symptoms from 15 years before (adults) or 10 years before (paediatric) until 10 years after a first recorded diagnosis of CFS/ME in cases and controls. **Table S5a**. GP consultations, tests, prescriptions and referrals from 10 years before until 10 years after a first recorded diagnosis of CFS/ME in female adult cases and controls. **Table S5b.** GP consultations, tests, prescriptions and referrals from 10 years before until 10 years after a first recorded diagnosis of CFS/ME in male adult cases and controls. **Table S6a.** GP consultations, tests, prescriptions and referrals from 10 years before until 10 years after a first recorded diagnosis of CFS/ME in top 3 IMD quintile adult cases and controls. **Table S6b.** GP consultations, tests, prescriptions and referrals from 10 years before until 10 years after a first recorded diagnosis of CFS/ME in bottom 2 IMD quintile adult cases and controls (DOCX 30 kb)

Abbreviations
CFS/ME: Chronic fatigue syndrome/myalgic encephalomyelitis; CPRD: Clinical Practice Research Datalink; FM: Fibromyalgia; GPRD: General Practice Research Database; IMD: Index of Multiple Deprivation; PVFS: Post viral fatigue syndrome; RR: Rate ratio; UTS: Up To Standard

Acknowledgements
Not applicable.

Funding
SC received funding from the National Institute for Health Research (NIHR) to conduct this study (PDF-2013-06-011).

Authors' contributions
SMC designed the study, analysed the data, drafted and revised the paper. IJB, IN, EC, and PDW provided guidance for the analysis, interpreted the results, and revised the draft paper. All authors have read and approved the final version.

Competing interests
EC receives NIHR funding (SRF-2013-06-013), runs the specialist CFS/ME service at Royal United Hospital NHS Foundation Trust, and has received one grant from the Medical Research Council. PDW is a member of the Independent Medical Experts Group, which advises the UK Ministry of Defence regarding its Armed Forces Compensation Scheme, and does consultancy for a re-insurance company.

Author details
[1]School of Social and Community Medicine, University of Bristol, Oakfield House, Oakfield Grove, Bristol BS8 2BN, UK. [2]Norwegian Institute of Public Health, PO Box 4404Nydalen, 0403 Oslo, Norway. [3]Primary Care and Population Science, UCL Department of Primary Care and Population Health, UCL Royal Free Campus, Rowland Hill Street, London NW3 2PF, UK. [4]Psychological Medicine, Wolfson Institute of Preventive Medicine, Barts, London School of Medicine and Dentistry, Queen Mary University of London, London, UK.

References
1. Collin SM, Nuevo R, van de Putte EM, Nijhof SL, Crawley E. Chronic fatigue syndrome (CFS) or myalgic encephalomyelitis (ME) is different in children compared to in adults: a study of UK and Dutch clinical cohorts. BMJ Open. 2015;5(10):e008830.
2. Collin SM, Crawley E, May MT, Sterne JA, Hollingworth W. The impact of CFS/ME on employment and productivity in the UK: a cross-sectional study based on the CFS/ME national outcomes database. BMC Health Serv Res. 2011;11(1):217.
3. McCrone P, Darbishire L, Ridsdale L, Seed P. The economic cost of chronic fatigue and chronic fatigue syndrome in UK primary care. Psychol Med. 2003;33(2):253–61.
4. Sabes-Figuera R, McCrone P, Hurley M, King M, Donaldson AN, Ridsdale L. The hidden cost of chronic fatigue to patients and their families. BMC Health Serv Res. 2010;10:56.
5. Herrett E, Gallagher AM, Bhaskaran K, Forbes H, Mathur R, van Staa T, Smeeth L. Data resource profile: clinical practice research datalink (CPRD). Int J Epidemiol. 2015;44(3):827–36.
6. Collin SM, Sterne JA, Hollingworth W, May MT, Crawley E. Equity of access to specialist chronic fatigue syndrome (CFS/ME) services in England (2008–2010): a national survey and cross-sectional study. BMJ Open. 2012;2(4):e001417.
7. Collin SM, Bakken IJ, Nazareth I, Crawley E, White PD: Trends in the incidence of chronic fatigue syndrome and fibromyalgia in the UK, 2001–2013: a Clinical Practice Research Datalink study. J R Soc Med. 2017. doi: 10.1177/0141076817702530.
8. Gallagher AM, Thomas JM, Hamilton WT, White PD. Incidence of fatigue symptoms and diagnoses presenting in UK primary care from 1990 to 2001. J R Soc Med. 2004;97(12):571–5.
9. Lewis JD, Bilker WB, Weinstein RB, Strom BL. The relationship between time since registration and measured incidence rates in the General Practice Research Database. Pharmacoepidemiol Drug Saf. 2005;14(7):443–51.
10. The English Indices of Deprivation 2010: Department for Communities and Local Government, London. 2011. The cited document is available from: https://www.gov.uk/government/collections/english-indices-of-deprivation and as PDF from: https://www.gov.uk/government/uploads/system/uploads/attachment_data/file/6871/1871208.pdf
11. Edwards CR, Thompson AR, Blair A. An 'overwhelming illness': women's experiences of learning to live with chronic fatigue syndrome/myalgic encephalomyelitis. J Health Psychol. 2007;12(2):203-14.
12. Gray ML, Fossey EM. Illness experience and occupations of people with chronic fatigue syndrome. Aust Occup Ther J. 2003:50(3):127-36.
13. Haney E, Smith ME, McDonagh M, Pappas M, Daeges M, Wasson N, Nelson HD. Diagnostic methods for myalgic encephalomyelitis/chronic fatigue syndrome: a systematic review for a national institutes of health pathways to prevention workshop. Ann Intern Med. 2015;162(12):834–40.
14. Holmes GP, Kaplan JE, Gantz NM, Komaroff AL, Schonberger LB, Straus SE, Jones JF, Dubois RE, Cunningham-Rundles C, Pahwa S, et al. Chronic fatigue syndrome: a working case definition. Ann Intern Med. 1988;108(3):387–9.
15. Fukuda K, Straus SE, Hickie I, Sharpe MC, Dobbins JG, Komaroff A. The chronic fatigue syndrome: a comprehensive approach to its definition and study. international chronic fatigue syndrome study group. Ann Intern Med. 1994;121(12):953–9.
16. Sharpe MC, Archard LC, Banatvala JE, Borysiewicz LK, Clare AW, David A, Edwards RH, Hawton KE, Lambert HP, Lane RJ, et al. A report–chronic fatigue syndrome: guidelines for research. J R Soc Med. 1991;84(2):118–21.
17. Carruthers BM, Jain AK, De Meirleir KL, Peterson DL, Klimas NG, Lerner AM, Bested AC, Flor-Henry P, Joshi P, Powles ACP, et al. Myalgic encephalomyelitis/chronic fatigue syndrome. J Chron Fatigue Syndr. 2003; 11(1):7–115.
18. Jason LA, Evans M, Porter N, Brown M, Brown A, Hunnell J, Anderson V, Lerch A, De Meirleir KL, Friedberg F. The development of a revised canadian myalgic encephalomyelitis chronic fatigue syndrome case definition. Am J Biochem Biotechnol. 2010;6(2):15.
19. Committee on the Diagnostic Criteria for Myalgic Encephalomyelitis/Chronic Fatigue Syndrome, Board on the Health of Select Populations, Institute of Medicine. Beyond Myalgic Encephalomyelitis/Chronic Fatigue Syndrome: Redefining an Illness. Washington (DC): National Academies Press (US); 2015.
20. National Institute for Health and Care Excellence (NICE). Chronic fatigue syndrome/myalgic encephalomyelitis (or encephalopathy): diagnosis and management [Clinical Guideline CG53]. London: NICE; 2007.

21. Crawley EM, Emond AM, Sterne JA. Unidentified chronic fatigue syndrome/myalgic encephalomyelitis (CFS/ME) is a major cause of school absence: surveillance outcomes from school-based clinics. BMJ Open. 2011;1(2):e000252.
22. Hamilton WT, Hall GH, Round AP. Frequency of attendance in general practice and symptoms before development of chronic fatigue syndrome: a case–control study. Br J Gen Pract. 2001;51(468):553–8.
23. Hughes G, Martinez C, Myon E, Taieb C, Wessely S. The impact of a diagnosis of fibromyalgia on health care resource use by primary care patients in the UK - An observational study based on clinical practice. Arthritis Rheum. 2006;54(1):177–83.
24. CFS/ME Service Investment Programme Report 2004–2006. Pinching AJ, Noons PA, editors. Peninsula Medical School; 2006.
25. Crawley E, Collin SM, White PD, Rimes K, Sterne JA, May MT, CMNO Database. Treatment outcome in adults with chronic fatigue syndrome: a prospective study in England based on the CFS/ME national outcomes database. QJM. 2013;106(6):555–65.
26. Crawley E. The epidemiology of chronic fatigue syndrome/myalgic encephalitis in children. Arch Dis Child. 2014;99(2):171–4.
27. Horton SM, Poland F, Kale S, Drachler Mde L, de Carvalho Leite JC, McArthur MA, Campion PD, Pheby D, Nacul L. Chronic fatigue syndrome/myalgic encephalomyelitis (CFS/ME) in adults: a qualitative study of perspectives from professional practice. BMC Fam Pract. 2010;11:89.
28. Chew-Graham C, Dowrick C, Wearden A, Richardson V, Peters S. Making the diagnosis of chronic fatigue syndrome/myalgic encephalitis in primary care: a qualitative study. BMC Fam Pract. 2010;11:16.
29. Devasahayam A, Lawn T, Murphy M, White PD. Alternative diagnoses to chronic fatigue syndrome in referrals to a specialist service: service evaluation survey. JRSM Short Rep. 2012;3(1):4.
30. Newton JL, Mabillard H, Scott A, Hoad A, Spickett G. The newcastle nhs chronic fatigue syndrome service: not all fatigue is the same. J R Coll Physicians Edinb. 2010;40(4):304–7.
31. Lloyd AR, Meer JW. The long wait for a breakthrough in chronic fatigue syndrome. BMJ. 2015;350:h2087.
32. Bakken IJ, Tveito K, Aaberg KM, Ghaderi S, Gunnes N, Trogstad L, Magnus P, Stoltenberg C, Haberg SE. Comorbidities treated in primary care in children with chronic fatigue syndrome/myalgic encephalomyelitis: A nationwide registry linkage study from Norway. BMC Fam Pract. 2016;17(1):128.

Impact of heart failure and other comorbidities on mortality in patients with chronic obstructive pulmonary disease

Elzbieta Kaszuba[1,2*], Håkan Odeberg[2], Lennart Råstam[2] and Anders Halling[2]

Abstract

Background: Multimorbidity has already become common in primary care and will be a challenge in the future. Primary care in Sweden participates to a great extent in the care of patients with two severe, chronic conditions: chronic obstructive pulmonary disease (COPD) and heart failure. Both conditions are characterized by high mortality and often coexist. Age, sex, heart failure and other comorbidities are considered to be the major predictors of mortality in patients with COPD. We aimed to study the impact of heart failure, other comorbidities, age and sex on mortality in patients with COPD.

Methods: A register-based, prospective cohort study conducted in Blekinge County in Sweden with about 150,000 inhabitants. The study population was comprised of people aged ≥35 years. The data about diagnoses of COPD and heart failure came from the 2007 health care register, in which we found 984 individuals with a diagnosis of COPD. Date of death was collected from January 1st, 2008 –August 31st, 2015. The diagnosis-based Adjusted Clinical Groups (ACG) Case-Mix System 7.1 was used to describe comorbidity. Each individual was assigned one of six comorbidity levels called resource utilization bands (RUB) graded from 0 to 5.

Results: Estimated eight year mortality in patients with COPD and coexisting heart failure was seven times higher than in patients with COPD alone - odds ratio 7.06 (95% CI 3.88–12.84). Adjusting for age and male sex resulted in odds ratio 3.75 (95% CI 1.97–7.15). Further adjusting for other comorbidities resulted in odds ratio 3.26 (95% CI 1.70–6.25). The mortality was strongly associated with the highest comorbidity level – RUB 5 where the odds ratio was 5.19 (95% CI 2.59–10.38).

Conclusion: Heart failure has an important impact on mortality in patients with COPD. The mortality in patients with COPD and coexisting heart failure was strongly associated with age, male sex and other comorbidities. Of those three predictors, only other comorbidities can be influenced. Heart failure and other comorbidities should be recognized early and properly treated in order to improve survival in patients with coexisting COPD and heart failure.

Keywords: Chronic obstructive pulmonary disease, Heart failure, Mortality, Age, Sex, Comorbidity

* Correspondence: elzbieta.kaszuba@med.lu.se
[1]Samaritens Primary Health Care Centre, 374 80 Karlshamn, Sweden
[2]Department of Clinical Sciences in Malmö General Practice, Center for Primary Health Care Research, Lund University, 205 02, Malmö, Sweden

Background

General practitioners nowadays seldom encounter patients with only one disease in daily practice. With an aging population there is, therefore, an increased likelihood of having two or more chronic diseases simultaneously among this population [1]. Multimorbidity has already become the norm and will be a challenge for future primary care. Our previous study showed that primary care in Sweden participates to a great extent in the care of patients with two severe, chronic conditions: chronic obstructive pulmonary disease (COPD) and heart failure [2]; both conditions are common in the Swedish population [3–5]. Prevalence of COPD is still high despite a decrease in the number of smokers in Sweden [6]. By the year 2030, COPD is predicted to be the third most common cause of death and disability worldwide [7]. High mortality is not caused by respiratory failure, which from the pathophysiological point of view can be considered a natural consequence of COPD due to disturbances in gas exchange [8]. Respiratory failure was a leading cause of death only in patients with advanced COPD and could explain mortality in only a third of these patients [9]. The major independent predictors of mortality in COPD were comorbidity and sex [10–12]. Heart failure occurs with high prevalence in patients with COPD [13]. Although the strategies in management of heart failure have improved during recent decades, the prognosis remains poor [14–16]. Comorbidities, age and sex are independent indicators for the prognosis in heart failure [17, 18]. Despite an increased understanding that COPD and heart failure often coexist [19], both have mostly been studied separately in prior studies. It is a matter of course that the more disorders an individual has the worse the outcome will be. However, it is not clear if one plus one makes two in medical practice. The aim of this study was to find how much coexisting heart failure increases the probability of death in patients with COPD and to describe the impact of age, sex and other comorbidities on mortality in patients with coexisting COPD and heart failure. Thereby we wanted to find what coexisting heart failure and other comorbidities mean for the survival of an individual with COPD, which is of special importance in primary care where the patient is the main focus.

Methods

This was a register-based, prospective, observational study. The study was conducted in Blekinge County in Sweden, which has about 150,000 inhabitants. The study population was comprised of people aged ≥35 years.

Data were obtained from the Blekinge County council health care register; a register that collects data concerning diagnosis at each consultation in all public and private health care units in both primary- and secondary health care. Diagnoses were recorded according to the International Statistical Classification of Diseases and Related Health Problems version 10 (ICD 10). We analyzed data from January 1st till December 31st, 2007.

An individual was identified as having COPD if the diagnosis code J44 was recorded on at least one consultation in primary- or secondary care including hospitalization. The code J44 comprised the following: J44 chronic obstructive lung disease, J44.0 chronic obstructive lung disease with acute infection in lower airways, J44.1 chronic obstructive lung disease with acute exacerbation, unspecified, J44.8 other specified chronic obstructive lung disease including chronic bronchitis with emphysema. The register did not contain information on the severity of COPD.

Coexisting heart failure was identified if the diagnosis code I50 was recorded.

The code I50 comprised: I50.0- chronic heart failure including congestive heart failure, right heart failure secondary to left heart failure, I50.1- left ventricular failure with or without lung oedema and asthma cardiale, I50.9 heart failure, unspecified. Occurrence of other diagnoses in medical records is referred to as other comorbidities.

The diagnosis-based Adjusted Clinical Groups (ACG) Case-Mix System 7.1 was used to measure other comorbidities [20, 21]. Each individual was assigned one of six comorbidity levels called resource utilization bands (RUB) graded from 0 to 5, where 5 means very high morbidity and need for care.

The date of death was collected from January 1st, 2008 – August 31st, 2015 and was obtained from the Blekinge County council. Individuals who left the Blekinge County during the observation time were excluded from the study.

Statistics

Data were analyzed in the STATA version 13 (Stata Corporation, Texas, USA).

Distribution of categorical variables was presented as numbers. Distribution of continuous variables was presented as a mean and 95% Confidence Interval (CI).

Univariate analysis was used to calculate odds ratios of mortality for different variables. Logistic regression was used to calculate adjusted odds ratios step-by-step. Thereafter, multiple logistic regression was performed in order to adjust the estimated odds ratio for the influence of age, sex and other comorbidities.

Results

The study population consisted of 91,227 individuals aged ≥35 years of which 51.07% were female and 48.93% were male. The diagnosis of COPD was registered in 1011 individuals of which 27 (2.67%) moved from the county during the observation time and were thus excluded from the study. The final analyses were made based on data from 984 individuals; 53% female and 47% male. The mean age in patients with the diagnosis of COPD was 71.1 (95% CI 70.4–71.8). The mean age for women was 69.4 (95% CI 68.5–70.4) and for men 72.9 (95% CI 72.0–73.8).

Comorbidity levels described by RUB were distributed as follows: RUB 3–71.14% ($n = 700$), RUB 4–21.65% ($n = 213$), RUB 5–7.22% ($n = 71$).

We found the diagnosis of heart failure in 10.06% ($n = 99$) of patients with the diagnosis of COPD.

Univariate analysis resulted in an odds ratio of mortality in patients with COPD and coexisting heart failure of 7.06 (95% CI 3.88–12.84). The highest level of other comorbidities was the next important variable that influenced mortality (Table 1).

Adjusting for age resulted in odds ratio 3.76 (95% CI 1.98–7.16) and for age and male sex in odds ratio 3.75 (95% CI 1.79–3.26 (1.70–6.25). Further adjusting for other comorbidities resulted in odds ratio 3.26 (95% CI 1.70–6.25). Adjusted odds ratios are presented in Table 2.

Multiple logistic regression showed that the mortality was associated with age and male sex but the strongest risk factor for mortality was the highest comorbidity level – RUB 5 where the odds ratio was 5.19 (95% CI 2.59–10.38) (Table 3). The most common comorbid diagnoses in our material were: hypertension (20%), ischaemic heart disease (12.7%), diabetes mellitus (12.6%) and atrial fibrillation (7.9%). The odds ratio was the highest for RUB 5,even after adjusting for those comorbid diagnoses (Table 4).

Discussion

We found that the odds of eight year mortality in patients with COPD and coexisting heart failure were seven times higher than in patients with COPD alone. Other comorbidities were found to be a very important factor affecting mortality in patients with COPD and coexisting heart failure.

Heart failure was previously reported as the most common comorbidity noted in deceased patients that had been hospitalized with COPD exacerbation [22]. The mortality risk in patients with COPD in primary care was more than doubled when heart failure occurred as a comorbidity [23]. Our study confirmed that heart failure considerably increases the probability of death in patients with COPD in the general population. This is not surprising when taking into consideration that COPD is associated with an increased risk of cardiovascular diseases [24] due to smoking as a common risk factor and systemic inflammation, oxidative and physiologic stress and vascular dysfunction as a common mechanism [25]. Age and male sex were associated with higher mortality in patients with COPD and coexisting heart failure, as expected when taking into consideration data on heart failure [17] and COPD alone [22]. A wide spectrum of comorbidities was previously reported as factors associated with mortality for patients with heart failure and COPD alone. The comorbidities with the highest impact on mortality in patients with heart failure were: COPD, stroke, renal disease, anemia, diabetes [15] and for patients with COPD: respiratory failure, pneumonia, heart failure, ischaemic heart disease, hypertension and lung cancer [26]. The importance of comorbidity for mortality was shown in a Swedish study in patients with severe COPD treated with long-term oxygen therapy [27]. We showed the same effect of comorbidity in a whole population of patients with COPD. The main aim in our study, however, was not to find out if but how much heart failure, age, sex and other comorbidities influence mortality in patients with COPD. It is known that prognosis in heart failure is poorer than in COPD [28, 29] and higher mortality in patients with coexisting COPD and heart failure was expected. By adjusting odds ratios for heart failure we wanted to show importance of other comorbidities; early identifying and proper management of those may decrease mortality.

Other comorbidity in our study was calculated as an individual measure using diagnoses analyzed with the ACG Case Mix system. The severity and chronicity of the different diagnoses in an individual led to a higher level of comorbidity (RUB). RUB is a categorization of

Table 1 Odds ratios of mortality in patients with COPD – univariate analyses of different variables used

OR (95%CI)	OR (95%CI)
Heart failure	7.06 (3.88–12.84)
Age	1.13 (1.11–1.14)
Male sex	1.78 (1.38–2.30)
RUB 4	2.03 (1.48–2.78)
RUB 5	4.78 (2.61–8.74)

Table 2 Odds ratios (OR) of mortality in heart failure in patients with COPD adjusted for different variables used

Variables	OR (95%CI)
Heart failure	7.06 (3.88–12.84)
Heart failure, age	3.76 (1.98–7.16)
Heart failure, age, male sex	3.75 (1.97–7.15)
Heart failure, age, male sex, other comorbidities	3.26 (1.70–6.25)

Table 3 Importance of different variables for mortality in patients with COPD. Odds ratios (OR) were adjusted for all other variables

Variables	Adjusted OR (95%CI)
Heart failure	3.26 (1.70–6.25)
Age	1.12 (1.10–1.14)
Male sex	1.37 (1.02–1.85)
RUB 4	1.82 (1.26–2.65)
RUB 5	5.19 (2.59–10.38)

Table 4. Importance of different variables including the most common comorbid diagnoses for mortality in patients with COPD. Odds ratios (OR) were adjusted for all other variable

Variables	Adjusted OR (95% CI)
Heart failure	3.79 (1.94 -7.43)
Hypertension	0.56 (0.39 - 0.81)
Ischemic heart disease	0.94 (0.58 - 1.51)
Diabetes mellitus	1.76 (1.12 - 2.78)
Atrial fibrillation	2.07 (1.08 - 3.96)
Age	1.08 (1.07-1.10)
Male sex	1.56 (1.16 - 2.09)
RUB 4	1.82 (1.26 - 2.62)
RUB 5	5.22 (2.64 -10.32)

the individual patient's morbidity and describes the sum of all comorbidities in an individual. We showed that the higher the level of comorbidity, the higher the odds ratio of mortality even when presence of heart failure was adjusted for. Odds ratio of mortality adjusted for age and male sex in the group with the highest level of other comorbidity was five times higher. Adjusting for the most common comorbidities: hypertension, ischaemic heart disease, diabetes mellitus and atrial fibrillation did not considerably change the importance of RUB as a summarizing measurement of all other comorbidities.

This means that other comorbidities are an important independent predictor of mortality;

this should be recognized when treating patients with COPD and coexisting heart failure.

An interesting finding when adjusting for major comorbidities was that the presence of the diagnosis of hypertension lowered odds ratio of mortality. Hypertension was previously reported as an important comorbid condition which contributed to a higher risk of mortality in patients with COPD [30]. A possible explanation of this finding can be benefits associated with more extensive cardiovascular medication in patients with known hypertension [31]. This would be worth looking into in more detail in further studies.

Strengths and limitations

Our study was register-based and the primary source of information in the register was the patient's medical record, which limited baseline characteristics to age and sex. The register collected data concerned diagnosis at each consultation in all public and private care units. The limitations that we had to deal with were completeness of data and validity of the diagnoses. Due to the listing system in primary care in the Blekinge County we could study the whole population, which is a strength of our study. Each inhabitant was either actively or passively listed with a primary care center. Data from both primary- and secondary care were collected in order to increase completeness of data. COPD and heart failure are heterogeneous diagnoses. In order to capture as many cases as possible we used all codes which are available under the main codes for COPD and heart failure according to ICD 10 classification. The limitation of our study is validity of diagnoses of COPD and heart failure in the register. Validating of diagnoses against the medical records at an individual level was not possible for ethical reasons. Previous studies, however, showed that both diagnoses in Swedish registers had an acceptable level of validity for being used in epidemiological research [32, 33]. Other studies showed that data from Swedish registers can be used in estimating prevalence of chronic diseases such as hypertension, ischaemic heart disease, COPD or diabetes [34].

Conclusion

Coexisting heart failure considerably increases the odds of mortality in patients with COPD.

The mortality in patients with COPD and coexisting heart failure is strongly associated with age, male sex and other comorbidities. Of those three predictors, only other comorbidities can be influenced. It is important to recognize other comorbidities early and to treat them adequately in patients with COPD and coexisting heart failure since they significantly influence survival.

Abbreviations

ACG: Adjusted clinical groups; CI: Confidence interval; COPD: Chronic obstructive pulmonary disease; RUB: Resource utilization band

Acknowledgments

Not applicable.

Funding

The study was supported by the Blekinge- and Skåne County Councils, which are non- commercial, local Swedish government organizations, financing the health care in Blekinge and Skåne counties. The role of these funding bodies was to approve funding and provide financial resources of the research project. They were not involved in the design of the study, data collection, analysis, interpretation of the data, or in writing the manuscript.

Authors' contribution

EK participated in the design of the study, statistical analysis, data interpretation and drafted the manuscript. HO and LR made contribution to the study design and critically revised the manuscript. AH designed the study, performed the statistical analysis, handled the data set, interpreted the data and participated in drafting the manuscript. All the authors gave final approval of the version to be published.

Ethics approval and consent to participate

The study has been approved by the Research Ethics Committee at Lund University.

No 2015/169.

The data from the Blekinge County Council health care register were used after special permission. The individual consent to participate was waived by the ethics committee in agreement with Swedish law and national guidelines regarding large register studies. Thus, presumed consent to participate was used. Detailed information about the study was published in two major local newspapers with contact information to the first author. The participants could have their data excluded from the study without giving a reason for this by contacting the first author through e-mail or telephone.

Consent for publication

Obtained by presumed consent in accordance with decision of the Research Ethics Committee at Lund University No 2015/169. No data were published at an individual level.

Competing interests

All the authors declare that they have no competing interests.

References

1. Marengoni A, Angleman S, Melis R, Mangialasche F, Karp A, Garmen A, Meinow B, Fratiglioni L. Aging with multimorbidity: a systematic review of the literature. Ageing Res Rev. 2011;10(4):430–9.
2. Kaszuba E, Odeberg H, Rastam L, Halling A. Heart failure and levels of other comorbidities in patients with chronic obstructive pulmonary disease in a Swedish population: a register-based study. BMC Res Notes. 2016;9:215–016–2008-4.
3. Swedish national care program for COPD [http://slmf.se/kol/huvudpunkter/].
4. RiksSvikt. Swedish National Heart Failure Register [http://www.ucr.uu.se/rikssvikt/].
5. Eriksson H, Svardsudd K, Larsson B, Ohlson LO, Tibblin G, Welin L, Wilhelmsen L. Risk factors for heart failure in the general population: the study of men born in 1913. Eur Heart J. 1989;10(7):647–56.
6. Backman H, Eriksson B, Ronmark E, Hedman L, Stridsman C, Jansson SA, Lindberg A, Lundback B. Decreased prevalence of moderate to severe COPD over 15 years in northern Sweden. Respir Med. 2016;114:103–10.
7. Chronic respiratory diseases [http://www.who.int/respiratory/copd/burden/en/].
8. Harada T, Yamasaki A, Fukushima T, Hashimoto K, Takata M, Kodani M, Okazaki R, Takeda K, Watanabe M, Kurai J, Shimizu E. Causes of death in patients with asthma and asthma-chronic obstructive pulmonary disease overlap syndrome. Int J Chron Obstruct Pulmon Dis. 2015;10:595–602.
9. Zielinski J, MacNee W, Wedzicha J, Ambrosino N, Braghiroli A, Dolensky J, Howard P, Gorzelak K, Lahdensuo A, Strom K, Tobiasz M, Weitzenblum E. Causes of death in patients with COPD and chronic respiratory failure. Monaldi Arch Chest Dis. 1997;52(1):43–7.
10. Groenewegen KH, Schols AM, Wouters EF. Mortality and mortality-related factors after hospitalization for acute exacerbation of COPD. Chest. 2003; 124(2):459–67.
11. de Torres JP, Cote CG, Lopez MV, Casanova C, Diaz O, Marin JM, Pinto-Plata V, de Oca MM, Nekach H, Dordelly LJ, Aguirre-Jaime A, Celli BR. Sex differences in mortality in patients with COPD. Eur Respir J. 2009;33(3):528–35.
12. Hasegawa W, Yamauchi Y, Yasunaga H, Sunohara M, Jo T, Matsui H, Fushimi K, Takami K, Nagase T. Factors affecting mortality following emergency admission for chronic obstructive pulmonary disease. BMC Pulm Med. 2014; 14:151–2466-4-151.
13. Rutten FH, Cramer MJ, Grobbee DE, Sachs AP, Kirkels JH, Lammers JW, Hoes AW. Unrecognized heart failure in elderly patients with stable chronic obstructive pulmonary disease. Eur Heart J. 2005;26(18):1887–94.
14. Jhund PS, Macintyre K, Simpson CR, Lewsey JD, Stewart S, Redpath A, Chalmers JW, Capewell S, McMurray JJ. Long-term trends in first hospitalization for heart failure and subsequent survival between 1986 and 2003: a population study of 5.1 million people. Circulation. 2009;119(4):515–23.
15. Maggioni AP, Dahlstrom U, Filippatos G, Chioncel O, Leiro MC, Drozdz J, Fruhwald F, Gullestad L, Logeart D, Metra M, Parissis J, Persson H, Ponikowski P, Rauchhaus M, Voors A, Nielsen OW, Zannad F, Tavazzi L. Heart failure association of ESC (HFA): EURObservational research Programme: the heart failure pilot survey (ESC-HF pilot). Eur J Heart Fail. 2010;12(10):1076–84.
16. Joffe SW, Webster K, McManus DD, Kiernan MS, Lessard D, Yarzebski J, Darling C, Gore JM, Goldberg RJ. Improved survival after heart failure: a community-based perspective. J Am Heart Assoc. 2013;2(3):e000053.
17. Jong P, Vowinckel E, Liu PP, Gong Y, Tu JV. Prognosis and determinants of survival in patients newly hospitalized for heart failure: a population-based study. Arch Intern Med. 2002;162(15):1689–94.
18. Simon T, Mary-Krause M, Funck-Brentano C, Jaillon P. Sex differences in the prognosis of congestive heart failure: results from the cardiac insufficiency Bisoprolol study (CIBIS II). Circulation. 2001;103(3):375–80.
19. Rutten FH, Cramer MJ, Lammers JW, Grobbee DE, Hoes AW. Heart failure and chronic obstructive pulmonary disease: an ignored combination? Eur J Heart Fail. 2006;8(7):706–11.
20. Starfield B, Kinder K. Multimorbidity and its measurement. Health Policy. 2011;103(1):3–8.
21. Orueta JF, Lopez-De-Munain J, Baez K, Aiarzaguena JM, Aranguren JI, Pedrero E. Application of the ambulatory care groups in the primary care of a European national health care system: does it work? Med Care. 1999;37(3):238–48.
22. Almagro P, Calbo E, Ochoa de Echaguen A, Barreiro B, Quintana S, Heredia JL, Garau J. Mortality after hospitalization for COPD. Chest. 2002;121(5):1441–8.
23. Boudestein LC, Rutten FH, Cramer MJ, Lammers JW, Hoes AW. The impact of concurrent heart failure on prognosis in patients with chronic obstructive pulmonary disease. Eur J Heart Fail. 2009;11(12):1182–8.
24. Feary JR, Rodrigues LC, Smith CJ, Hubbard RB, Gibson JE. Prevalence of major comorbidities in subjects with COPD and incidence of myocardial infarction and stroke: a comprehensive analysis using data from primary care. Thorax. 2010;65(11):956–62.
25. Maclay JD, MacNee W. Cardiovascular disease in COPD: mechanisms. Chest. 2013;143(3):798–807.
26. Sin DD, Anthonisen NR, Soriano JB, Agusti AG. Mortality in COPD: role of comorbidities. Eur Respir J. 2006;28(6):1245–57.
27. Ekstrom MP, Jogreus C, Strom KE. Comorbidity and sex-related differences in mortality in oxygen-dependent chronic obstructive pulmonary disease. PLoS One. 2012;7(4):e35806.
28. Global initiative for chronic obstructive lung disease [http://goldcopd.org/gold-2017-global-strategy-diagnosis-management-prevention-copd/].
29. Ponikowski P, Voors AA, Anker SD, Bueno H, Cleland JG, Coats AJ, Falk V, Gonzalez-Juanatey JR, Harjola VP, Jankowska EA, Jessup M, Linde C, Nihoyannopoulos P, Parissis JT, Pieske B, Riley JP, Rosano GM, Ruilope LM, Ruschitzka F, Rutten FH, van der Meer P. Authors/task force members, document reviewers: 2016 ESC guidelines for the diagnosis and treatment of acute and chronic heart failure: the task force for the diagnosis and treatment of acute and chronic heart failure of the European Society of Cardiology (ESC). Developed with the special contribution of the heart failure association (HFA) of the ESC. Eur J Heart Fail. 2016;18(8):891–975.
30. Mannino DM, Thorn D, Swensen A, Holguin F. Prevalence and outcomes of diabetes, hypertension and cardiovascular disease in COPD. Eur Respir J. 2008;32(4):962–9.
31. Hansson L, Lindholm LH, Ekbom T, Dahlöf B, Lanke J, Scherstén B, Wester P, Hedner T, de Faire U. STOP-Hypertension-2 study group: randomised trial of old and new antihypertensive drugs in elderly patients: cardiovascular mortality and morbidity the Swedish trial in old patients with Hypertension-2 study. Lancet. 1999;354(9192):1751–6.
32. Inghammar M, Engstrom G, Lofdahl CG, Egesten A. Validation of a COPD diagnosis from the Swedish inpatient registry. Scand J Public Health. 2012; 40(8):773–6.
33. Ingelsson E, Arnlov J, Sundstrom J, Lind L. The validity of a diagnosis of heart failure in a hospital discharge register. Eur J Heart Fail. 2005;7(5):787–91.
34. Wirehn AB, Karlsson HM, Carstensen JM. Estimating disease prevalence using a population-based administrative healthcare database. Scand J Public Health. 2007;35(4):424–31.

8

Protocol for a Delphi consensus exercise to identify a core set of criteria for selecting health related outcome measures (HROM) to be used in primary health care

Pasqualina Santaguida[1*], Lisa Dolovich[2,3], Doug Oliver[4], Larkin Lamarche[2], Anne Gilsing[5], Lauren E. Griffith[6], Julie Richardson[7], Dee Mangin[8], Monika Kastner[9] and Parminder Raina[10]

Abstract

Background: Promoting the collection and use of health related outcome measures (HROM) in daily practice has long been a goal for improving and assessing the effectiveness of care provided to patients. However, there has been a lack of consensus on what criteria to use to select outcomes or instruments, particularly in the context of primary health care settings where patients present with multiple concurrent health conditions and interventions are whole-health and person-focused. The purpose of this proposed study is to undertake a formal consensus exercise to establish criteria for selecting HROM (including patient-reported (PRO or PROM), observer-reported (ObsR)), clinician-reported (ClinRO) and performance related outcomes (PerfO) for use in shared decision-making, or in assessing, screening or monitoring health status in primary health care settings.

Methods: A Delphi consensus online survey will be developed. Criteria for the Delphi panel participants to consider were selected from a targeted literature search. These initial criteria ($n = 35$) were grouped into four categories within which items will be presented in the Delphi survey, with the option to suggest additional items. Panel members invited to participate will include primary health care practitioners and administrators, policy-makers, researchers, and experts in HROM development; patients will be excluded. Standard Delphi methodology will be employed with an expectation of at least 3 rounds to achieve consensus (75% agreement). As the final list of criteria for selecting HROM emerges, panel members will be asked to provide opinions about potential weighting of items. The Delphi survey was approved by the Ethics Committee in the Faculty of Health Sciences at McMaster University.

Discussion: Previous literature establishing criteria for selecting HROM were developed with a focus on patient reported outcomes, psychological/ behavioural outcomes or outcomes for minimum core outcome sets in clinical trials. Although helpful, these criteria may not be applicable and feasible for application in a primary health care context where patients with multi-morbidity and complex interventions are typical and the constraints of providing health services differ from those in research studies. The findings from this Delphi consensus study will address a gap for establishing consensus on criteria for selecting HROM for use across primary health care settings.

Keywords: Delphi consensus, Selection of outcomes, Primary health care, Protocol

* Correspondence: santag@mcmaster.ca
[1]Department of Health Research Methods, Evidence and Impact, McMaster University HSC 3N50-G, 1280 Main Street West, Hamilton, Ontario L8S 4L7, Canada
Full list of author information is available at the end of the article

Background

Collection of outcomes for use in evaluation of health care, quality improvement, clinical decision-making or effectiveness research continues to be promoted and encouraged. Routine collection of health related outcomes can occur in more formal contexts, for example in developing patient or disease registries, or less formal where findings are documented in individual patient charts. Collection of health related outcomes can be used at a system level or for individual patient management. In either case, the dilemma remains as to which health related outcomes to select that accurately captures the intended purposes for collection. There are a large number of criteria that could be considered to select outcomes which makes the process challenging.

Several attempts to establish a minimum or core set of criteria used to evaluate or select outcomes have been reported [1–6]. However, there are important limitations in these previous recommendations. Some focus predominately on patient reported [1] or psychological/ behavioural outcomes [2, 3]; there are many other types of measures used to assess the impact of care. Another attempt was developed in the context of comparing clinical trials and using an agreed upon set of common outcomes [4]. Similarly another is to be considered broadly at a systems level and not readily operationalized with consistency [5, 6]. Although helpful, these previous criteria recommended to select outcomes may not be applicable for all types of outcomes or in other contexts in which they were developed.

This paper will detail a protocol to establish criteria for selecting health related outcome measures (HROM) in the context of primary health care (PHC). PHC is characterized by patients with multifactorial health problems and accordingly the interventions are multilayered and complex. We propose a Delphi consensus study that includes experts in HROM development and clinical research. We provide background information around definitions and use of HROM, previous attempts to establish criteria to select measures, hypothesized benefits and use of HROM in clinical settings, the relevance to the PHC context and evaluation of complex interventions generally. The proposed research protocol details are specified and previous gaps in the literature are addressed. The overall goal of this research is to contribute to the development of a transparent and reproducible process to select HROM that will be used across different sites that are implementing and adapting complex PHC interventions.

Purpose and definition of outcomes and health related outcome measures

Apart from the practical and logistical aspects of routine collection of health related outcomes for evaluation purposes, there are some challenges conceptually in defining what is and is not an outcome. This is related to the variation in definitions of an outcome generally, as well as, definitions of an outcome measure and an outcome assessment [7–23]. The term outcome is often used in a global sense to connect the expected impact of an intervention. It is also used frequently to refer to instruments or scales used to assess or evaluate interventions or patient status at any point in the health care trajectory. The term outcome may be confused with the term endpoint (which sometimes is defined as a group of outcomes used to establish the benefit or harm of an intervention).

For the purposes of this paper we have adopted the definition of an outcome as one that captures a "measureable characteristic that is influenced or affected by an individuals' baseline state or an intervention as in a clinical trial or other exposure" [8, 19]. An outcome could reflect both the benefit or harm to a patient who receives an intervention and exposure [10]. This definition is in keeping with the Donabedian framework for quality improvement which defines outcome as the "effects of care on the health status of patients and populations" [11]. Outcome assessment is considered to be the most important of three categories of assessment of quality of care (including structure (context where care is delivered and including buildings, equipment, staffing, etc.) and process (interactions between patients, providers, system) [11, 24, 25]. In this quality improvement framework, the focus of outcomes is on the impact of care on the person receiving it. Ideally the assessment of outcome of care should always reflect what patients actually experience and consider important [26]. Thus HROM are measures or scales or instruments that are designed to capture outcomes (domains and constructs) in a health care context.

What is key in this definition of outcomes and HROM is that it is not the specific type of measure or instrument or test that is used in the assessment but rather the intended purpose of the outcome measurement and the timing of the collection during care receiving. For example, consider hemoglobin A1c in the care of patients with diabetes. Capture of the frequency of measurement of hemoglobin A1c can be used to assess health service processes; estimation of the mean level (or mean change) can be used to assess the impact of the health services outcome (on the recipient). The influential Food and Drug Administration (FDA) in the United States considers a *clinical* outcome *assessment* as one that may use any of four primary types of "outcome measures" that would reflect domains important to relevant stakeholders and these include: patient reported outcome measures (PROM) or (PRO), observer reported outcomes (ObsRO), clinician reported outcomes (ClinRO), and performance outcomes (PerfO). In the FDA regulatory process, laboratory tests, biomarkers, and even mortality/survival are also important types of outcomes that can be used to assess the effectiveness of interventions (in their regulatory capacity, this refers to drugs, devices and biomarkers) for which approval is sought. This broad understanding of HROM and their potential classification are useful in understanding outcome assessment generally.

Use of HROM as an intervention

Promoting the capture of HROM in daily practice has long been a goal for assessing the effectiveness of care provided to patients [27]. However, it is only recently that there is increasing recognition that the routine collection and interpretation of HROM in practice can be shown to influence ongoing care, such that it becomes an intervention in and of itself. Greenhalgh [28, 29] hypothesized pathways of influence and impact of using PROM in clinical settings. Within this hypothesized model, the use of PROM (a type of HROM) will prompt clinicians to discuss health related quality of life concerns, it will enable clinicians to detect unrecognised problems, and will likely change the way in which a clinician will respond (as the findings from the PROM may show a change in the health related quality of life . The act of reviewing or using PROM serves to monitor treatment potentially resulting in changes to the patient's behaviour and improvement in the patient's overall health status or satisfaction with care. Thus, outcome assessment by collecting HROM not only evaluates the impact of an intervention at the resolution or end of a particular episode of care, but it can be considered an added "intervention" that serves to direct or modify care. For example, the rate of screening for depression is one outcome that could be used to demonstrate the impact of a routine visit to a family doctor. However, if the screening result is positive, then the physician will now direct care to address this previously undetected health problem. In the context of PHC, like other areas of health care provision, a wide spectrum of HROM are used to assess both simple and complex interventions and single and comorbid health conditions. Added to this complexity is that most visits to PHC are for symptoms or complaints rather than diseases so the range of available HROM related to single diseases are less appropriate [30].

It is not clear which of types of HROM should be selected to provide useful information to assess the impact of care or to allow clinicians and decision-makers to direct or modify care. What is an ideal HROM in one context may not be so in another context and in part reflects the intended purpose of the outcome assessment. The challenge for clinicians, researchers and decision-makers is to select the most appropriate HROM in light of the fact that likely several well established HROM currently exist and are candidates for selection. Although there have been some attempts to set some general guidelines for selecting HROM for outcome assessment, these criteria have several key limitations that have been noted and none provide recommendations for dealing with equally valid but competing measures.

Hypothesized benefits of using HROM in clinical settings

Donabedian was one of the first to propose that structure, process and outcomes are seminal to evaluating quality of care [24, 25]. Since the late 1960s there has been great emphasis on the selection and use of HROM in quality assessment but also in effectiveness research and even directing clinical decision-making for individual patients. As noted previously, Greenhalgh [28, 29] hypothesized pathways of influence and impact of using PROM in clinical settings. Within this model, PROM can be considered as having multiple purposes that include "clinical tests", "interventions" and "outcomes". Table 1 details how the model specifies the clinical goal when using PROM and the potential impact of using these in clinical settings. Note that this model may be applied to HROM, as the definition of HROM includes PROM (as well as, ObsRO, ClinRO, PerfO).

When considering the clinical goals (i.e., assess change, monitor, detect, etc.) for using an HROM, it is not clear if the criteria used to select measures will vary as a function of the specific purpose. It is likely that the criteria may vary not only as a function of the clinical purpose for using the HROM, but also the health domain being assessed by the tool and for other administrative concerns. Soliciting expert opinions on this issue would add to the knowledge of how to apply HROM for clinical, administrative, or research purposes.

Table 1 Greenhalgh [24] model hypothesizing pathways of influence and impact in using PROM in clinical settings

Clinical Goal of PROM	Impact of PROM use
Change the content and nature of the communication between the family doctor/ primary health care team and the patient/consumer to improve patient centered care	Changes to patient behaviour
Monitor health status or response to treatment	Changes to the clinical management of patient's/ consumers
Detect unrecognized problems or screen for disease problems in those at high risk	Improved health outcomes and satisfaction of patient
	Facilitation of communication amongst multidisciplinary teams
	Evaluation of the effectiveness of routine care and assessing the quality of care

Primary health care context and complex interventions

In the context of PHC, there is increasing recognition that most interventions are complex. The Medical Research Council (United Kingdom) has been instrumental in conceptualizing the issues related to developing, evaluating, and reporting on complex interventions [31]. Complex interventions are characterized by having a number of interactions between components and requiring a number of different behaviours by those delivering or receiving the intervention [31]. Adding to this definition is that a number of groups and organizational levels are affected by the intervention. Although some would make the distinction between the complexity of the intervention versus the complexity of the health system [32] the two components interact. Flexibility and adaptation characterize complex interventions [31]. Practically this means that changes in implementation of an intervention are to be expected. More importantly, it follows that a number of outcomes may be required, as well as variability in outcomes assessing the same attribute of interest [31]. This would suggest that adaptations of interventions in one component of a health system may result in the need to select different or modify existing HROM relative to that context. The benefit of this is that it reflects the varying and flexible aspects of PHC interventions and therefore reflects strengths of the interventions in different settings.

The development of this Delphi consensus study is considered in the context of such a complex intervention. Health TAPESTRY is a novel intervention currently being implemented in Canadian PHC settings and undergoing evaluation in a randomized trial. The intervention components involve patients, volunteers, health care teams, and researchers, as well as, the use of an electronic patient health record accessed by all relevant stakeholders [33]. There are several affiliates of Health TAPESTRY across different sites in Canada that vary in their patient populations and focus in PHC services. As expected, each Health TAPESTRY site currently uses different HROM (or will need to select new HROM), and this may present challenges for evaluating benefits and quality of this complex intervention. One overriding goal of Health TAPESTRY is to integrate new and old functionality within and across each of these centres. As the Health TAPESTRY intervention is being adapted and implemented it did not seem feasible to enforce standardization of HROM. However, stakeholders acknowledge that there is a need to guide selection of key HROM to be used in evaluating the impact of the Health TAPESTRY intervention across implementation sites. Health TAPESTRY serves as a quintessential example of PHC issues and the complexity of evaluation. Recognizing the potential for differences across Health TAPESTRY sites, a valid and trustworthy process to review and accept suggestions for HROM is needed to allow for evaluation of effectiveness and impact across sites. To our knowledge there is no guideline or consensus on criteria to select HROM within a PHC setting.

Study purposes

Our primary purpose for the Delphi consensus exercise is to derive a minimum core criteria set (CCS) of items to be used to select HROM when faced with many different measures that can be used within PHC settings. Related to this we will solicit opinions about the relative weighting of criteria groups to be used when selecting HROM.

Additional purposes for the Delphi survey are to consider core areas and domains of HROM that are important to collect in PHC and reflecting the complex interventions that are flexible and adaptable (such as Health TAPESTRY). The CCS will assist in selecting HROM but it will not provide guidance as to the core health areas of importance for PHC. Therefore, a second purpose of this study is to elicit opinions about core areas and domains and HROM that effectively capture the attributes of interest within these core areas/domains that are optimal for use within PHC settings.

Methods/design

General approach

The stated objectives of this study require consensus on criteria for selecting HROM and opinions about areas and types of outcomes to be used in PHC settings and Health TAPESTRY. There are a number of methods used to solicit group opinion and consensus and these include nominal techniques, Delphi consensus, and consensus development conferences [34]. From these approaches we selected the Delphi consensus as the most appropriate for the purposes of this study. The global aim of the Delphi consensus exercise is to achieve consensus on a CCS for selecting HROM relevant to PHC and Health TAPESTRY. Figure 1 shows the expected rounds of the survey to achieve consensus for CCS.

Health TAPESTRY centres will also need to consider what key health areas or domains should be captured (for example physical function is a core area of health and within this there are several domains that might include activities of daily living and physical activity levels). We will solicit the opinions of the Delphi panel about core areas and domains and important HROM that they feel meet the CCS and are relevant for PHC settings and complex interventions such as Health TAPESTRY. We will not require consensus with regards to core areas and domains suggested by participants.

Key assumptions and definitions

Defining HROM

The types of HROM we are considering in this Delphi consensus study are likely standardized measures of

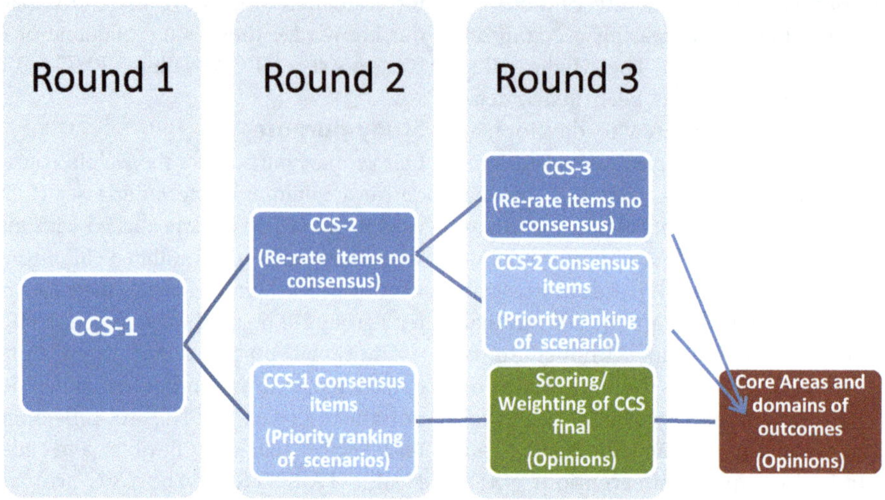

Fig. 1 Anticipated rounds of the Delphi consensus exercise and timing of soliciting opinions on clinical scenarios and core outcomes

health status, disability, impairment, or handicap, as well as other clinical tests. They assess specific dimensions of a disease or a health problem (e.g., depression or frailty or fasting glucose levels). Many of these measures can be uni-dimensional (reflecting a single health construct) or multi-dimensional (several health constructs).

A number of different measures reflecting the patients' health experiences can be used in the PHC setting and these include:

1. PROM (e.g., visual analogue scale [VAS], Short Form 36 [SF36]): PROM's are measures that are reported or collected directly from the patient. PRO/PROM may be collected via self-administered questionnaires completed by the patient themselves or via interviews of the patients ensuring their views are adequately captured.
2. PerfO (e.g., Timed up and go test): PerfO are those that require assessment of the patient's capacity to perform pre-specified tasks. Typical performance-based measures include the Berg Balance Scale or the 50 ft Walking Test.
3. ClinRO/ ObsRO (e.g., Edmonton Frailty Index, Functional Index Measure [FIM]): Outcomes that include clinical scales are measures where clinicians/ outcome assessors evaluate the health construct of interest. This can include laboratory tests.

Defining primary health care

We have selected the PHC care context for our study, as it encompasses a general approach to health policy and service provision that reflect the core principles espoused by the World Health Organization (universal access, health equity, community participation, inter-sectoral approaches to health) [35] and recognizes the importance of the broad determinants of health [36]. PHC focuses on patient and provider relationship, as well as organized care. Thus, PHC embraces a wide suite of services and involves a broad range of health care providers [37, 38] that include the following: i) family physicians/general practitioners; ii) nurses, nurse practitioners; iii) rehabilitation professionals (e.g., occupational therapist); iv) physician assistants; v) nutritionists and; vi) behaviour counselors (e.g., social work).

The selection of HROM in the context of PHC can encompass a variety of outcomes reflecting domains of efficacy, effectiveness, patient engagement, patient satisfaction, and other aspects of care. Given the range of health care providers, the intended purposes of the use of the outcome may also vary. Further the selection of outcomes may need to reflect the series of complex interactions and interventions that are part of the services provided in PHC.

Selecting core areas and domains from which to map outcomes

Core areas and domains represent the key aspects of health that the HROM attempts to capture. For example, physical function is a core area of health. Domains within the core area of physical function could include physical activity or lower extremity mobility. It is anticipated that a community adapting an intervention or putting a new intervention in place may choose different HROM that capture important core areas and domains relevant to PHC. As noted previously, our literature review identified one initiative to develop criteria for selecting outcomes in the context of clinical trials and the need for developing a core outcome set (COS) [38]. This review stemmed from the recent work from Core Outcome Measures in Effectiveness Trials (COMET) [39, 40] and OMERACT [39, 41–44] suggesting approaches to developing core areas and domains for selecting outcomes. The aim of this approach is to establish key areas of health and then select HROM to consistently assess across different research and clinical initiatives. The challenge with selecting a core set of HROM is that most initiatives are centred on a single disease and in the PHC context there are multiple health conditions often for the same patient.

We have specified a broad set of core areas (see Fig. 2). The literature suggests that the selection of HROM is related to the purpose and core area/domain of health that is of interest. At this time there is no literature specifying core areas/domain of relevance to PHC. Therefore a secondary aim of the Delphi consensus survey is to solicit opinions of the Delphi panel on the relative value of the core areas, domains and subdomains that has been preselected by Health TAPESTRY investigators. Additionally, we will solicit opinions on important HROM that would capture the aspects of health of interest and meet the core set of selection criteria established through the Delphi consensus exercise. Opinions about core areas, domains and subdomains, as well as suggested HROM will assist different Health TAPESTRY centres in selecting these measures (once the core criteria are established).

Development of the Delphi questionnaire for CCS

Literature review

The investigators assembled potentially relevant criteria for selection of outcomes from a targeted literature review. We searched Pubmed using terms related to outcomes (i.e., *outcome measures, Patient reported outcomes, Comparative effectiveness, Patient-centered outcomes research, Psychometrics, Measurement properties, Questionnaire, Patient Registry, Methods*). We also searched specific websites (i.e. FDA and others listed below) related to outcome measures. The citations listed below were important sources of from which our criteria was selected and these included:

1) Consensus-based Standards for the selection of health Measurement Instruments (COSMIN) checklist) [45–49]; the checklist establishes which measurement properties should be evaluated in health related patient-reported outcomes and is used to evaluate studies that attempt to establish the properties of a health related patient-reported outcomes.
2) International Society for Quality of Life Research (ISOQOL) which recently set minimum standards for patient-reported outcome measures used in patient-centered outcomes and comparative effectiveness research [1].
3) Theoretical paper discussing outcome measure assessment [50].
4) Examples of systematic reviews evaluating outcome measures [51, 52].
5) Criteria used on the GEM wiki (www.gem-measures.org) [3]
6) Issues related to harmonizing patient reported data elements in registries and health records [2, 53].
7) Reports on registries for reporting patient outcomes [26].
8) Patient Reported Outcome and Quality of Life Instruments Database (PROQOLID) (database identifies and describes clinical outcome assessments [COA's]) to help choose appropriate instruments and facilitate access to them [54].

Structure of the consensus survey

The criteria derived from the targeted literature search (detailed above) were grouped into four primary categories

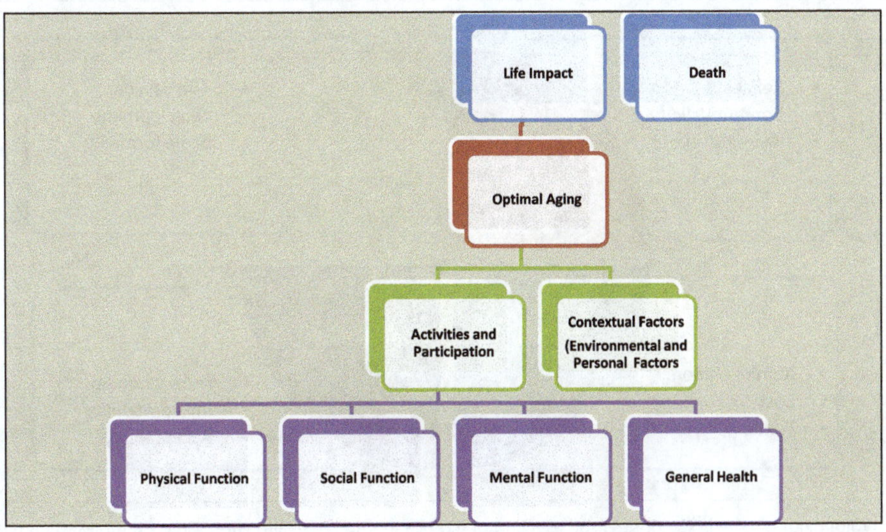

Fig. 2 Core areas for health-related outcome measures (HROM) to be used in primary health care

reflecting aspects of the outcome and these included: 1) gold standard measurement properties; 2) purpose and structure; 3) applicability; and 4) feasibility. Figure 3 shows some examples of subcategories of criteria within the four broad categories. Table 2 shows the criteria proposed to Delphi panel members for their consideration.

From the targeted literature search a total of 35 criteria have been identified for Panel members to consider in Round 1 (see Table 2). In Round 1 panel members are asked to rate whether they view the criterion as one that could be used to select amongst different HROM and then asked to comment on their reasons. For each criterion, Delphi participants can view a short description of the conceptual basis/definitions and where possible references or sources associated with it were noted.

For criteria that has reached consensus, Delphi participants are asked additional questions in Round 2. Delphi participants are asked to comment on potential for differences in inclusion or exclusion of criterion relative to the four clinical goals/scenarios (i.e., engage, assess, screen, monitor). Prior to launch of the Delphi consensus survey pre-testing will be undertaken to ensure correct functioning of the survey online screens and for wording of the questions and notes provided to participants.

General approach for soliciting opinions about core areas in round 3

Developing questions related to core areas and domains of outcomes

Figure 4 shows core areas and domains that the investigators selected after review of the literature of frameworks for core outcome measures [38]. The investigators believe these core areas are comprehensive and important to PHC. We will solicit opinions from the Delphi panel regarding suitable domains and subdomains to be captured consistently in primary care. We will also solicit opinions about HROM suitable for primary care settings within the suggested domains.

General structure of questions about the weighting of core items

These questions will be open ended and will be determined based on the results of the previous 2 rounds.

Selection of stakeholder groups and nominated participants

Our general approach is to select individuals who have knowledge of the outcome and outcome assessment and with clinical or research experience in PHC [55]; the goal is also to have representation of different perspectives with respect to the use of HROM or the professional role of those who use the HROM [55]. For this reason we will use a purposive sampling approach. The selection of Delphi panel members should reflect the population that is intended to use the CCS or be informed by the research. In order to ensure validity of the final CCS, the panelists should reflect a diverse range of stakeholders, and likely from representing different geographic regions within Canada or internationally.

Identifying relevant stakeholders

There are two sets of issues to consider when selecting participants in the Delphi exercise to achieve consensus for the selection of criteria for choosing outcome measures in PHC settings and Health TAPESTRY. The first is with regards to the stakeholders and potential areas of expertise or representation from which to recruit potential panel members. We will identify key stakeholder

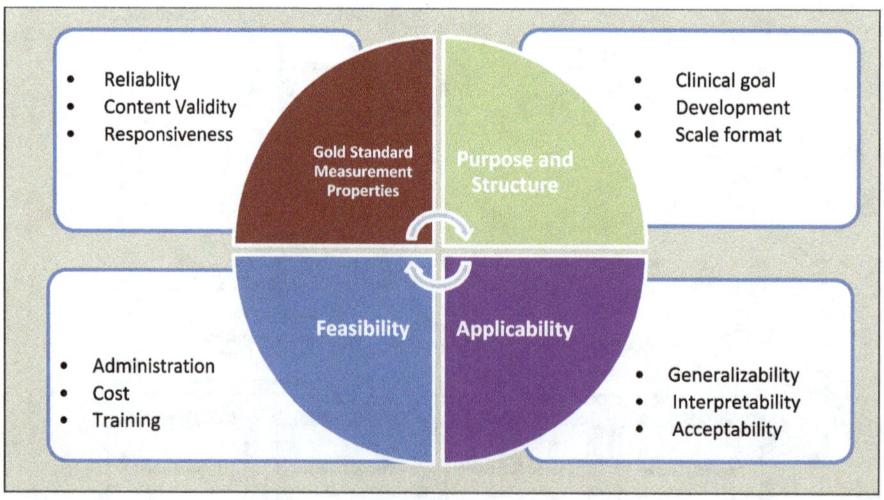

Fig. 3 Categorization (grouping) of criteria to consider for selecting outcomes in primary health care; some examples of criteria within each categorization are shown

Table 2 Criteria found in targeted literature search and the items identified as potential criteria to be used when selecting HROM in clinical settings

Gold standard properties (*N* = 8)	Purpose, development & structure (*N* = 10)
1) Reliability	1) Clinical goal
2) Content validity	2) Specificity of the measure (disease/ generic)
3) Construct validity	3) Theoretical framework
4) Criterion validity	4) Modifications since original development
5) Cross-cultural validity	5) Number of items and subscales
6) Responsiveness	6) Recall period/ Time interval
7) Population norms	7) Scoring method
8) Diagnostic accuracy	8) Direction of effect
9) Missed any criterion	9) Literacy level
	10) Translation to different languages
Feasibility (*N* = 9)	**Applicability (*N* = 8)**
1) Mode of administration	1) Setting and population used in validation
2) Format	2) Validation of measure for use with proxy participants
3) Time to complete	3) Interpretability by patients
4) Potential for harm	4) Interpretability by clinicians (and policymakers and researchers)
5) Need for specific skills for those that administer	5) Burden to patients
6) Specialized equipment required	6) Burden to clinicians/staff/ data collectors (volunteers)
7) Cost	7) Value added
8) Accessibility	8) Recognized or frequently used
9) Harmonization potential	

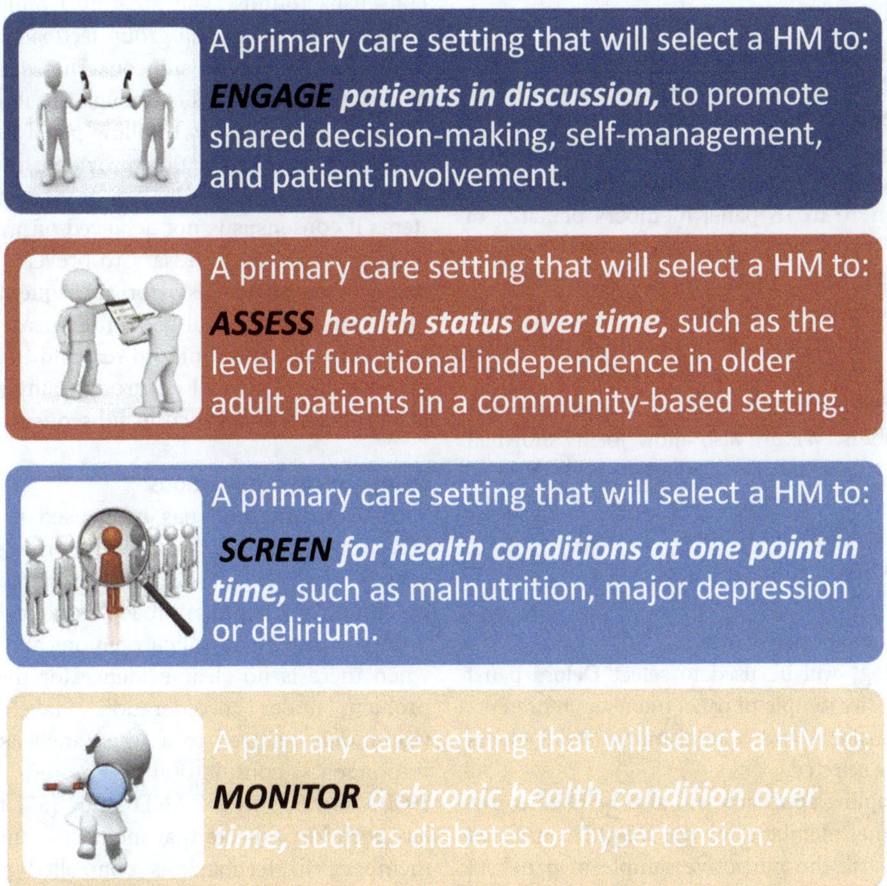

Fig. 4 Four clinical purposes of using outcomes and these include activities that Engage, Assess, Screen, and Monitor primary health care patients

groups and these include: i) PHC team members (all health professional disciplines of relevance) including those likely to be involved in the Health TAPESTRY across Canada (including sites in Ontario, Quebec, Saskatchewan, NFLD, and British Columbia); ii) management or administration team members in PHC clinical care sites; iii) health and health services researchers with experience in primary care HROM (including quality indicators); iv) experts in administrative issues related to collecting measures (including harmonization related issues); v) methodologists working in outcomes-related and questionnaire development research; and vi) community service organizations involved in patient care or support. Patients and volunteers will not be represented in the Delphi panel membership.

Invitation and reminder to Delphi panel participants

All Delphi participants identified will be invited to complete each Delphi round, unless they indicate withdrawal from the study. Continuation of the Delphi participant (by linking to the survey) will be assumed as consent to participate. Reminders will be sent every 14 days following distribution of the survey. Round 1 will be closed after 12 weeks.

Sample size for the Delphi panel

There is no set standard for sample size of a panel but it is generally agreed that the more members will increase the reliability of group judgments [34]. In has been suggested that a minimum number of panel members [56] would range from 10 to 18 panel members per area of expertise. Given the complexity of the criteria and the number of different health professionals likely with multiple areas of expertise, we will aim towards a minimum sample size of 50 participants. We will send email invitations to approximately 60 potential panel members assuming a 20% rejection rate, yielding a final sample size of 50 panel members. We are also allow for a "snowball sampling" approach, which we anticipate will increase our sample; we will encourage the pool of potential panel members to send invitations to other potential relevant participants.

Sampling strategy and response rate

A combined strategy will be used to select Delphi panel members. A purposive sample of panel members representing relevant professional and administrative stakeholders within PHC will be selected.

A snowball sampling approach will also be used to recruit potential panel members for the Delphi consensus exercise. We will ask the purposive sample of panelists to suggest names (and email contact) of other relevant stakeholders. Potential panel members who have experience in PHC practice or outcome measurement research will be considered.

A response of 75% is suggested for each round to achieve or maintain rigour [57] and we will monitor response rate for each round. There is the potential to introduce "withdrawal bias" if participants choose to withdraw after the first round. If Delphi panel members choose to not continue participation, we will attempt to solicit reasons for withdrawal (e.g., not enough time, too complicated, not interested) in order to assess possible threats to validity of the Delphi process [58].

Invitation, reminders and data management of panel member information

Each participant will be allocated a random identification number and analysis of results through LimeSurvey 2.0. Demographic data (collected at the end of Round 1) will be collated and summarized as exported by LimeSurvey 2.0.

Selection role of the Steering Committee members

Steering committee members will be selected from our team of investigators. The Steering Committee will function to summarize responses from the iterative Delphi consensus rounds. The Steering Committee will be responsible for preparing group feedback to panel respondents, and to identify any concerns with moving forward to reaching consensus. Although the intent of the Delphi consensus exercise is to allow panel members to judge and filter the information provided, the Steering Committee may need to make some decisions to reduce items if consensus is not achieved on many criteria. This approach may be necessary to prevent risk of over burden to Delphi panelists for subsequent rounds [57]. A reduction in items will be communicated to panel members and the opportunity to respond to the feedback will be provided. This will ensure that any potential for bias is identified and rectified in subsequent rounds [57].

Delphi consensus methods

The Delphi method has been used in a variety of research contexts to achieve both consensus [34] and dissensus [59] when soliciting stakeholder or expert opinion. The Delphi approach, is typically selected as an unbiased process to solicit opinions and reach consensus when there is no clear evidence for the solution to the problem under consideration. Stakeholder or expert (commonly referred to as the panellists, participants or respondents) consultation is required. Developed in the 1950's and 60's in a RAND study [57] the methodology has been key aspects that include: i) anonymity of panel members; ii) feedback is controlled and fed back to panelists; iii) survey and feedback is iterative (usually 3 successive rounds); and iv) iteration of rounds until consensus is achieved (or the law of diminishing returns sets in). The advantages of the Delphi process are that opinions of experts and other stakeholders are collected in a non-confrontational manner, free from group pressures, while group opinions are fed back to panelists. The process may help to identify aspects of the problem or solution under consideration that may have been missed or may have thought to be of limited relevance.

Defining and achieving final consensus and timeline

For the purpose of this study, consensus is defined as general agreement of a substantial majority (75% or greater) of Delphi panelists. Re-evaluation of items would continue with iterations of Delphi rounds (a minimum of 2) or until consensus is reached on all criteria within the four groupings. If consensus cannot reached after 5 rounds, the Steering Committee will stop rounds and finalize the items within the CCS. In accordance with improved reporting standards, consensus is thus defined a priori, with specific quantitative thresholds to achieve consensus, with rounds specified as an expected 3 and up to 5, criteria for excluding and including criteria and feedback on why items were dropped or added [60]. We have specified how we will invite and select Delphi participants in a manner that is reproducible [60].

It is anticipated that we will require three rounds and expect analysis between the rounds will take up to 12 months. Round 1 commenced on January 15 2016.

First round

As the Delphi method involves a series of rounds in order to achieve consensus, different activities will occur at each successive round. In the first round, panel members will link to a web-based version of the Delphi questionnaire in LimeSurvey 2.0, which includes background information, instructions to the survey, and help files for specific questions. In this Round 1 Delphi panelists will be asked to rate: the appropriateness of the criterion for selecting HROM, and 2) the reason why the item would be selected or not.

We will ask Delphi panel members to suggest rephrasing, provide any rationale for their choices (each item in the survey has a comment box), and suggest missing or new items. Panel members will be given up to 12 weeks to respond. To enhance response rate, panelists will be sent a reminder notice after 2 weeks of the initial email requesting participation.

Second round

The responses from Round 1 will be aggregated, and analysed. The aggregated information will be fed back to panel members anonymously as part of the introductory material for the second round. Items where there is consensus to include in the CCS will be identified. Conversely, items for which there is consensus to exclude will also be identified. Finally, items for which there is a lack of consensus will be identified. Panel members will then be asked to reconsider the criteria for which consensus will not have been reached. Delphi panel members will be asked to review these findings and provide any comments.

Additionally, in the second round respondents will be asked if priority ranking of the criterion will change as a consequence of the clinical goal (see Fig. 1). Figure 4 identifies four clinical goals (adapted from Greenhalgh [28, 29]) that are related to the HROM being used. This will be asked for items for which there is consensus that the criteria should be included. Note that consensus is not necessary in these responses to priority ranking. Our aim is to solicit opinions with regards to ranking as a function of the clinical goal of the HROM. We will ask Delphi panel members to suggest rephrasing, provide any rationale for their choices (each item in the survey has a comment box), and suggest missing or new items.

Third round (or greater)

Criteria that remain indeterminate from Round 2 will be brought back into the third round or for continued series of iterations until consensus is achieved (see Fig. 1). Panel members will re-evaluate criteria for which there is insufficient consensus for inclusion/exclusion. Conversely, a third round will be omitted if consensus (on all remaining items) is reached following the second round. We will ask Delphi panel members to suggest rephrasing, provide any rationale for their choices (each item in the survey had a comment box), and suggest missing or new items.

We will add additional questions regarding the relative weighting of the four groupings of items for a final CCS for which consensus has been reached. These questions will be developed as the CCS emerges following the Delphi rounds. The aim of these questions is to solicit opinions only and not achieve consensus.

Finally, we will solicit opinions about the core areas and domains and outcomes that meet the CCS final criteria within these domains.

Discussion

There are several important gaps in the literature with respect to how to select criteria to choose HROM and in which contexts. We consider several of these gaps here.

Previous attempts to establish criteria for selecting HROM and their limitations

There have been several attempts to establish criteria for selecting HROM. If the focus of the outcome assessment is on matters of importance to patients, then it is clear that measures evaluating health related quality of life are important to consider. The ISOQOL has provided one such effort with the goal to establish minimum standards for the design and selection of PROM suitable for comparative effectiveness reviews and for patient centered outcomes research [1]. They assembled potential criteria from a targeted literature review identifying existing guidance ($n = 28$ guidance documents) on the selection of PROM in patient-centred outcomes research, followed by an online survey of their membership. Their recommended criteria focused on a succinct list ($n = 7$) of measurement properties (i.e., reliability, validity, etc.) and practical attributes (i.e., interpretability, acceptable burden, etc.). Although an important initial step, these criteria were developed with consideration of PROM and multidimensional instruments reflecting health related quality of life; they did not take into account the specific health setting or clinical context for use (i.e., screening, monitoring, etc.).

A second attempt to establish criteria for selecting HROM did take into account the PHC context; the criteria for selecting outcomes was considered with respect to use of the electronic health record to record PROM specifically measuring health behaviours and psychosocial concerns [2, 3]. In the inaugural phases of this initiative, content experts (i.e., expertise in physical activity, goal setting, patient literacy, anxiety and depression, etc.) were instructed to consider a set of proposed scientific and practical criteria for recommending outcomes to capture attributes of health promotion and disease prevention. From these a core set of criteria ($n = 12$) that were grouped according to "scientific" attributes and "practical considerations" were proposed. A grid-enabled measures (GEM) portal on a wiki site provided a repository of recommended psychosocial outcome instruments and allowed other stakeholders (researchers, practitioners, administrators) to continue to make suggestions and recommendations on the use of these measures in the context of these criteria. Although the focus of these criteria was targeting only selection of PROM for behavioural and psychosocial issues and considering the electronic health record in PHC, real world contexts were considered and reflected in the "practical considerations" components of the criteria.

A third set of core criteria were developed by the Core Outcome Measurement Instrument Selection (COMIS) [4, 20] in cooperation with the COMET Initiative and the COSMIN. The criteria was derived using a Delphi consensus exercise (that included both research and clinical experts) with the intended goal of developing a guideline on how to select measurement instruments included in a Core Outcome Set (COS). A COS is an agreed minimum set of outcomes that should be measured and reported in all clinical trials of a specific disease or trial population. The definition of an outcome considered in this research is one that conceptualizes outcome as the "what" is being measured and defined as a "construct or domain". It follows then that an outcome measurement instrument captures these constructs. Prinsen et al., (2016) [4] did not restrict their criteria to any type of instrument (e.g. included PROM but is all inclusive) and included experts with both clinical and research experience. However, the focus during development of these criteria was to develop a minimum set of outcomes for use in clinical trials for a disease or patient population rather than a health service or setting.

The fourth initiative to identify criteria to select health related measures generally and HROM was developed by the Institute of Medicine (IOM) which examined core measures used within the American health care system and considered some criteria for core measures and core sets. The IOM committee aimed to decrease inconsistent and duplicative efforts to collect HROM when assessing system level quality and established criteria for core measures [5, 6]. For individual patient outcomes these included: consideration of the measures' importance to health, strength of linkage to progress, understandability of the measure, technical integrity, potential for broader system impact, and utility at multiple levels. Additional consideration was given to system related issues and these included: systemic reach, outcomes oriented, person meaningful, parsimonious, representative, and utility at multiple levels [6]. The IOM effectively considered both individual and system level categories that could be applied to PHC and likely capturing complex interventions.

These previous attempts to establish criteria to select PROM/HROM demonstrate the growing interest in establishing criteria and also justification for selecting outcomes. These previous attempts provide important context for what criteria have been considered and how these were developed. There are areas of overlap across these four different sets of recommended criteria which reflect a convergence of key attributes that may be grouped into those reflecting measurement properties and practical aspects. However, there are differences in items within these broad categories across criteria sets, which may in part reflect the specific purposes of each of their respective development processes. The influence of the health care setting, particularly PHC and the complex nature of this environment, is not clear in the development of these criteria and would merit further exploration.

Although helpful, these previous attempts at establishing a CCS may not be applicable and feasible for application in PHC settings where patients with multiple health conditions and complex interventions are the typical and the constraints of providing health services differ from those in research studies. We have proposed a methodology to conduct a Delphi and constructed an online survey which we pilot tested for comprehension and pre-tested to ensure adequate functioning of the survey set up. Although we did not undertake cognitive debriefing but believe the pre-testing will take this into account.

Understanding the context of primary care and primary health care

There is some inconsistency in understanding differences between primary care and PHC [35] and the differences are typically around the types of services provided. For the purposes of this paper we refer to primary care where there are interactions and services with clinicians (usually general practitioners) as first line of service. [35]. In contrast PHC is broader in scope and encompasses a general approach to health policy and service provision (i.e. core principles that include universal access, health equity, community participation, inter-sectoral approaches to health promoted by the World Health Organization) [35]. Effective PHC is community-based, promotes healthy lifestyles to prevent illnesses, considers ongoing care for chronic conditions and acknowledges the importance of the broad determinants of health [36]. There is evidence to show that PHC helps prevent morbidity and mortality and is associated with more equitable distribution of health in the populations [21].

PHC also reflects the first contact with the health care system and coordination and integration thereby ensuring access to care (diverse services and health providers) [36, 37] that include the following: i) family physicians/ general practitioners; ii) nurses, nurse practitioners; iii) rehabilitation professionals (e.g., occupational therapist); iv) physician assistants; v) nutritionists and; vi) behaviour counselors (e.g., social work).

Understanding the role of PHC in the health of a population, the rationale for selecting HROM is compelling. The selection of HROM in the context of PHC can encompass a variety of outcomes reflecting domains of efficacy, effectiveness, patient engagement, patient satisfaction, and other aspects of care. Given the range of health care providers, the intended purposes of the use of the outcome may also vary. Further the selection of outcomes may need to reflect the series of complex interactions and interventions that are part of the services provided in PHC.

Availability of multiple HROM

We anticipate that there are many HROM that possess good aspects and this presents a new dilemma; that is, selecting from several HROM attempting to capture the same health attribute of interest that meet the established criteria for selection. The stakeholder is faced with having a rationale for their choice. One potential strategy to address this issue is to consider "weighting" some items as more important over others; soliciting opinions from the Delphi panel on the final set of criteria for which consensus is achieved may provide some practical direction for implementation.

Soliciting opinions about important core domains for outcomes may also assist stakeholders in making choices amongst different HROM that meet the CCS. The conceptual models that underpin some complex or multi-dimensional HROM may need to be compared to core areas deemed appropriate or ideal for the PHC context. As noted previously, primary care patients reflect heterogeneous population with a variety of health conditions. There is limited discussion in the literature about the core areas and subdomains that ideally should be captured. Opinions from panel members will be collated and reflected back in the guidance document of for implementation of the CCS.

Because of these gaps, we developed this protocol to undertake a Delphi consensus online survey to establish criteria for a broader array of types of outcomes (i.e., HROM) specific to the context of PHC settings. A Delphi consensus exercise is a preferred method when consensus is lacking and in this case the literature suggests some lack of overlap in possible criteria. The advantages of the Delphi which include anonymity, provision of controlled feedback, and avoidance of face to face meetings will minimize potential biases due to personalities and other types of influences. Our selection of sample members will not be random and is influenced by current members of different Health TAPESTRY affiliates; the sample therefore may reflect these perspectives and not be truly representative of all primary health care contexts. The findings from this Delphi study will address a gap for establishing consensus on criteria for selecting HROM for use across PHC settings and complex interventions.

Abbreviations

CCS: Core criteria set; ClinRO: Clinician reported outcome; COA: Clinical Outcome Assessment; COS: Core outcome set; FIM: Functional Index Measure; HROM: Health related outcome measures; ObsRO: Observer reported outcome; PerfO: Performance outcome; PHC: Primary health care; PRO: Patient reported outcome; PROM: Patient reported outcome measure; PROQOLID: Patient Reported Outcome and Quality of Life Instruments Database; SF36: Short Form 36; VAS: Visual analogue scale

Funding

Funding for this study is from Health Canada and the Canadian Institutes of Health. Thes agencies had no role in the design of this protocol and will not be involved in the future data collection, analysis and interpretation of data, nor in the writing of the manuscript.

Authors' contributions

PLS, LD, AG, and LL were responsible for the initial methods development and all authors contributed to refining these and comments on the results. All authors (PLS, LD, AG, LL, DO, LG, JR, DM, MK and PR were responsible for reviewing drafts of the manuscript. All authors read and approved the final manuscript.

Competing interests
Research.

1) Parminder Raina holds a Tier 1 Canada Research Chair in Geroscience and the Raymond and Margaret Labarge Chair in Research and Knowledge Application for Optimal Aging
2) Lauren Griffith PhD is supported by a Canadian Institutes of Health Research New Investigators Award and the McLaughlin Foundation Professorship in Population and Public Health
3) The other authors declare that they have no competing interests.

Author details
[1]Department of Health Research Methods, Evidence and Impact, McMaster University HSC 3N50-G, 1280 Main Street West, Hamilton, Ontario L8S 4L7, Canada. [2]Department of Family Medicine, DBHSC, McMaster University, 5th Floor 100 Main St West, Hamilton, ON L8P 1H6, Canada. [3]Leslie Dan Faculty of Pharmacy, University of Toronto, Toronto, Ontario M5S 3M2, Canada. [4]Department of Family Medicine, DBHSC, McMaster University, 3rd Floor, 100 Main St West, Hamilton, ON L8P 1H6, Canada. [5]Department of Health Research Methods, Evidence and Impact, McMaster University, 175 Longwood Rd. S. Suite 207A, Hamilton, ON L8P 0A1, Canada. [6]Department of Health Research Methods, Evidence and Impact, McMaster University, 175 Longwood Rd. S. Suite 309A, Hamilton, ON L8P 0A1, Canada. [7]School of Rehabilitation Sciences, McMaster University, 1400 Main St. W. IAHS 443, Hamilton, ON L8S 1C7A, Canada. [8]Department of Family Medicine, DBHSC, McMaster University, 5th Floor, 100 Main St West, Hamilton, Ontario L8P 1H6, Canada. [9]Institute of Health Policy, Management and Evaluation, University of Toronto, 155 College Street, Toronto, ON M5T 3M6, Canada. [10]Department of Health Research Methods, Evidence and Impact, McMaster University, 175 Longwood Rd. S. Suite 309A, Hamilton, ON L8P 0A1, Canada.

References
1. Reeve BB, Wyrwich KW, Wu AW, Velikova G, Terwee CB, Snyder CF, Schwartz C, Revicki DA, Moinpour CM, McLeod LD, et al. ISOQOL recommends minimum standards for patient-reported outcome measures used in patient-centered outcomes and comparative effectiveness research. Qual Life Res. 2013;22(8):1889–905.
2. Estabrooks PA, Boyle M, Emmons KM, Glasgow RE, Hesse BW, Kaplan RM, Krist AH, Moser RP, Taylor MV. Harmonized patient-reported data elements in the electronic health record: supporting meaningful use by primary care action on health behaviors and key psychosocial factors. J Am Med Inform Assoc. 2012;19(4):575–82.
3. Rabin BA, Purcell P, Naveed S, Moser RP, Henton MD, Proctor EK, Brownson RC, Glasgow RE. Advancing the application, quality and harmonization of implementation science measures. Implement Sci. 2012;7:119.
4. Prinsen CAC, Vohra S, Rose MR, Boers M, Tugwell P, Clarke M, Williamson PR, Terwee CB. How to select outcome measurement instruments for outcomes included in a "Core outcome set" - a practical guideline. Trials. 2016;17:449.
5. Blumenthal D, McGinnis J. Measuring vital signs: an IOM report on core metrics for health and health care progress. JAMA. 2015;313(19):1901–2.
6. IOM. Vital signs: Core metrics for health and health care progress. In: Blumenthal D, Malphrus E, McGinnis JM, editors. . Washington, DC: National Academies Press; 2015.
7. Guidance FDA. Guidance for industry: patient-reported outcome measures: use in medical product development to support labeling claims: draft guidance. BMC Med Res Methodol. 2006;4(1):1–20.
8. BEST (Biomarkers, EndpointS, and other tools) Resource [Internet] [https://www.ncbi.nlm.nih.gov/books/NBK326791/pdf/Bookshelf_NBK326791.pdf].
9. Physiopedia [http://www.physio-pedia.com/Outcome_Measures].
10. Clinical Outcome Assessment (COA): Glossary of Terms. http://wayback.archive-it.org/7993/20180424212148/https://www.fda.gov/Drugs/DevelopmentApprovalProcess/DrugDevelopmentToolsQualificationProgram/ucm370262.htm#pro. https://www.fda.gov/Drugs/DevelopmentApprovalProcess/DrugDevelopmentToolsQualificationProgram/ucm284077.htm.
11. Donabedian A. The quality of care. How can it be assessed? JAMA. 1988; 260(12):1743–8.
12. Fawcett AL. Principles of assessment and outcome measurement for occupational therapists and physiotherapists: theory, skills and application. West Sussex: John Wiley and Sons; 2007.
13. FDA PRO. Guidance for industry: patient-reported outcome measures: use in medical product development to support Labelling claims. In: Food and Drug Administration, U S Department of Health and Human Resources; 2009.
14. Gleeson H, Calderon A, Swami V, Deighton J, Wolpert M, Edbrooke-Childs J. Systematic review of approaches to using patient experience data for quality improvement in healthcare settings. BMJ Open. 2016;6(8)
15. In H, Rosen JE. Primer on outcomes research. J Surg Oncol. 2014;110(5):489–93.
16. Global perspective on patient experience movement [http://www.theberylinstitute.org/?page=PXBENCHMARKING2015]. Accessed 20 Aug 2018.
17. Lipscomb J, Gotay CC, Snyder CF. Patient-reported outcomes in cancer: a review of recent research and policy initiatives. CA Cancer J Clin. 2007;57(5): 278–300.
18. Lipscomb J, Reeve BB, Clauser SB, Abrams JS, Bruner DW, Burke LB, Denicoff AM, Ganz PA, Gondek K, Minasian LM, et al. Patient-reported outcomes assessment in cancer trials: taking stock, moving forward. J Clin Oncol. 2007; 25(32):5133–40.
19. McLeod LD, Coon CD, Martin SA, Fehnel SE, Hays RD. Interpreting patient-reported outcome results: US FDA guidance and emerging methods. Expert Rev Pharmacoecon Outcomes Res. 2011;11(2):163–9.
20. Prinsen CA, Vohra S, Rose MR, King-Jones S, Ishaque S, Bhaloo Z, Adams D, Terwee CB. Core outcome measures in effectiveness trials (COMET) initiative: protocol for an international Delphi study to achieve consensus on how to select outcome measurement instruments for outcomes included in a 'core outcome set. Trials. 2014;15:247.
21. Starfield B: Primary care: an increasingly important contributor to effectiveness, equity, and efficiency of health services. SESPAS report 2012. Gac Sanit. 2012; 26(Suppl 1):20–26.
22. Starfield B, Shi L, Macinko J. Contribution of primary care to health systems and health. Milbank Q. 2005;83(3):457–502.
23. Zarin DA. Factual errors about ClinicalTrials.gov and other federal mandates in special report by Shuster. Clin Transl Sci. 2012;5(2):217.
24. Donabedian A: Evaluating the quality of medical care. Milbank Mem Fund Q 1966, 44(3):Suppl-206.
25. Donabedian A. The quality of medical care: a concept in search of a definition. J Fam Pract. 1979;9(2):277–84.
26. AHRQ. Registries for Evaluating Patient Outcomes: A User's Guide. Third edition. In: Gliklich RE, Dreyer NA, Leavy MB, Rockville (MD), editors. Agency for Healthcare Research and Quality (US); 2014.
27. The Outcome of Outcomes Research at AHCPR: Final Report [http://archive.ahrq.gov/research/findings/final-reports/outcomes-research/index.html].
28. Greenhalgh J. The applications of PROs in clinical practice: what are they, do they work, and why? Qual Life Res. 2009;18(1):115–23.
29. Greenhalgh J, Long AF, Flynn R. The use of patient reported outcome measures in routine clinical practice: lack of impact or lack of theory? Soc Sci Med. 2005;60(4):833–43.
30. Sanders AR, van W, I, Vogelaar M, Verheul W, Pieters RH, de Wit NJ, Bensing JM: Effects of improved patient participation in primary care on health-related outcomes: a systematic review. Fam Pract 2013, 30(4):365–378.
31. Developing and Evaluating Complex Interventions; New Guidance [http://www.mrc.ac.uk/documents/pdf/complex-interventions-guidance].
32. Shiell A, Hawe P, Gold L. Complex interventions or complex systems? Implications for health economic evaluation. BMJ. 2008;336(7656): 1281–3.
33. Dolovich L, Oliver D, Lamarche L, Agarwal G, Carr T, Chan D, Cleghorn L, Griffith L, Javadi D, Kastner M, et al. A protocol for a pragmatic randomized controlled trial using the health teams advancing patient experience: strengthening quality (health TAPESTRY) platform approach to promote person-focused primary healthcare for older adults. Implement Sci. 2016;11:49.
34. Murphy MK, Black NA, Lamping DL, McKee CM, Sanderson CF, Askham J, Marteau T: Consensus development methods, and their use in clinical guideline development. Health Technol Assess 1998, 2(3):i-88.
35. Muldoon LK, Hogg WE, Levitt M. Primary care (PC) and primary health care (PHC). What is the difference? Can J Public Health. 2006;97(5):409–11.
36. Kingston-Reichers J, Ospina M, Jonsson E, Childs P, MacLeod L, Maxted J. Patient Safety in Primary Care. In: Alberta E, editor. Canadian Patient Safety Institute:BC Patient safety & Quality Control; 2010.

37. Canadian Institute for Health Information: Pan-Canadian primary health care indicators. Report 1, Volume 1. In.: Canadian Institute of Health Information (CIHI); 2006.
38. Idzerda L, Rader T, Tugwell P, Boers M. Can we decide which outcomes should be measured in every clinical trial? A scoping review of the existing conceptual frameworks and processes to develop core outcome sets. J Rheumatol. 2014;41(5):986–93.
39. Gargon E, Williamson PR, Altman DG, Blazeby JM, Clarke M. The COMET initiative database: progress and activities from 2011 to 2013. Trials. 2014;15:279.
40. Williamson PR, Altman DG, Blazeby JM, Clarke M, Devane D, Gargon E, Tugwell P. Developing core outcome sets for clinical trials: issues to consider. Trials. 2012;13:132.
41. Boers M, Idzerda L, Kirwan JR, Beaton D, Escorpizo R, Boonen A, Magasi S, Sinha I, Stucki G, Tugwell P. Toward a generalized framework of core measurement areas in clinical trials: a position paper for OMERACT 11. J Rheumatol. 2014;41(5):978–85.
42. Boers M, Kirwan JR, Gossec L, Conaghan PG, D'Agostino MA, Bingham CO III, Brooks PM, Landewe R, March L, Simon L, et al. How to choose core outcome measurement sets for clinical trials: OMERACT 11 approves filter 2. 0. J Rheumatol. 2014;41(5):1025–30.
43. Boers M, Kirwan JR, Wells G, Beaton D, Gossec L, D'Agostino MA, Conaghan PG, Bingham CO III, Brooks P, Landewe R, et al. Developing core outcome measurement sets for clinical trials: OMERACT filter 2.0. J Clin Epidemiol. 2014;67(7):745–53.
44. Kirwan JR, Boers M, Hewlett S, Beaton D, Bingham CO III, Choy E, Conaghan PG, D'Agostino MA, Dougados M, Furst DE, et al. Updating the OMERACT filter: core areas as a basis for defining core outcome sets. J Rheumatol. 2014;41(5):994–9.
45. Mokkink LB, Terwee CB, Gibbons E, Stratford PW, Alonso J, Patrick DL, Knol DL, Bouter LM, de Vet HC. Inter-rater agreement and reliability of the COSMIN (COnsensus-based standards for the selection of health status measurement instruments) checklist. BMC Med Res Methodol. 2010;10:82.
46. Mokkink LB, Terwee CB, Knol DL, Stratford PW, Alonso J, Patrick DL, Bouter LM, de Vet HC. The COSMIN checklist for evaluating the methodological quality of studies on measurement properties: a clarification of its content. BMC Med Res Methodol. 2010;10:22.
47. Mokkink LB, Terwee CB, Patrick DL, Alonso J, Stratford PW, Knol DL, Bouter LM, de Vet HC. The COSMIN study reached international consensus on taxonomy, terminology, and definitions of measurement properties for health-related patient-reported outcomes. J Clin Epidemiol. 2010;63(7):737–45.
48. Mokkink LB, Terwee CB, Patrick DL, Alonso J, Stratford PW, Knol DL, Bouter LM, de Vet HC. The COSMIN checklist for assessing the methodological quality of studies on measurement properties of health status measurement instruments: an international Delphi study. Qual Life Res. 2010;19(4):539–49.
49. Terwee CB, Mokkink LB, Knol DL, Ostelo RW, Bouter LM, de Vet HC. Rating the methodological quality in systematic reviews of studies on measurement properties: a scoring system for the COSMIN checklist. Qual Life Res. 2012;21(4):651–7.
50. Guyatt GH, Kirshner B, Jaeschke R. Measuring health status: what are the necessary measurement properties? J Clin Epidemiol. 1992;45(12):1341–5.
51. Jolles BM, Buchbinder R, Beaton DE. A study compared nine patient-specific indices for musculoskeletal disorders. J Clin Epidemiol. 2005;58(8):791–801.
52. Stevens A, Beurskens A, Koke A, van der Weijden T. The use of patient-specific measurement instruments in the process of goal-setting: a systematic review of available instruments and their feasibility. Clin Rehabil. 2013;27(11):1005–19.
53. National Quality Forum (NFQ). Guidance for Measure Harmonization: A consensus Report [http://www.qualityforum.org/Publications/2016/03/Value_Set_Harmonization_-_Final_Report.aspx].
54. Patient Reported Outcome and Quality of Life Instruments Database (PROQOLID). [https://eprovide.mapi-trust.org/search?form[searchText]=&form[ezxform_token]=MpVNPeOrCC2Kmnr8qFukURaqGtklLmrfVUsSPnE9ap0)].
55. Hasson F, Keeney S. Enhancing rigour in the Delphi technique research. In: Technological Forecasting and Social Change, The Delphi technique: Past, present, and future prospects. Vol. 78; 2011. p. 1695–704.
56. Okoli C, Pawlowski SD. The Delphi method as a research tool: an example, design considerations and applications. Information & Management. 2004;42:15–29.
57. Hasson F, Keeney S, McKenna H. Research guidelines for the Delphi survey technique. J Adv Nurs. 2000;32(4):1008–15.
58. Keeney S, Hasson F, McKenna H. Consulting the oracle: ten lessons from using the Delphi technique in nursing research. J Adv Nurs. 2006;53(2):205–12.
59. van de Linde E, van der Duin P. The Delphi method as early warning: linking global societal trends to future radicalization and terrorism in the Netherlands. In: Technological Forecasting and Social Change, The Delphi technique: Past, present, and future prospects. Vol. 78; 2011. p. 1557–64.
60. Diamond IR, Grant RC, Feldman BM, Pencharz PB, Ling SC, Moore AM, Wales PW. Defining consensus: a systematic review recommends methodologic criteria for reporting of Delphi studies. J Clin Epidemiol. 2014;67(4):401–9.

9

Controlled trial of the impact of a BC adult mental health practice support program (AMHPSP) on primary health care professionals' management of depression

Bianca Lauria-Horner[1*], Tara Beaulieu[1], Stephanie Knaak[2,5], Rivian Weinerman[3], Helen Campbell[4] and Scott Patten[5]

Abstract

Background: Depression affects over 400 million people globally. The majority are seen in primary care. Barriers in providing adequate care are not solely related to physicians' knowledge/skills deficits, but also time constraints, lack of confidence/avoidance, which need to be addressed in mental health-care redesign. We hypothesized that family physician (FP) training in the Adult Mental Health Practice Support Program (AMHPSP) would lead to greater improvements in patient depressive symptom ratings (a priori primary outcome) compared to treatment as usual.

Methods: From October 2013 to May 2015, in a controlled trial 77 FP practices were stratified on the total number of physicians/practice as well as urban/rural setting, and randomized to the British Columbia AMHPSP a multi-component contact-based training to enhance FPs' comfort/skills in treating mild-moderate depression (intervention), or no training (control) by an investigator not operationally involved in the trial. FPs with a valid license to practice in NS were eligible. FPs from both groups were asked to identify 3–4 consecutive patients > 18 years old, diagnosis of depression, Patient Health Questionnaire (PHQ-9) score ≥ 10, able to read English, intact cognitive functioning. Exclusion criteria: antidepressants within 5 weeks and psychotherapy within 3 months of enrollment, and clinically judged urgent/emergent medical/psychiatric condition. Patients were assigned to the same arm as their physician. Thirty-six practices recruited patients (intervention $n = 23$; control $n = 13$). The study was prematurely terminated at 6 months of enrollment start-date due to concomitant primary health-care transformation by health-system leaders which resulted in increased in-office demands, and recruitment failure. We used the PHQ-9 to assess between-group differences at baseline, 1, 2, 3, and 6 months follow-up. Outcome collectors and assessors were blind to group assignment.

Results: One hundred-and-twenty-nine patients (intervention $n = 72$; control $n = 57$) were analysed. A significant improvement in depression scores among intervention group patients emerged between 3 and 6 months, time by treatment interaction, likelihood ratio test (LR) chi2(3) = 7.96, $p = .047$.

Conclusions: This novel skill-based program shows promise in translating increased FP comfort and skills managing depressed patients into improved patient clinical outcomes even in absence of mental health specialists availability.

Keywords: Primary care, Skill-based training, Depressive disorders, Mental disorders, Patient-centered outcomes

* Correspondence: Bianca.Horner@dal.ca
[1]Department of Psychiatry, Dalhousie University, Halifax, Nova Scotia, Canada
Full list of author information is available at the end of the article

Background

The World Health Organization (WHO) recognizes mental illness as becoming the number one cause of years-lived with disability worldwide by 2020 [1–3]. Depression is one of the most prevalent and costly conditions, affecting over 400 million people globally [4–6]. Concurrent with other physical and psychiatric conditions, there is higher morbidity and cost to the healthcare system [7]. These facts underscore the need for evidence-based strategies that promote early recognition and treatment, thereby improving patient outcomes [1, 6]. Thus, integration of mental health in primary care is ideal and has been an area of focus in mental healthcare redesign that strengthens patient-centered, evidence-based, sustainable care. Family physicians (FPs) see over 85% of these patients, and the majority can be handled early and effectively in this setting [8–15]. Most patients experience less stigma and increased comfort sharing problems with their doctor with whom they have established trust [16–18]. However, even when the diagnosis is made, less than 20% receive adequate treatment [19]. In one study conducted in 21 countries, respondents who met DSM-IV criteria for major depressive disorder (MDD) within 12 months before the interview, only 16.5% received minimally adequate treatment as defined by evidenced-based guidelines [i.e. receiving either pharmacotherapy (for a minimum of 1 month, plus 4 visits with any type of medical doctor) or psychotherapy (for a minimum of 8 visits with any professional including religious or spiritual advisor, social worker or counsellor)]. Other studies have shown that although FPs commonly prescribe antidepressants, [20] in mild/moderate cases antidepressants are not necessarily associated with improved long-term outcomes, [21–24]. Studies suggest that cognitive behaviour therapy (CBT) has an enduring effect with lower rates of relapse, that many patients prefer non-drug options, [25] and where clinically appropriate, patient choice of evidence-based options improves outcomes [26].

The extent to which training programs lead to practice changes or improved clinical outcomes remains questionable [27–31]. Barriers in providing adequate care are not solely related to physicians' knowledge deficits, but as a result of complex interdependent factors. There are physician factors, e.g., in-office time constraints, a large number of domains to which they extend care, mental and physical health conditions being intertwined and thereby confusing symptoms; systems support factors, e.g., lack of mental health specialists, ineffective interdisciplinary teams, funding, legislation [32, 33]; and patient factors, e.g., stigma as a barrier to help-seeking, patients lack of disclosure sensing physicians' time pressures, costly uninsured services [10, 31, 34, 35].

Training programs with top-down and bottom-up approaches such as the British Columbia (BC) Adult Mental Health Practice Support Program (AMHPSP) show the most promise as the program expands well beyond a simple education program or workshop [36, 37]. Physicians are trained to manage mild-moderate depression and anxiety disorders on their own within office time constraints by coaching patients through supported CBT-based self-management strategies. They flexibly use tools and strategies with or without antidepressants, reflecting a "real world" scenario, [38–40] and the program is based on the quality improvement framework of plan-do-study-act shown to effectively affect change [41–48] by offering FP opportunities to practice new skills immediately after the training sessions within the scope of their practice. A practice support coordinator provides on-site, in-practice support during action periods to help implement and sustain these changes [31, 49–51]. Patients are engaged through guided self-management strategies, which is key for effective chronic illness care [52–57]. Finally, physicians are compensated to attend training. In a realistic context where physicians are responsible on their own to manage these patients, or while patients wait to be seen by specialty services, we —were looking to evaluate—in a real-world environment—if training in the AMHPSP improves patient clinical outcomes. The training would provide physicians another feasible non-drug treatment option in their armamentarium.

While qualitative evaluations of the AMHPSP conducted in BC report a positive impact on several key outcomes [37], the program *has not been rigorously evaluated* through a controlled trial The NS Department of Health & Wellness and Mental Health Commission of Canada therefore sponsored a trial to evaluate its effectiveness.

The first published part of our study shows a significant improvement (diminishment) in intervention-group physicians' preference for social distance, and significant increases in perceived confidence and comfort managing mental illness [58]. In this part of the study, we sought to determine whether training FPs in the AMHPSP would lead to greater improvements in patient depression scores (primary outcome in this part of the study) compared to the control group. This paper also focuses on patients' satisfaction with care received, and physicians' antidepressants prescribing. A third part of the study consisting of a health economic analysis is underway.

We chose a cluster RCT design (randomized practices) as the impact of intervention might bring about practice pattern changes. In the component of the study looking at patient outcomes we planned an individual-level analysis of depressive symptoms, accounting for the clustering of patients within practices, since this seemed more clinically salient than practice-level outcomes in this part of the analysis. An implication of this decision, however, is that the full benefits of randomization are lost since the unit of analysis differs from the unit of randomization.

Methods

Aim, study design and setting

The aim of this study was to evaluate whether training family physicians (FPs) in the AMHPSP would lead to greater improvements in patients' depression scores (primary outcome) compared to the control group.

This was a multicentre two-parallel group, controlled trial in which practices were randomly allocated to the intervention arm (INT) or control arm and allocation was masked in the outcome assessment. Physicians in practices assigned to the intervention group attended the AMHPSP training whereas physicians assigned to the control group continued with treatment as usual (TAU).

Participant eligibility

Physician practices

Seventy-seven NS community-based family practices identified through associations, presentations, and promotional letters. Interested physicians provided written informed consent and enrolled between October 2013 and January 2014 (111 FP). Physicians actively seeing patients remunerated by any method (fee-for-service/alternative funding program etc.) with a NS practice license were eligible to participate.

Eligible patients were identified by their physician. Inclusion criteria included over 18 years of age, diagnosis of depression, PHQ-9 score $\geq$ 10, ability to read/speak English (grade 6 level), intact cognitive functioning (physician judgment). Exclusion criteria included active treatment with antidepressants within 5 weeks and psychotherapy within 3 months of enrollment, urgent/emergent medical or psychiatric condition (physician judgment). Patients were enrolled between June 2014 and May 2015, with the last follow-up visit in November 2015.

Procedure

Practice recruitment, randomization and masking

Seventy-seven practices (111 community-based FP) were enrolled. Practice allocation was concealed at cluster level through a unique practice number (1–77) assigned by the principal Investigator (PI): B.L-H. Practices were stratified on number of physicians/practice, as well as urban and rural setting before randomization. An investigator (SP) not involved in trial operations assigned the randomization sequence. STATA, version 12 (College Station, TX, 2012) was used to generate the randomization sequence from a binomial distribution—probability of success of 0.5.

Patients and physicians'—assigned unique identifier codes—were linked to their corresponding practice number. The PI kept a master file containing participant names with ID codes in a secure location. Study databases contained de-identified information. We could not conceal arm allocation from physicians for obvious reasons. However, the RC (data collector) and outcome assessors (independent researchers) were blinded to group assignment. In addition—although we could not guarantee patient blinding—physicians were asked not to disclose group allocation to their patients.

Practices ranged from 1 to 6 physicians (INT), and 1–8 physicians (Control). Thirty-nine practices were allocated to the intervention group, and 38 to the control group. Nine percent of targeted practices withdrew prior to intervention delivery. The main reason; lack of time for study specific requirements. Only 23 of 36 (64%) of intervention and 13 of 34 (38%) of control practices recruited patients for the same reason (Fig. 1). Physician baseline characteristics such as age, gender, years of practice, pattern of work (full-time, part-time etc.), practice size, number of unique annual patients were collected.

Intervention

Between February–June 2014, physicians in practices assigned to the intervention group attended three half-day interactive workshops delivered by the BC team, the Adult Mental Health Practice Support Program (AMHPSP). The AMHPSP consists of three half-day interactive workshops delivered by the BC team, interspaced by 5–6 week action periods during which physicians practiced what they learned. The program introduces an organized approach that takes learners through a problem and strength-based assessment to the development of an action plan. Key components included 3 supported self-management strategies for mild to moderate depression and anxiety meant to help shift responsibility from primary care provider to a shared responsibility with the patients engaging them in illness management and their recovery; the Cognitive Behavioral Interpersonal Skills workbook incorporating a comprehensive mental illness screening tool and patient user friendly supported self-management handouts based on evidence-based cognitive behavioural therapy principles; the Canadian Mental Health Association (CMHA) Bounce Back program, a telephone guided CBT-based service; and an Antidepressant Skills Workbook [59]. Contact-based education occurred through first-voice advocates sharing their journey [60]. Office staff members attended the training and Mental Health First Aid [61] to increase their comfort caring for patients. Local psychiatrists and allied health professionals (counsellors, psychologists, clinicians etc.) attended training solely to familiarize themselves with the program. During action

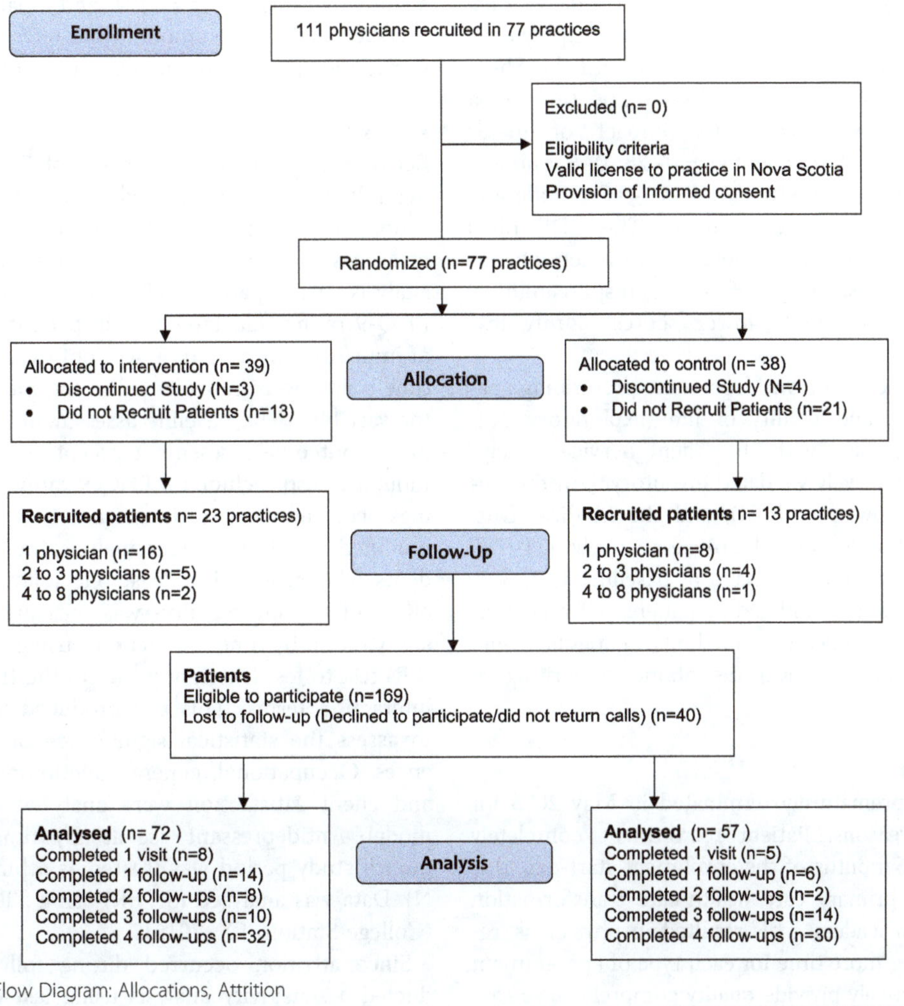

Fig. 1 Participant Flow Diagram: Allocations, Attrition

periods, a coordinator offered on-site guidance on practical office redesign to enhance the implementation of new learnings and tools, and shares experiences, challenges, and recommendations with stakeholders. Physicians had flexibility to use tools and strategies as clinically judged. Intervention group FPs received a learning stipend (CAN$3274.20) to participate in workshops and action periods but remunerated through usual methods to manage their patients. The control group practices received the training November 2015 (at study end) including the learning stipend.

Patient recruitment

Once the intervention group completed the training (June 2014), all FPs from both intervention and control groups were asked to identify 3–4 consecutive patients with a clinical diagnosis of depression, and a Patient Health Questionnaire PHQ-9 score ≥ 10. To minimize damaging the doctor/patient relationship (patients refusing or feeling-pressured to participate [62]), willing patients' were contacted by the research coordinator (RC) who described the study, administered and obtained written consent, and assessed study eligibility. Eligible patients were assigned to the same arm as their physician. Once enrolled, patients' own FP continued to manage the depression. A total of 169 patients were eligible to participate. Forty of 169 (24%) declined or did not return calls to complete baseline data. We enrolled 129 patients (intervention $n = 72$, control $n = 57$) all included in the analysis (Fig. 1).

Outcome measures

For depression scores (primary outcome), we used the PHQ-9. The PHQ-9 covers the nine DSM-5 symptom-based criteria for major depressive disorder. Total score range: 0–27; 0–4 not depressed; 5–9 mild; 10–14 moderate; 15–19 moderate-severe; 20–27 severe [63–66]. (Score ≥ 10; sensitivity 88%, specificity; 88%; positive likelihood ratio, 7.1). During scale development, criterion validity was assessed against the Structured Clinical Interview (SCID) [66, 67].

Occupational/general functioning (secondary outcomes) were assessed with the Lam Employment Absence and Productivity Scale (LEAPS) and the Sheehan Disability Scale (SDS) respectively. The LEAPS a 7-item scale assesses workplace impact of major depression [68]. Total score range = 0–28; 0–5 = none--minimal impairment; 6–10 = mild; 11–16 = moderate; 17–22 = severe; 23–28 = very severe. The SDS rates disruption (0–10) in each domain work/school; social/leisure activities; family life/home responsibilities, (Total score range = 0–30; lower scores signify less disruption) [69].

Physician frequency of antidepressant prescribing, patient satisfaction, and quality of life (exploratory outcomes), were assessed with the Client Service Receipt Inventory, an extensively validated inventory, [70] the Client Satisfaction Inventory (CSI), and the Medical Outcomes Study Short-Form (SF-36) respectively [71–73]. Outcome measures were collected at baseline, 1, 2, 3, 6 months. All scales are validated as patient self-report, as well as telephone-collection methods. Patients could complete questionnaires over the phone, in writing or digitally online.

Early termination

The study was prematurely terminated in May 2015 for the following reasons. Patient recruitment completely stopped within 6 months of the enrollment start-date due to concomitant primary care health-care transformation by health-system leaders. This resulted in physicians' reports of requiring more time for each type of appointment in order to effectively provide quality comprehensive care within in-office time constraints, thus reducing available time they could allocate to the study. The research team's substantial efforts to re-engage physicians through evidenced-based recruitment "Best-Practices" had minimal impact. We therefore choose to report results and our challenges as useful information for future study designs, and as an exploratory assessment of the intervention.

Ethics statement

The NS Multisite and University of Calgary Research Ethics Boards approved this study, registration www.clinicaltrials.gov #NCT01975948.

Statistical methods

Sample size

We calculated a sample size of 100 evaluable patients/arm to achieve 80% power to detect between-group differences in PHQ-9 mean of 2 points, with a significance level (α) of .05, 2-sided test, and assumed standard deviation of 5 points. A compensatory increase to 166 patients/arm was needed using a design effect of 1.1 (intra cluster correlation of 0.05 for patient outcomes based on a study by Murphey et al., [74] and 3 patients/practice on average), and the assumption that 66% of patients would provide adequate follow-up data, accounting for attrition.

Analysis

Between-group mean differences of PHQ-9 scores during follow-up were assessed as a group-by-time interaction. In order to take advantage of the multiple measures of data, we used a multi-level mixed-model analysis with patients clustered within practices and PHQ-9 ratings clustered within patients. As the pattern of improvement over time was not expected to be linear, time points were represented in the model using indicator variables. The baseline assessment was not included in the outcome assessment except as a covariate (even though it also included a PHQ-9 rating) since these ratings occurred prior to the intervention. We conducted a modified intention to treat analysis, including all respondents who provided at least one follow-up rating. The effect of the intervention was measured as series of 3 study group by time interactions, using a likelihood ratio (LR) test to test the significance of the treatment by time interaction terms. This test produced the p-value used to assess the statistical significance of observed differences. Occupational, general functioning, quality of life, and client satisfaction were analyzed using the same model. Antidepressant use at any time during the 6 month study period was treated as a binary variable (Y/N). Data was analysed (SP, SK) using STATA, version 14 (College Station, TX, 2015).

Since attrition occurred during follow-up, we conducted a sensitivity analysis using last observation carried forward imputation of post-attrition PHQ-9 ratings and also conducted an analysis of completers only.

Results

Practice characteristics

One between-group difference was observed. Physicians assigned to intervention group were more likely to work in small practices due to one large practice being randomly assigned to the control group. Twenty-four of 36 practices (67%) who recruited patients were individual-practice FPs (Table 1).

Patient characteristics

Patients were predominantly female, employed, and post-secondary educated. There were no clinically meaningful between-group differences, except that a higher proportion of control group participants were employed as compared to intervention group participants (Table 2). Also, participants with complete follow-up data tended to be in smaller practices, had somewhat lower baseline PHQ-9 scores, and were more likely to identify as married/common-law.

Table 1 Practice Characteristics

	Intervention (n = 23)	Control (n = 13)	p	Patient recruitment by practices size: Yes (n = 36)	No (n = 41)	P
Practice size						
1 physician	16	8		24	37	0.11
2 to 3 physicians	5	4	0.647	9	3	
4 to 8 physicians	2	1		3	1	
Urban Setting						
	14	9	0.727	23	29	0.627
Percentage	39%	35%		64%	71%	
# patients recruited/ practice						
1 to 2	11	4		–	–	–
3 to 4	7	5	0.252	–	–	–
5 or more	5	4		–	–	–
# patients with complete f/u data						
1 to 2	13	6		–	–	–
3 to 4	6	3	0.538	–	–	–
5 or more	4	4		–	–	–

Table 2 Patient Baseline Characteristics: Intervention group, control group, completed all follow-up time points versus those who missed one or more follow-up time points

Patient Characteristics	Intervention Group	Control Group	Completed all Follow-Up		P^
	n = 72	n = 57*	Yes (n = 62)	No (n = 67)**	
Gender					
Female	49 (68.1%)	43 (76.8%)	44 (71.0%)	48 (72.7%)	.33, .85
Marital status					
Married/common-law	38 (52.8%)	37 (66.1%)	42 (67.7%)	33 (50.0%)	.15, .05
Not married/single/divorced/ separated/widowed	34 (47.2%)	19 (33.9%)	20 (32.3%)	33 (50.0%)	
Age					
18–39	31 (43.1%)	31 (55.4%)	26 (41.9%)	36 (54.5%)	
40–59	26 (36.1%)	18 (32.1%)	26 (41.9%)	18 (27.3%)	.33, .20
60+	15 (20.8%)	7 (12.5%)	10 (16.1%)	12 (18.2%)	
Employment status					
Employed (full or part time)	38 (52.8%)	43 (78.2%)	43 (69.4%)	38 (58.5%)	
Unemployed	9 (12.5%)	3 (5.5%)	4 (6.5%)	8(12.3%)	.01, .37
Retired/student/at-home/other	25 (34.7%)	9 (16.4%)	15 (24.2%)	19 (29.2%)	
Education					
Some elementary or High school	9 (12.5%)	3 (5.4%)	5 (8.1%)	7 (10.6%)	
High school/some post-secondary	23(31.9%)	21 (37.5%)	18 (29.0%)	26 (39.4%)	.40, .32
Post-secondary diploma/degree +	40 (55.6%)	32 (75.0%)	39 (62.9%)	33 (50.0%)	
Mother tongue					
English	66 (91.7%)	55 (98.2%)	59 (95.2%)	62 (93.9%)	
Other	6 (8.3%)	1 (1.8%)	3 (4.8%)	4 (6.1%)	.14, 1.0

*One respondent did not provide demographic data. Percentages based on n = 56. Two respondents did not provide employment status data
**One respondent did not provide demographic data. Percentages based on n = 66. Two respondents did not provide employment status data
^Fisher's exact test was used
First p value pertains to INT/control comparison, the second for completed vs not comparison

Primary outcome

PHQ-9 scores diminished in both groups (Fig. 2). The treatment group, however, had a progressive diminishment in mean PHQ-9 scores, whereas the control group did not continue to decrease after the 3-month follow-up visit. The multi-level mixed model results were reflective of a significant treatment effect (LR for treatment group by time interactions, chi2(3) = 7.96, p = .047), which was essentially unchanged after adjusting for baseline depressive symptoms (LR Chi2(3) = 9.04, p = 0.029). Addition of age categories and sex to the model (the age categories were depicted in the dataset using indicator variables representing six age groups) did not change the result (LR for treatment group by time interactions terms, chi2(3) =10.40, p = 0.006). Consistent with the pattern seen in Fig. 2, which suggests that differences were only evident in the final time interval, removal of the first 2 time-by-treatment group interactions did not significantly affect the fit of the models, e.g. for the model with adjustments for age, sex and baseline depressive symptoms (LR comparing the original to the reduced model, chi2(1) = 1.07, p = 0.301), indicating no significant loss of fit with removal of the two interaction terms.

Because of the imbalance in employment observed in Table 2, the analysis was repeated including an indicator term for full time employment status. The results were unchanged: LR chi2(3) = 10.37, Prob > chi2 = 0.0157.

Secondary outcomes

Between-group changes on LEAPS and SDS, SF-36, and CSI were not significantly different (See Additional file 1).

	Intervetion	Control	
0	16.67	17.47	0.01
1	11.25	10.39	1.01
2	9.73	8.46	2.01
3	8.44	7.55	3.01
6	6.81	8.42	6.01

Intervention
mean=16.7, sd=4.80, n=67
mean=11.25, sd=5.82, n=55
mean=9.73, sd=6.28, n=44
mean=8.44, sd=6.16, n=45
mean=6.79, sd=5.41, n=47

Time (months)

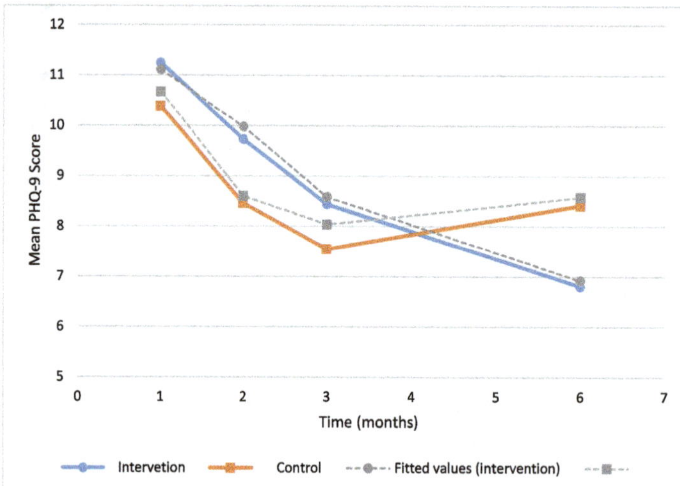

grp	-0.4391262	1.189685	-0.37	0.712	-2.77087	1.892614
T2	-1.136177	0.773507	-1.47	0.142	-2.65222	0.379869
T3	-2.527956	0.771049	-3.28	0.001	-4.03919	-1.01673
T6	-4.191764	0.772055	-5.43	0	-5.70496	-2.67856
int2	-0.9343796	1.122222	-0.83	0.405	-3.1339	1.265136
int3	-0.1085238	1.128795	-0.1	0.923	-2.32092	2.103874
int6	2.100621	1.103378	1.9	0.057	-0.06196	4.263202
_cons	11.1109	0.790915	14.05	0	9.560732	12.66106

Fitted values (intervention)		Fitted values (control)	
1	11.1109	1	10.67177
2	9.974723	2	8.601217
3	8.582944	3	8.035294
6	6.919136	6	8.580631

Fig. 2 Between-group mean differences of PHQ-9 scores, group-by-time interaction

Exploratory outcomes

Antidepressant use at any time during the 6 months study period was significantly lower in the intervention group compared to the control group Fisher's exact test, $p = 0.003$. (Control group = 68.4%; Intervention group = 41.7%). In a sensitivity analysis using LOCF imputation there was no evidence of a treatment effect as assessed by the three group by time interactions (LR for the treatment group by time interactions, chi2(3) = 5.28, Prob > chi2 = 0.153). However, in the completer analysis, the effect remained significant: LR for the treatment group by time interactions chi2(3) = 7.96, Prob > chi2 = 0.047. Fifty-one percent of INT patients used program tools/strategies. The top 3 were CBT-based with BounceBack being highest (51% of patients who used tools, 26% of INT patients) (Table 3).

Discussion

Results of this study provide tentative evidence of the AMHPSP's effectiveness in improving patient depression scores. A large majority of INT patients (71%) reported using the program tools and strategies, the most frequently used was the BounceBack program (Table 3). Anecdotal FP reports suggested that BounceBack program offers increased support by shared patient management. PHQ-9 scores diminished in both groups from baseline to 3 months due to the episodic nature of depression expected to cause regression to the mean, and possibly as a result of placebo responders through repeated encounters with the research data collector. In psychiatric disorders such as depression, this non-specific treatment effect is a well-recognized component in all psychotherapeutic encounters [75]. The treatment group, however, had a progressive diminishment in mean PHQ-9 scores, whereas the control group did not continue to decrease after the 3-month follow-up visit (Fig. 1).

Further research is needed in this area as our study did not achieve its pre-planned sample size, lending to the possibility of Type II error. Also, the effect observed was small only evident at a single time interval, between 3 and 6 months, a finding that may have occurred as a result of Type I error. There was substantial attrition, and LOCF imputation did not result in preservation of the effect. However, the pattern of between-group change in mild/moderate depression scores over time is suggestive of a possible treatment effect. Furthermore, these changes occurred despite reduced prescribing of medication by FPs. (Table 3) Participants with complete follow-up data had somewhat lower baseline PHQ-9 scores, which is consistent with the AMHPSP's target population: mild to moderate depression, hence future studies should consider including only this group. Future studies should also strongly consider using a practice-level unit of analysis since randomization in such trials must by necessity occur at the practice level.

In a context where collaborative care has proven difficult, (e.g., where primary care is delivered in independent practice settings and/or no funding mechanisms for collaborative care arrangements, we were looking at ways of implementing time-efficient evidence-based strategies to increase physicians' comfort and skills, decreasing anxiety/avoidance treating highly prevalent depression conditions. We do not feel there are or will ever be enough mental health physicians/clinicians to support FPs especially in rural and remote areas. Therefore, responsibility to care for the mentally ill largely rests with family physicians. We hear time and again that primary care knowledge gaps contribute to unrecognized and undertreated mental illness. However, training efforts aimed to improve mental health management and patient outcomes remain questionable [30]. Training efforts need to include time efficient tools FPs can feasibly implement in the realistic context of a busy practice.

Table 3 Antidepressant Prescribing at 6 months: Intervention and control groups Strategies used: Intervention

Antidepressant Use (%)	INT			CONTROL
	41.7%			68.4%
Specific tools used	N	% of participants (n = 37)	% of all INT participants (n = 72)	
Referral to BB	19	51.4%	26.4%	0
ASW resources	11	29.7%	15.3%	0
CBIS resources	9	24.3%	12.5%	0
BB DVD provided	6	16.2%	8.3%	0
Physician telephone follow-up	3	8.1%	4.2%	0
DAI administered	3	8.1%	4.2%	0
Total*	51	116%	71%	0

*patients used 1 or more tools

*Mentioned tools: Diagnostic Assessment Interview (DAI) administered; Antidepressant Skills Workbook (ASW) provided; Referral to Bounce Back (BB); Bounce Back DVD provided; Cognitive Behavioural Interpersonal Skills (CBIS) resources provided; physician follow-up by telephone

The AMHPSP cannot address all barriers, however it is novel recognizing that FPs need in-practice support that expand well beyond a simple education program or workshop. It includes many theoretically crucial ingredients required to fill knowledge gaps, through organized training that creates a substantial sustainable change, in the delivery of patient-centered respectful care, by FPs that fits their busy schedule, targets stigma, and supports physicians and patients through incentives, resources, and tools engaging patients in recovery efforts. Most patients want to participate in their recovery. Where better to learn the skills than in a trusted, safe place with their physician, even in settings where access to specialty care is difficult or unavailable?

To our knowledge, this study is the first RCT of its kind specifically evaluating a practice support program focusing on mental health as it is meant to be used in a real-world environment. We believe this provides insight on the potential impact of the AMHPSP training on patients' clinical outcomes and practical applicability of delivering the program in primary care. Furthermore improvement in depression scores occurred despite reduced prescribing of medication by FPs which suggests possible cost offsets due to reduced prescribing costs (Table 3). Also, prior analyses indicated reductions in social distance preferences and increased confidence and comfort with the training, beneficial effects not captured by the analysis of patient-reported outcomes presented here[58].

Limitations

First, this was a controlled trial, but randomization occurred at the practice level rather than individual patients. Because the analysis occurred at the level of patients, the benefits of randomization (equal distribution of confounding variables) cannot be assumed to have fully manifested in the analysis. Indeed, as some practices failed to recruit patients at all, the patient data analysis may have been influenced by selection bias despite the randomization. Whereas the random assignment would help ensure that the practices assigned to each group had similar characteristics, including unmeasured ones, it does not ensure that the ones that recruited patients were comparable on such characteristics. The significant difference in PHQ-9 scores was observed later in follow-up, at which point some physician and patient attrition had occurred, and this attrition may have caused bias. The lack of significant effects in a sensitivity analysis using LOCF imputation heightens these concerns. In addition, the there was an imbalance in patient group sizes (intervention $n = 72$, Control $n = 57$) which could have further affected the specific effects of the intervention compared to TAU (Fig. 1). However, the mixed model analysis methods permits the use of all data (e.g. data points from earlier in follow-up even when lost to follow-up), and may help to control bias that may arise due to attrition.

As noted above, future studies randomizing such interventions by practice should consider the use of practice-level outcome measures that would allow the analysis to derive full benefit from the randomization, a larger sample size and employ effective strategies to prevent attrition, especially since the benefits of this type of intervention may unfold over a time frame of several months. Third, physician participants were volunteers receiving a learning stipend, therefore may not be representative of FPs in general, may have a special interest in the subject matter. Although some aspects of the study could not be blinded, performance bias was minimized by data collector and outcome assessors blinding as well as the use of widely validated scales more specifically the PHQ-9 for our primary outcome. We took measures also to minimize the risk of patient selection bias by asking physicians to identify 3 consecutive patients with a diagnosis of depression.

Finally, a longer patient follow-up period may be important to shed light if divergence of depression scores would further increase, or reveal a significant difference in quality of life/occupational functioning as these outcomes may take longer to improve. Since the study sample consisted mostly of white, married, middle-age females, there should be caution in generalizing results beyond this group. However, the approach is applicable to all prepaid health insurance plans in the US and to Canada's single payer system [42].

In assessing satisfaction, most patients reported high baseline physician satisfaction ceiling effect. An outcome measure specific to mental healthcare would have been a better choice.

Conclusion

This study provides preliminary evidence that well-designed novel skills-based PSPs that promote integration of mental health into primary care may contribute to mental health strategies in improving mental health care. It also highlights the difficulties in evaluating community-delivered interventions.

Abbreviations

AMHPSP: Adult mental health practice support program; BC: British Columbia; CBT: cognitive behaviour therapy; CMHA: Canadian mental health association; CSI: Client satisfaction inventory; FP: Family physician; LEAPS: Lam employment absence and productivity scale; LOCF: last observation carried forward; LR: likelihood ratio t; NS: Nova Scotia; PHQ-9: Patient health questionnaire-9; PI: Principal investigator; RC: Research coordinator; SCID: Structured clinical interview; SDS: Sheehan disability scale; SF-36: Medical outcomes study short-form; TAU: Treatment as usual

Acknowledgements

The authors would like to thank the primary care providers and patients who participated as part of this trial.

Upon completion of the project Ms. Beaulieu's affiliation changed. She held the position of Research Coordinator, British Columbia Centre for Excellence in HIV/AIDS.

Funding
This project was made possible through funding from the Nova Scotia Department of Health and Wellness and the Mental Health Commission of Canada. The DOH&W covered the time and expenses of the research coordinator/practice support coordinator, participants, psychiatrists, mental health clinicians and first voice individuals. The DOH&W also covered costs associated with the Bounce Back program, the Mental Health First Aid training, and costs related to training facilities, equipment, and materials. The MHCC covered travel expenses related to meetings as well as the remuneration for RW, HC and those responsible for delivery of the intervention. As the lead research institution, Dalhousie University, Department of Psychiatry contributed in-kind services for the Principal Investigator, BLH, as well as related institutional overhead costs. The MHCC and the DOH&W did not influence any aspect of the research or publication.

Authors' contributions
BLH led the design and implementation of the research study, wrote the main paper, and was responsible for the approval of the final version submitted for publication. BLH had full access to all the data in the study and responsible for the integrity of the data. SK (employed by the MHCC) and SP were responsible for the accuracy of data analysis, and preparation of evaluation reports. TB was central to ongoing collaboration across professionals, research team members, and stakeholders, and contributed in critically revising the manuscript for important intellectual content. RW, HC and their team led the design of the Adult Mental Health Practice Support Program. All authors contributed substantially to critically revising the paper. All authors read and approved the final manuscript.

Consent for publication
Not applicable.

Competing interest
The authors declare that they have no competing interests.

Author details
[1]Department of Psychiatry, Dalhousie University, Halifax, Nova Scotia, Canada. [2]Opening Minds Anti-Stigma Initiative, Mental Health Commission of Canada, Ottawa, ON, Canada. [3]University of British Columbia, Medical Staff Honorary Status Island Health Authority, Victoria, Canada. [4]Department of Psychiatry, University of British Columbia, Vancouver, Canada. [5]University of Calgary, Calgary, Alberta, Canada.

References
1. Murray CJL, Barber RM, Foreman KJ, Ozgoren AA, Abd-Allah F, Abera SF, et al. Global, regional, and national disability-adjusted life years (DALYs) for 306 diseases and injuries and healthy life expectancy (HALE) for 188 countries, 1990–2013: quantifying the epidemiological transition. Lancet. 2015;386: 2145–91.
2. Whiteford HA, Degenhardt L, Rehm J, Baxter AJ, Ferrari AJ, Erskine HE, et al. Global burden of disease attributable to mental and substance use disorders: findings from the global burden of disease study 2010. Lancet. 2013;382:1575–86.
3. Depression in Europe [Internet]. 2012 [cited 2018 May 26]. Available from: http://www.euro.who.int/en/health-topics/noncommunicable-diseases/mental-health/news/news/2012/10/depression-in-europe
4. Lim K-L, Jacobs P, Ohinmaa A, Schopflocher D, Dewa CS. A new population-based measure of the economic burden of mental illness in Canada. Chronic Dis Can. 2008;28:92–8.
5. Kessler RC, Aguilar-Gaxiola S, Alonso J, Chatterji S, Lee S, Ormel J, et al. The global burden of mental disorders: an update from the WHO world mental health (WMH) surveys. Epidemiol Psichiatr Soc. 2009;18:23–33.
6. Principaux repères sur la dépression [Internet]. World Health Organ. [cited 2018 May 25]. Available from: http://www.who.int/fr/news-room/fact-sheets/detail/depression
7. Naylor C. SP0115 the link between long-term conditions and mental health. Ann Rheum Dis. 2013;71:28–9.
8. Barr MS. The need to test the patient-centered medical home. JAMA. 2008; 300:834–5.
9. Iglehart JK. No place like home--testing a new model of care delivery. N Engl J Med. 2008;359:1200–2.
10. Unützer J, Park M. Strategies to improve the management of depression in primary care. Prim Care. 2012;39:415–31.
11. Kauye F, Jenkins R, Rahman A. Training primary health care workers in mental health and its impact on diagnoses of common mental disorders in primary care of a developing country, Malawi: a cluster-randomized controlled trial. Psychol Med. 2014;44:657–66.
12. Butler M, Kane RL, McAlpine D, Kathol RG, Fu SS, Hagedorn H, et al. Integration of mental health/substance abuse and primary care. Evid Rep Technol Assess. 2008:1–362.
13. Unutzer J, Katon WJ, Fan M-Y, Schoenbaum MC, Lin EHB, Della Penna RD, et al. Long-term cost effects of collaborative care for late-life depression. Am J Manag Care. 2008;14:95–100.
14. WHO | Integrating mental health into primary care: a global perspective [Internet]. WHO. [cited 2018 May 26]. Available from: http://www.who.int/mental_health/policy/services/integratingmhintoprimarycare/en/
15. Mental Health and Addictions Strategy | novascotia.ca [Internet]. [cited 2018 May 26]. Available from: https://novascotia.ca/dhw/mental-health/mental-health-addiction-strategy.asp
16. Orleans CT, George LK, Houpt JL, Brodie HK. How primary care physicians treat psychiatric disorders: a national survey of family practitioners. Am J Psychiatry. 1985;142:52–7.
17. Azrin ST. Integrated care: high-impact mental health-primary care research for patients with multiple comorbidities. Psychiatr Serv Wash DC. 2014;65: 406–9.
18. Jorm AF, Korten AE, Jacomb PA, Christensen H, Rodgers B, Pollitt P. "Mental health literacy": a survey of the public's ability to recognise mental disorders and their beliefs about the effectiveness of treatment. Med J Aust. 1997;166: 182–6.
19. Mulsant BH, Whyte E, Lenze EJ, Lotrich F, Karp JF, Pollock BG, et al. Achieving long-term optimal outcomes in geriatric depression and anxiety. CNS Spectr. 2003;8:27–34.
20. Kendrick T, King F, Albertella L, Smith PW. GP treatment decisions for patients with depression: an observational study. Br J Gen Pract. 2005;55: 280–6.
21. Schulberg HC, Block MR, Madonia MJ, Rodriguez E, Scott CP, Lave J. Applicability of clinical pharmacotherapy guidelines for major depression in primary care settings. Arch Fam Med. 1995;4:106–12.
22. Schulberg HC, Block MR, Madonia MJ, Scott CP, Lave JR, Rodriguez E, et al. The "usual care" of major depression in primary care practice. Arch Fam Med. 1997;6:334–9.
23. Fournier JC, DeRubeis RJ, Hollon SD, Dimidjian S, Amsterdam JD, Shelton RC, et al. Antidepressant drug effects and depression severity: a patient-level meta-analysis. JAMA. 2010;303:47–53.
24. Kirsch I, Deacon BJ, Huedo-Medina TB, Scoboria A, Moore TJ, Johnson BT. Initial severity and antidepressant benefits: a meta-analysis of data submitted to the Food and Drug Administration. PLoS Med. 2008;5:e45.
25. van Schaik DJF, Klijn AFJ, van Hout HPJ, van Marwijk HWJ, Beekman ATF, de Haan M, et al. Patients' preferences in the treatment of depressive disorder in primary care. Gen Hosp Psychiatry. 2004;26:184–9.
26. Sherbourne CD, Wells KB, Duan N, Miranda J, Unützer J, Jaycox L, et al. Long-term effectiveness of disseminating quality improvement for depression in primary care. Arch Gen Psychiatry. 2001;58:696–703.
27. van Os TW, Ormel J, van den Brink RH, Jenner JA, Van der Meer K, Tiemens BG, et al. Training primary care physicians improves the management of depression. Gen Hosp Psychiatry. 1999;21:168–76.
28. Kroenke K, Taylor-Vaisey A, Dietrich AJ, Oxman TE. Interventions to improve provider diagnosis and treatment of mental disorders in primary care. A critical review of the literature. Psychosomatics. 2000;41:39–52.
29. Kalet AL, Gillespie CC, Schwartz MD, Holmboe ES, Ark TK, Jay M, et al. New measures to establish the evidence base for medical education: identifying educationally sensitive patient outcomes. Acad Med J Assoc Am Med Coll. 2010;85:844–51.
30. Sikorski C, Luppa M, König H-H, van den Bussche H, Riedel-Heller SG. Does GP training in depression care affect patient outcome? - a systematic review and meta-analysis. BMC Health Serv Res. 2012;12:10.
31. Crabtree BF, Nutting PA, Miller WL, McDaniel RR, Stange KC, Jaen CR, et al. Primary care practice transformation is hard work: insights from a 15-year developmental program of research. Med Care. 2011; 49(Suppl):S28–35.

32. Phillips RL, Miller BF, Petterson SM, Teevan B. Better integration of mental health care improves depression screening and treatment in primary care. Am Fam Physician. 2011;84:980.
33. Chomienne M-H, Grenier J, Gaboury I, Hogg W, Ritchie P, Farmanova-Haynes E. Family doctors and psychologists working together: doctors' and patients' perspectives. J Eval Clin Pract. 2011;17:282–7.
34. Unützer J, Schoenbaum M, Druss BG, Katon WJ. Transforming mental health care at the interface with general medicine: report for the presidents commission. Psychiatr Serv Wash DC. 2006;57:37–47.
35. Pereira B, Andrew G, Pednekar S, Kirkwood BR, Patel V. The integration of the treatment for common mental disorders in primary care: experiences of health care providers in the MANAS trial in Goa, India. Int J Ment Health Syst. 2011;5:26.
36. Fortney J, Enderle M, McDougall S, Clothier J, Otero J, Altman L, et al. Implementation outcomes of evidence-based quality improvement for depression in VA community based outpatient clinics. Implement Sci IS. 2012;7:30.
37. Weinerman R, Campbell H, Miller M, Stretch J, Kallstrom L, Kadlec H, et al. Improving mental healthcare by primary care physicians in British Columbia. Healthc Q Tor Ont. 2011;14:36–8.
38. Greenhalgh T, Robert G, Macfarlane F, Bate P, Kyriakidou O. Diffusion of innovations in service organizations: systematic review and recommendations. Milbank Q. 2004;82:581–629.
39. Miller WL, Crabtree BF, McDaniel R, Stange KC. Understanding change in primary care practice using complexity theory. J Fam Pract. 1998;46:369–76.
40. Plsek P. Complexity and the Adoption of Innovation in Health Care. Paper presented at Accelerating Quality Improvement in Health Care: Strategies to Accelerate the Diffusion of Evidence-Based Innovations. Washington, D.C.: National Institute for Healthcare Management Foundation and National Committee for Quality in Health Care; 2003.
41. Ruggles B. The improvement guide: a practical approach to enhancing organizational performance. Qual Prog Milwaukee. 1998;31:108.
42. MacCarthy D, Weinerman R, Kallstrom L, Kadlec H, Hollander MJ, Patten S. Mental health practice and attitudes of family physicians can be changed! Perm J. 2013;17:14–7.
43. Alweis R, Greco M, Wasser T, Wenderoth S. An initiative to improve adherence to evidence-based guidelines in the treatment of URIs, sinusitis, and pharyngitis. J Community Hosp Intern Med Perspect [Internet]. 2014 [cited 2018 May 25];4. Available from: https://www.ncbi.nlm.nih.gov/pmc/articles/PMC3937558/
44. Ginsburg LR, Lewis S, Zackheim L, Casebeer A. Revisiting interaction in knowledge translation. Implement Sci IS. 2007;2:34.
45. Stange KC, Goodwin MA, Zyzanski SJ, Dietrich AJ. Sustainability of a practice-individualized preventive service delivery intervention. Am J Prev Med. 2003;25:296–300.
46. Parker LE, Kirchner JE, Bonner LM, Fickel JJ, Ritchie MJ, Simons CE, et al. Creating a quality-improvement dialogue: utilizing knowledge from frontline staff, managers, and experts to foster health care quality improvement. Qual Health Res. 2009;19:229–42.
47. Rubenstein LV, Mittman BS, Yano EM, Mulrow CD. From understanding health care provider behavior to improving health care: the QUERI framework for quality improvement. Quality Enhancement Research Initiative. Med Care. 2000;38:I129–41.
48. Mendel P, Meredith LS, Schoenbaum M, Sherbourne CD, Wells KB. Interventions in organizational and community context: a framework for building evidence on dissemination and implementation in health services research. Admin Pol Ment Health. 2008;35:21–37.
49. Walters ST, Matson SA, Baer JS, Ziedonis DM. Effectiveness of workshop training for psychosocial addiction treatments: a systematic review. J Subst Abus Treat. 2005;29:283–93.
50. Tamburrino MB, Nagel RW, Lynch DJ. Managing antidepressants in primary care: physicians' treatment modifications. Psychol Rep. 2011;108:799–804.
51. Davis DA, Thomson MA, Oxman AD, Haynes RB. Changing physician performance. A systematic review of the effect of continuing medical education strategies. JAMA. 1995;274:700–5.
52. Nicholas MK, Asghari A, Corbett M, Smeets RJEM, Wood BM, Overton S, et al. Is adherence to pain self-management strategies associated with improved pain, depression and disability in those with disabling chronic pain? Eur J Pain Lond Engl. 2012;16:93–104.
53. Turner A, Anderson JK, Wallace LM, Bourne C. An evaluation of a self-management program for patients with long-term conditions. Patient Educ Couns. 2015;98:213–9.
54. Sevick MA, Trauth JM, Ling BS, Anderson RT, Piatt GA, Kilbourne AM, et al. Patients with complex chronic diseases: perspectives on supporting self-management. J Gen Intern Med. 2007;22(Suppl 3):438–44.
55. Theeboom T, Beersma B, Van Vianen A. Does coaching work? A meta-analysis on the effects of coaching on individual level outcomes in an organizational context. J Posit Psychol. 2013;9(1):1–18.
56. Linden A, Butterworth SW, Prochaska JO. Motivational interviewing-based health coaching as a chronic care intervention. J Eval Clin Pract. 2010;16:166–74.
57. Butterworth S, Linden A, McClay W, Leo MC. Effect of motivational interviewing-based health coaching on employees' physical and mental health status. J Occup Health Psychol. 2006;11:358–65.
58. Beaulieu T, Patten S, Knaak S, Weinerman R, Campbell H, Lauria-Horner B. Impact of skill-based approaches in reducing stigma in primary care physicians: results from a double-blind, parallel-cluster, randomized controlled trial. Can J Psychiatry Rev Can Psychiatr. 2017;62:327.
59. Antidepressant Skills Workbook - CARMHA - Centre for Applied Research in Mental Health & Addiction - Simon Fraser University [Internet]. [cited 2018 May 25]. Available from: https://www.sfu.ca/carmha/publications/antidepressant-skills-workbook.html
60. Healthy Minds Cooperative: [Internet]. [cited 2018 May 25]. Available from: https://www.healthyminds.ca/.
61. Mental Health First Aid | Mental Health Commission of Canada [Internet]. [cited 2018 May 25]. Available from: https://www.mentalhealthcommission.ca/English/resources/mental-health-first-aid
62. Hellman S, Hellman DS. Of mice but not men. Problems of the randomized clinical trial. N Engl J Med. 1991;324:1585–9.
63. Mulrow CD, Williams JW, Gerety MB, Ramirez G, Montiel OM, Kerber C. Case-finding instruments for depression in primary care settings. Ann Intern Med. 1995;122:913–21.
64. Martin A, Rief W, Klaiberg A, Braehler E. Validity of the brief patient health questionnaire mood scale (PHQ-9) in the general population. Gen Hosp Psychiatry. 2006;28:71–7.
65. Löwe B, Schenkel I, Carney-Doebbeling C, Göbel C. Responsiveness of the PHQ-9 to psychopharmacological depression treatment. Psychosomatics. 2006;47:62–7.
66. Kroenke K, Spitzer RL. The PHQ-9: a new depression diagnostic and severity measure. Psychiatr Ann. 2002;32:509–15.
67. Kroenke K, Spitzer RL, Williams JB. The PHQ-9: validity of a brief depression severity measure. J Gen Intern Med. 2001;16:606–13.
68. Lam RW, Michalak EE, Yatham LN. A new clinical rating scale for work absence and productivity: validation in patients with major depressive disorder. BMC Psychiatry. 2009;9:78.
69. Sheehan DV, Harnett-Sheehan K, Raj BA. The measurement of disability. Int Clin Psychopharmacol. 1996;11(Suppl 3):89–95.
70. Chisholm D, Knapp M, Knudsen H, Amaddeo F, Gaite L, Van Wijngaarden B. Client socio-demographic and service receipt inventory - European Version: Development of an instrument for international research - EPSILON Study 5. Br J Psychiatr. 2000;177:S28–33.
71. Ware JE, Sherbourne CD. The MOS 36-item short-form health survey (SF-36). I. Conceptual framework and item selection. Med Care. 1992;30:473–83.
72. McHorney CA, Ware JE, Raczek AE. The MOS 36-item short-form health survey (SF-36): II. Psychometric and clinical tests of validity in measuring physical and mental health constructs. Med Care. 1993;31:247–63.
73. McHorney CA, Ware JE, Lu JF, Sherbourne CD. The MOS 36-item short-form health survey (SF-36): III. Tests of data quality, scaling assumptions, and reliability across diverse patient groups. Med Care. 1994;32:40–66.
74. Murphy AW, Esterman A, Pilotto LS. Cluster randomized controlled trials in primary care: an introduction. Eur J Gen Pract. 2006;12:70–3.
75. Schoemaker JH, Kilian S, Emsley R, Vingerhoets AJJM, Medical and Clinical Psychology. Factors associated with placebo response in depression trials. Neurol Psychiatry Brain Res. 2017;30:12–21.

10

Characteristics of patients with acute myocardial infarction contacting primary healthcare before hospitalisation

Per O. Andersson[1,4*], Sofia Sederholm Lawesson[2], Jan-Erik Karlsson[3], Staffan Nilsson[1], Ingela Thylén[2] and on behalf of the SymTime Study Group

Abstract

Background: The characteristics of patients with on-going myocardial infarction (MI) contacting the primary healthcare (PHC) centre before hospitalisation are not well known. Prompt diagnosis is crucial in patients with MI, but many patients delay seeking medical care. The aims of this study was to 1) describe background characteristics, symptoms, actions and delay times in patients contacting the PHC before hospitalisation when falling ill with an acute MI, 2) compare those patients with acute MI patients not contacting the PHC, and 3) explore factors associated with a PHC contact in acute MI patients.

Methods: This was a cross-sectional multicentre study, enrolling consecutive patients with MI within 24 hours of admission to hospital from Nov 2012 until Feb 2014.

Results: A total of 688 patients with MI, 519 men and 169 women, were included; the mean age was 66±11 years. One in five people contacted PHC instead of the recommended emergency medical services (EMS), and 94% of these patients experienced cardinal symptoms of an acute MI; i.e., chest pain, and/or radiating pain in the arms, and/or cold sweat. Median delay time from symptom-onset-to-decision-to-seek-care was 2:15 hours in PHC patients and 0:40 hours in non-PHC patients ($p<0.01$). The probability of utilising the PHC before hospitalisation was associated with fluctuating symptoms (OR 1.74), pain intensity (OR 0.90) symptoms during off-hours (OR 0.42), study hospital (OR 3.49 and 2.52, respectively, for two of the county hospitals) and a final STEMI diagnosis (OR 0.58).

Conclusions: Ambulance services are still underutilized in acute MI patients. A substantial part of the patients contacts their primary healthcare centre before they are diagnosed with MI, although experiencing cardinal symptoms such as chest pain. There is need for better knowledge in the population about symptoms of MI and adequate pathways to qualified care. Knowledge and awareness amongst primary healthcare professionals on the occurrence of MI patients is imperative.

Keywords: Chest pain, Myocardial infarction, Primary healthcare, Pre-hospital delay

* Correspondence: per.o.andersson@liu.se
[1]Primary Health Care and Department of Medical and Health Sciences, Linköping University, Linköping, Sweden
[4]Ljungsbro Health Care Centre, Evastigen 9, 590 71 Ljungsbro, Ljungsbro, Sweden
Full list of author information is available at the end of the article

Background

About 1–3% of primary healthcare (PHC) patients experience chest pain [1, 2]. Chest pain can have many different causes; most of them are of non-cardiac origin. In 10–18% of cases, the chest pain is caused by ischaemic heart disease, of which 2–4% as the result of myocardial infarction (MI) or unstable angina [3–5], conditions that require immediate attention. In some countries, general practitioners (GP) play a major role in the early care of acute MI and are often the first to be contacted by patients [6]. In most settings, however, consultation with a GP, instead of a direct call to the emergency medical services (EMS), increases pre-hospital delay [4, 7, 8]. Many cases of sudden cardiac death occur outside a hospital. Therefore, prompt action when patients experience symptoms indicating acute cardiac ischemia is of great importance [7].

According to existing European clinical guidelines on cardiovascular disease prevention, the GP should evaluate the risk factors and clinical findings when a patient contacts PHC with chest pain, and decide if the patient should be transferred to hospital [9]. However, the low prevalence of acute MI can make the diagnosis difficult [10], particularly because the medical history, symptom presentation, and findings from an electrocardiogram (ECG) are not always indicative [11, 12].

A great deal of knowledge exists today about the reasons for patient [13, 14], as well as system, delay [15]. Similarly, studies have consistently reported that only half of the patients with MI use the EMS [16, 17]. Factors associated with underutilisation of the EMS have previously been explored [18, 19]. However, the reasons for contacting the PHC for symptoms suggestive of acute MI, as a contributory factor to prolonged pre-hospital delay, have not yet been examined.

Therefore, the aims of this study were to 1) describe background characteristics, symptoms, actions and delay times in patients contacting the PHC before hospitalisation when falling ill with an acute MI, 2) compare those patients with acute MI patients not contacting the PHC, and 3) explore factors associated with a PHC contact in acute MI patients.

Methods

Setting

In Sweden, there are about 1300 PHC centres for a population of 10 million people. The PHC centres are staffed with approximately 6500 GPs (2000 patients per GP annually) [20]. In the Swedish emergency system, individuals with a suspected acute MI are urged to contact the EMS by telephone and describe their symptoms. Generally, when symptoms of MI are reported, an ambulance is sent. However, a substantial number of individuals experiencing MI symptoms self-transport to the ED (Emergency Department), contact their PHC or a national telephone-nurse advisement number (Swedish Healthcare Direct, SHD) as their first medical contact [8].

Study design

This Swedish multi-centre study (SymTime) was a cross-sectional study based on self-reported data and has been described in detail previously [8]. Participants were enrolled from five different hospitals: two university hospitals and three county hospitals. The university hospitals were located in Linköping (southeast) and Umeå (northeast), and the county hospitals in Sunderby (northeast), Jönköping (south) and Kalmar (southeast), respectively. The data were collected between November 2012 and January 2014 and the hospitals were selected by geographic location and size/type of hospital.

Participants and procedure

Within 24 hours after admittance to the coronary care unit (CCU), patients were included consecutively. The criteria for inclusion were as follows: diagnosed with acute MI [21], able to fill in the questionnaire, and willing to participate. Patients who were still clinically unstable 24 hours after admittance (i.e., with ongoing chest pain, shock or other severe symptoms) were excluded from the study, as were patients with difficulties reading and speaking Swedish. STEMI (ST-elevation myocardial infarction) patients were included at all five hospitals, while NSTEMI (non-ST-elevation myocardial infarction) patients were included at the two university hospitals.

Participants of interest were those stating in the questionnaire that they had been in contact with PHC (direct or by phone) before hospitalisation because of acute MI. In total, 694 acute MI patients were included in the SymTime study. Of those 688 (99%) had answered the question about being in contact with the PCH when falling ill. Those patients constituted the study population in the present study.

Data collection

Clinical variables

The CCU nurse in charge gathered information about co-morbidities and important time point variables from the medical records, as well as from the patient. Final diagnosis (non ST-elevation MI [NSTEMI] or [STEMI]) was obtained from medical records.

Symptoms and pre-hospital actions

A previously validated self-administrated survey covering 35 items was used to access data on symptoms, actions, and pre-hospital delay times and transport mode to the hospital [8, 22].

Statistical analysis

Proportions and frequencies were used to describe the patient's characteristics and the socio-demographic, clinical and contextual variables. Continuous variables were reported as means ± standard deviation (SD) or median (25th to 75th percentile) as appropriate. In the bivariate analyses, we used the Pearson χ^2 test (Fisher's exact test when cells had expected count less than five) for categorical data and the two-tailed Student t test (for normally distributed variables) or Mann-Whitney U test (for non-normally distributed variables) for continuous data when comparing MI patients contacting the PHC (direct or by phone) before hospitalisation with all other MI patients.

A logistic multiple regression model (Enter method) was used to determine factors associated with a contact with PHC. Variables in the regression model were chosen based on results from bivariate analyses (*p*-value <. 10) or on clinical and theoretical relevance. Backward elimination was used to abort non-significant variables down to the significance level of $p<0.05$.

All tests were two tailed and a p value <0.05 indicated statistical significance. Statistical analyses were performed using SPSS software, version 25.0 (SPSS Inc, Chicago, Illinois, USA) for Windows.

Results

Demographics and clinical variables

A total of 688 patients with acute MI, 519 men and 169 women, were included; the mean age was 66±11 years. In total, 147 patients (21%) turned to PHC before hospitalisation when falling ill. A minority had previously experienced an MI (15%), nearly half of the participants had hypertension (47%), and 14% had diabetes. The majority (77%) were subsequently diagnosed with STEMI.

When comparing those contacting PHC before hospitalisation with patients who did not, the PHC patients more often lived in the north (i.e., more rural) areas of Sweden (46% vs. 36%, $p<0.05$) and were more often diagnosed with a NSTEMI, (31% vs. 21%, $p<0.01$). There were no significant differences with respect to age, gender, presence of time of symptom onset (time of day or weekday) or being alone or not when falling ill. The background characteristics are given in more detail in Table 1.

Symptoms when falling ill

Most of the participants experienced chest pain when falling ill (88%), and 97% experienced a combination of cardinal MI symptoms, i.e., chest pain and/or radiating pain in the arms and/or cold sweats. As well as those classic symptoms of an evolving MI, other symptoms such as weakness (39%), shortness of breath (32%), vertigo (23%) and fear (22%) were also commonly reported. The total number of symptoms reported was 5.19 (±2.49). One in five patients (n=141) had experienced prodromal symptoms in the previous 2 weeks. Most of the patients (66%) interpreted their acute symptoms as cardiac in origin.

When comparing those contacting PHC before hospitalisation with patients who did not, the PHC patients more seldom experienced cardinal symptoms (i.e., chest pain and/or radiating pain in the arms and/or cold sweat) (94% vs. 98%, $p<0.05$), cold sweats (44% vs. 56%, $p<0.01$), vertigo (16% vs. 25%, $p<0.05$), nausea (22% vs. 32%, $p<0.05$) or fear (15% vs. 24%, $p<0.05$). The PHC group described more worries (52% vs. 42%, $p<0.05$), a less severe pain ($p<0.00$), a lower symptom burden ($p<0.00$). There were no significant differences between groups in experiencing chest pain or prodromal symptoms. The symptoms are given in more detail in Table 2.

Factors associated with contacting the primary healthcare centre

The probability of utilising the PHC before hospitalisation was associated with fluctuating symptoms (OR 1.74), pain intensity (OR 0.90), symptoms during off-hours (OR 0.42), study hospital location (OR 3.49 for Sunderby county hospital and 2.52 for Jönköping county hospital with Linköping University hospital as reference) and a final STEMI diagnosis (OR 0.58). Gender, age, co-morbidities, symptoms, interpretation of symptoms, being alone when falling ill, or distance to hospital were not significantly associated with the outcome (Table 3).

Time interval from symptom onset to action

Median delay time from symptom onset to decision to seeking care was 2:15 hours in the PHC patients (P_{25} 0:30; P_{75} 11:15) and 0:40 hours (P_{25} 0:15; P_{75} 2:00) in the other patients ($p<0.01$). Twenty-three percent of the PHC patients and 6% of the other patients delayed >12 hours ($p<0.001$) before decision to seeking care. Median delay from decision until action was taken was 0:30 hours (P_{25} 0:10; P_{75} 1:07) in the PHC patients and 0:25 hours (P_{25} 0:10; P_{75} 0:40) in the other patients ($p<0.05$). When analysing the free text answers in the total group regarding reasons for not acting immediately after decision was taken, the most common reasons were; 1) waiting for the ambulance, 2) wanted to talk to a next-of-kin before going to hospital, or 3) trying self-care.

Patients that subsequently were diagnosed with STEMI (n=522) had a median time from symptom onset to diagnosis (i.e., ECG) of 2:02 hours (P_{25} 0:42; P_{75} 4:18). When comparing those STEMI patients contacting PHC before hospitalisation with patients who did not, those contacting the PHC had a median time from symptom onset to diagnosis of 3:15 hours (P_{25} 1:32; P_{75} 18:22) with the corresponding delay time for the non-PHC patients being 1:40 hours (P_{25}1:00; P_{75} 3:19), $p<0.001$).

Table 1 Background characteristics of patients contacting PHC before hospitalisation compared with those not contacting PHC when experiencing symptoms of an acute MI

	All *N*=688	PHC *n*=147	Other *n*=541	*p*-value
Socio-demographics				
Age, years[b]	66 ± 11	65 ± 11	66 ± 11	0.46
Gender, men	519 (75)	112 (76)	407 (75)	0.81
Education, ≤ 9 years	270 (39)	60 (41)	210 (39)	0.68
Current smoker	174 (26)	39 (28)	135 (25)	0.60
Living alone	162 (24)	36 (25)	126 (23)	0.76
Co-morbidities[a]				
Hypertension	366 (53)	82 (56)	284 (53)	0.48
Diabetes	101 (15)	20 (14)	81 (15)	0.68
Angina Pectoris	103 (15)	21 (15)	82 (16)	0.83
Atrial fibrillation	38 (6)	6 (4)	32 (6)	0.38
Heart failure	22 (3)	1 (1)	21 (4)	**0.06**
Previous myocardial infarction	109 (16)	16 (11)	93 (17)	**0.06**
Previous stroke	26 (4)	5 (3)	21 (4)	1.00
Contextual factors				
Falling ill at home	529 (77)	110 (14)	419 (77)	0.50
Symptom onset, off hours[*]	380 (56)	73 (50)	307 (57)	0.12
Living in the north part of Sweden	261 (38)	67 (46)	194 (36)	**0.03**
Distance to hospital, >50 km	105 (16)	22 (15)	84 (16)	0.93
Being alone at symptom onset	191 (28)	38 (26)	153 (28)	0.59
Diagnosis				
NSTEMI	160 (23)	46 (31)	114 (21)	**<0.01**

Some missing responses, which explains the differences in percentages
Data are presented as numbers (percentages) if not otherwise indicated
[a]Collected from the patients and validated against the medical records
[b]Data are presented as mean ± SD; [*]Evenings, nights and weekends
PHC=Primary Healthcare Centre; Other=not contacting the PHC before hospitalisation

Reasons for not contacting the emergency medical services when falling ill

About half of the patients (53%) had previous experience of being transported by an ambulance. The reason for not contacting the EMS as a first action was predominantly because the patients did not consider themselves sick enough; this applied to 57% of the PHC patients compared with 28% of the other patients ($p<0.00$), Table 4.

After contacting PHC, most (80%) subsequently arrived at the hospital by ambulance; 62% contacted the EMS by themselves or with the help by a bystander.

Discussion

The main observation of this study was that one in five people contacted PHC when experiencing symptoms suggestive of an acute MI, and this was more common in patients later diagnosed with NSTEMI. Fluctuating symptoms were predicative for PHC contact and onset of symptoms out of hours predicted other contacts than PHC. Furthermore, the PHC patients had a considerably longer delay time from symptom onset to decision to seek medical care with a median difference of 1:35 hours. A contact with the PHC also impacted on the total delay from symptom onset to diagnosis in STEMI patients. This is in line with another Swedish study that reported that patients with MI are delayed to hospital admission when they contact the PHC in the pre-hospital phase [23]. A rapid recognition and transportation of all patients with MI is crucial for their treatment. This has been well proven for STEMI, but patients with NSTEMI also benefit from reduced delay [24–26]. However, 20% of those contacting the PHC in our study did not arrive by ambulance to the hospital. For these reasons, triage of patients with chest pain is imperative. In addition to the existing clinical European guidelines on cardiovascular prevention in PHC [9], GPs are in need of validated diagnostic tools to help distinguish patients with chest pain for referral to the ED, particularly since the medical history, symptom presentation, and findings from the ECG are not always

Table 2 Symptoms when falling ill in acute myocardial infarction

	All *N*=688	PHC *n*=147	Other *n*=541	*p*-value
Cardinal symptoms[a]	667 (97)	138 (94)	529 (98)	**0.03**
Symptoms, pain				
Chest pain	607 (88)	124 (84)	483 (89)	0.10
Pain in neck or throat	143 (20)	24 (16)	119 (22)	0.13
Pain in the jaw or teeth	80 (12)	18 (12)	62 (12)	0.79
Back pain	116 (16.9)	26 (18)	90 (17)	0.76
Stomach pain	58 (8)	16 (11)	42 (8)	0.23
Shoulder pain	142 (21)	34 (23)	(108 (20)	0.40
Radiating pain in the arm(s)	379 (55)	75 (51)	304 (56)	0.26
Other symptoms				
Cold sweat	368 (53)	64 (44)	304 (56)	**<0.01**
Weakness	267 (39)	54 (37)	213 (39)	0.57
Tiredness	224 (33)	45 (31)	179 (33)	0.62
Shortness of breath	219 (32)	44 (30)	175 (32)	0.58
Nausea/vomiting	206 (30)	33 (22)	173 (32)	**0.03**
Numbness in the hands	205 (30)	36 (25)	169 (31)	0.11
Vertigo	160 (23)	23 (16)	137 (25)	**0.01**
Fear	150 (22)	22 (15)	128 (24)	**0.02**
Anxiety	91 (13)	15 (10)	76 (14)	0.22
General sick feeling	103 (15)	19 (13)	84 (16)	0.43
Prodromal symptoms, ≤ 2 weeks	141 (20)	39 (27)	102 (19)	0.28
Symptom burden *	5.19 (±2.49)	4.64 (±2.19)	5.33 (±2.54)	**<0.01**
Symptom character				
Oppressive feeling across the chest	231 (38)	56 (42)	175 (38)	0.40
Dull pain	99 (16)	26 (19)	73 (16)	0.32
Tightness across the chest	85 (14)	18 (13)	67 (14)	0.77
Cramp-like pain	64 (11)	12 (9)	52 (11)	0.46
Burning pain	41 (7)	5 (4)	36 (8)	0.10
Razor-sharp pain	22 (4)	5 (4)	17 (4)	0.97
Stinging pain	21 (4)	7 (5)	14 (3)	0.28
Tenderness pain	13 (2)	2 (2)	11 (2)	0.74
Stabbing pain	6 (1)	2 (2)	4 (1)	0.62
Experience of symptoms				
Unpleasant	386 (56)	80 (54)	306 (57)	0.64
Worrying	303 (44)	77 (52)	226 (42)	**0.03**
Troublesome	191 (28)	47 (32)	144 (27)	0.22
Unbearable	188 (27)	33 (22)	155 (29)	0.14
Frightening	177 (26)	27 (18)	150 (28)	**0.02**
Anxiety-ridden	134 (20)	33 (22)	101 (19)	0.35
Tiring	138 (20)	24 (16)	114 (21)	0.25
Stressful	91 (13)	23 (16)	68 (13)	0.34
Suffocating	78 (11)	13 (9)	65 (12)	0.31
Irritating	67 (10)	15 (10)	52 (10)	0.88

Table 2 Symptoms when falling ill in acute myocardial infarction *(Continued)*

	All *N*=688	PHC *n*=147	Other *n*=541	*p*-value
Pain intensity				
Numeric rating scale[b]	6.75 (±2.04)	6.29 (±2.02)	6.87 (±2.03)	**<0.01**
Passing	22 (3)	9 (6)	13 (3)	**0.04**
Fluctuating	168 (25)	52 (36)	116 (22)	**<0.01**
Constant	359 (54)	68 (47)	291 (55)	**<0.01**
Increasing	121 (18)	16 (11)	105 (20)	**0.01**
Interpretation of the symptoms				
Cardiac in origin	456 (66)	88 (60)	368 (68)	0.08

Some missing responses, which explains the differences in percentages
Data are presented as numbers (percentages) if not otherwise indicated
[a]Chest pain and/or radiating pain in the arms and/or cold sweat; [b]Data are presented as mean ± SD
PHC=Primary Healthcare Centre; Other=not contacting the PHC before hospitalisation

indicative [11, 27]. The use of troponin testing - a biomarker used to assess myocardial injury - may reduce emergency referrals but probably at the cost of an increased risk of overdiagnoses, especially among older patients with acute MI and often chronically increased troponin levels [2], and is therefore not encouraged in GP offices [28, 29]. However, a more in-depth medical history, detailed symptom assessment and physical examination using a clinical prediction score could possibly assist the GP to rule out coronary heart disease in PHC patients with chest pain [30, 31]. A previous study has shown that older age, male gender and a history of MI are useful predictors of ischaemic heart disease when evaluating patients with chest pain [32]. Likewise, the presence of IHD risk factors (i.e., diabetes, smoking, hyperlipidaemia) should also lead to an increased suspicion of acute cardiac ischemia, when evaluating patients with chest pain [9].

In our study, most patients contacting PHC had cardinal symptoms of MI, and no symptom was independently associated with PHC contact. Thus, symptoms do not discriminate MI patients taking contact with PHC from other MI patients. On the other hand, was symptoms waxing and waning strongly associated with PHC contact. Accordingly, a patient with cardinal MI symptoms but whose symptoms have not been constant but have instead been coming and going ought to lead to suspicion from the GP that this may be an acute MI. However, up to 80% of patients consulting a GP with chest pain have a non-cardiac diagnosis and do not need referral to the ED. Referral of all these patients would result in overcrowding of the ED [3]. Consequently, more studies are needed to discriminate factors between cardiac and non-cardiac chest pain.

Table 3 Predictors of contacting the primary healthcare centre before hospitalisation[a] *n*=648

Variable	OR	95% CI	*p*-value
Diagnosis, STEMI	0.58	0.36-0.94	**0.03**
Pain intensity	0.90	0.81-0.98	**0.02**
Fluctuating symptoms	1.74	1.14-2.64	**0.01**
Symptom onset, off-hours	0.42	0.29-0.62	**<0.001**
Study hospital location (Linkoping University as reference)	1.00		**<0.01**
Jonkoping county hospital vs. Linkoping university hospital	2.52	1.32-4.82	**<0.01**
Sunderby county hospital vs. Linkoping university Hospital	3.49	1.82-6.69	**<0.01**

[a]Regression conducted using multiple logistic regression (Enter method, backward elimination). Only significant variables are presented in the final model
OR=Odds Ratio, *CI*=Confidence Interval, NSTEMI=non-ST elevation myocardial infarction

Table 4 Reasons for not contacting the emergency medical services when falling ill

	All *N*=143	PHC *N*=42	Other *N*=101	*p*-value
Reason for not contacting the EMS				
Did not considered myself sick enough	52 (36)	24 (57)	28 (28)	**0.001**
My way was faster	45 (31)	12 (29)	33 (33)	0.69
Easier to take a taxi	32 (22)	6 (14)	26 (26)	0.18
Never thought about it	29 (20)	13 (31)	16 (16)	0.07
Unnecessary to call an ambulance	24 (17)	8 (19)	16 (16)	0.63
Easier to drive on my own	20 (14)	10 (24)	10 (10)	**0.03**
Others have greater needs	10 (7)	5 (12)	5 (5)	0.16
Would not like to draw attention to myself	7 (5)	0 (0)	7 (7)	0.10
Did not want to disturb the EMS	6 (4)	3 (7)	3 (3)	0.55
Thought being denied	4 (3)	1 (2)	3 (3)	1.00
Did not know the capability of the paramedics	2 (1)	1 (2)	1 (1)	0.50

EMS= emergency medical services, *PHC*=Primary Healthcare Centre, Other=not contacting the PHC before hospitalisation

We found that approximately half of the patients who contacted PHC did not consider themselves sick enough to contact the EMS. This finding is important since active care of patients with MI starts in the ambulance and the decision to claim expensive but necessary resources for transportation needs to be strengthened. Patient delay is the longest in the pre-hospital chain and a difficult aspect to modify, as previous public campaigns have shown [33], although a more recent mass media campaign in Australia demonstrated that an awareness of the campaign was significantly associated with shorter delay times [34]. Studies focusing on individual education programmes have been more successful than mass media campaigns [33, 35]. These interventions should take into account the complexity of translating knowledge into actions and tailor their message according to target groups. GPs are an important part of these pre-hospital interventions, since many patients with chest pain contact PHC. Clinicians should individualise their approach when educating patients with an increased risk of MI, such as those with hypertension, diabetes and hypercholesterolemia, and address relevant issues such as the various presentations of MI and the importance of a timely response to these symptoms [36]. Still, whatever we as clinicians do or say, some people will contact their PHC for symptoms suggestive of an acute MI, not because they are ignorant or unaware of the importance of a short delay, but just because it seems the right thing for them to do. And when they do contact the PHC, we need to respond constructively.

Strengths and limitations

The strengths of this study are the inclusion of a large number of patients from five different hospitals in different areas of Sweden, which emphasizes the external validity of the results. There were no differences in age or gender between the groups. The aim was to include consecutive patients and there were defined criteria for inclusion in the study. A limitation of this study could be that the number of cases of NSTEMI, who are probably more often seen by a GP, was lower than the number with STEMI due to the study design. The patients were enrolled at the CCU where the number of the very oldest with multi-morbidity not suitable for interventions is usually lower than it is on general medical wards. This could mean that a healthier and younger population were included, missing the experiences of older patients with NSTEMI who may have been hospitalised in other areas or wards. One of the inclusion criteria was knowledge of the Swedish language, thus excluding, e.g., recently arrived refugees this could impact on the generalizability of the study.

Conclusion

A substantial part of the patients contacts their PHC before they are diagnosed with MI, although experiencing cardinal symptoms such as chest pain and ambulance services are still underutilized in acute MI patients. There is need for better knowledge in the population about symptoms of MI and adequate pathways to qualified care. Knowledge and awareness amongst primary healthcare professional´s on the occurrence of MI patients is imperative.

Abbreviations

CCU: Coronary care unit; ECG: Electrocardiogram; ED: Emergency department; EMS: Emergency medical services; GP: General practitioners; MI: Myocardial infarction; NSTEMI: Non- ST-elevation myocardial infarction; PHC: Primary healthcare; SHD: Swedish healthcare direct; STEMI: ST-Elevation myocardial infarction

Acknowledgements

We are grateful to the all the participants who have made this work possible and also to the group of the Swedish multi-centre study (SymTime). (Thylen I, Ericsson M, Hellstrom Angerud K, Isaksson RM, Sederholm Lawesson S).

Funding

This study was funded with grants from the Medical Research Council of Southeast Sweden (FORSS) and the Region Östergötland, ALF.

Author's contributions

PA, SSL, IT, JEK and SN contributed to the conception and design of this study. PA conceptualized the research problem and PA, SSL and IT performed and contributed to the statistical analyses. PA, SSL, IT, JEK and SN discussed the interpretation of data. PA provided literature review and drafted the manuscript and PA, SSL, IT, JEK and SN contributed to manuscript preparation and revision. All authors read and approved the final manuscript.

Consent for publication

Not applicable

Competing interests

The authors declare that they have no competing interests.

Author details

[1]Primary Health Care and Department of Medical and Health Sciences, Linköping University, Linköping, Sweden. [2]Department of Cardiology and department of Medical and Health Sciences, Linköping University, Linköping, Sweden. [3]Department of Internal Medicine, Region Jönköping County, Jönköping, and Department of Medical and Health Sciences, Linköping University, Linköping, Sweden. [4]Ljungsbro Health Care Centre, Evastigen 9, 590 71 Ljungsbro, Ljungsbro, Sweden.

References

1. Verdon F, Burnand B, Herzig L, Junod M, Pecoud A, Favrat B. Chest wall syndrome among primary care patients: a cohort study. BMC Fam Pract. 2007;8:51.
2. Nilsson S, Andersson PO, Borgquist L, Grodzinsky E, Janzon M, Kvick M, et al. Point-of-Care Troponin T Testing in the Management of Patients with Chest Pain in the Swedish Primary Care. Int J Family Med. 2013;2013:532093.

3. Svavarsdottir AE, Jonasson MR, Gudmundsson GH, Fjeldsted K. Chest pain in family practice. Diagnosis and long-term outcome in a community setting. Can Fam Physician. 1996;42:1122–8.
4. Task Force on the management of STseamiotESoC, Steg PG, James SK, Atar D, Badano LP, Blomstrom-Lundqvist C, et al. ESC Guidelines for the management of acute myocardial infarction in patients presenting with ST-segment elevation. Eur Heart J. 2012;33(20):2569–619.
5. Ibanez B, James S, Agewall S, Antunes MJ, Bucciarelli-Ducci C, Bueno H, et al. 2017 ESC Guidelines for the management of acute myocardial infarction in patients presenting with ST-segment elevation: The Task Force for the management of acute myocardial infarction in patients presenting with ST-segment elevation of the European Society of Cardiology (ESC). Eur Heart J. 2018;39(2):119–77.
6. Steg PG, James SK, Gersh BJ. 2012 ESC STEMI guidelines and reperfusion therapy: Evidence-based recommendations, ensuring optimal patient management. Heart. 2013;99(16):1156–7.
7. Hoglund H, Jansson JH, Forslund AS, Lundblad D. Prodromal symptoms and health care consumption prior to out-of-hospital cardiac arrest in patients without previously known ischaemic heart disease. Resuscitation. 2014;85(7):864–8.
8. Thylen I, Ericsson M, Hellstrom Angerud K, Isaksson RM, Sederholm Lawesson S, SymTime study g. First medical contact in patients with STEMI and its impact on time to diagnosis; an explorative cross-sectional study. BMJ Open. 2015;5(4):e007059.
9. Piepoli MF, Hoes AW, Agewall S, Albus C, Brotons C, Catapano AL, et al. 2016 European Guidelines on cardiovascular disease prevention in clinical practice. Rev Esp Cardiol (Engl Ed). 2016;69(10):939.
10. Buntinx F, Truyen J, Embrechts P, Moreel G, Peeters R. Chest pain: an evaluation of the initial diagnosis made by 25 Flemish general practitioners. Fam Pract. 1991;8(2):121–4.
11. Haasenritter J, Aerts M, Bosner S, Buntinx F, Burnand B, Herzig L, et al. Coronary heart disease in primary care: accuracy of medical history and physical findings in patients with chest pain--a study protocol for a systematic review with individual patient data. BMC Fam Pract. 2012;13:81.
12. Fanaroff AC, Rymer JA, Goldstein SA. JAMA Patient Page. Acute Coronary Syndrome. JAMA. 2015;314(18):1990.
13. Kaul P, Armstrong PW, Sookram S, Leung BK, Brass N, Welsh RC. Temporal trends in patient and treatment delay among men and women presenting with ST-elevation myocardial infarction. Am Heart J. 2011;161(1):91–7.
14. McKee G, Mooney M, O'Donnell S, O'Brien F, Biddle MJ, Moser DK. Multivariate analysis of predictors of pre-hospital delay in acute coronary syndrome. Int J Cardiol. 2013;168(3):2706–13.
15. Ting HH, Bradley EH, Wang Y, Lichtman JH, Nallamothu BK, Sullivan MD, et al. Factors associated with longer time from symptom onset to hospital presentation for patients with ST-elevation myocardial infarction. Arch Intern Med. 2008;168(9):959–68.
16. Kerr D, Holden D, Smith J, Kelly AM, Bunker S. Predictors of ambulance use in patients with acute myocardial infarction in Australia. Emerg Med J. 2006; 23(12):948–52.
17. Kirchberger I, Amann U, Heier M, Thilo C, Peters A, Meisinger C. Factors Associated With Emergency Services Use by Patients With Recurrent Myocardial Infarction: From the Monitoring Trends and Determinants in Cardiovascular Disease/Cooperative Health Research in the Region of Augsburg Myocardial Infarction Registry. J Cardiovasc Nurs. 2016.
18. Boothroyd LJ, Lambert LJ, Segal E, Ross D, Kouz S, Maire S, et al. Comparison of outcomes of ambulance users and nonusers in ST elevation myocardial infarction. Am J Cardiol. 2014;114(9):1289–94.
19. Austin D, Yan AT, Spratt JC, Kunadian V, Edwards RJ, Egred M, et al. Patient characteristics associated with self-presentation, treatment delay and survival following primary percutaneous coronary intervention. Eur Heart J Acute Cardiovasc Care. 2014;3(3):214–22.
20. http://www.socialstyrelsen.se/statistik/statistikdatabas/halsoochsjukvardspersonal. 2015
21. Windecker S, Kolh P, Alfonso F, Collet JP, Cremer J, Falk V, et al. 2014 ESC/EACTS guidelines on myocardial revascularization. EuroIntervention. 2015; 10(9):1024–94.
22. Johansson I, Stromberg A, Swahn E. Factors related to delay times in patients with suspected acute myocardial infarction. Heart Lung. 2004;33(5):291–300.
23. Nilsson G, Mooe T, Soderstrom L, Samuelsson E. Pre-hospital delay in patients with first time myocardial infarction: an observational study in a northern Swedish population. BMC Cardiovasc Disord. 2016;16(1):93.
24. Katritsis DG, Siontis GC, Kastrati A, van't Hof AW, Neumann FJ, Siontis KC, et al. Optimal timing of coronary angiography and potential intervention in non-ST-elevation acute coronary syndromes. Eur Heart J. 2011;32(1):32–40.
25. Milasinovic D, Milosevic A, Marinkovic J, Vukcevic V, Ristic A, Asanin M, et al. Timing of invasive strategy in NSTE-ACS patients and effect on clinical outcomes: A systematic review and meta-analysis of randomized controlled trials. Atherosclerosis. 2015;241(1):48–54.
26. Navarese EP, Gurbel PA, Andreotti F, Tantry U, Jeong YH, Kozinski M, et al. Optimal timing of coronary invasive strategy in non-ST-segment elevation acute coronary syndromes: a systematic review and meta-analysis. Ann Intern Med. 2013;158(4):261–70.
27. Fanaroff AC, Rymer JA, Goldstein SA, Simel DL, Newby LK. Does This Patient With Chest Pain Have Acute Coronary Syndrome?: The Rational Clinical Examination Systematic Review. JAMA. 2015;314(18):1955–65.
28. Andersson PO, Karlsson JE, Landberg E, Festin K, Nilsson S. Consequences of high-sensitivity troponin T testing applied in a primary care population with chest pain compared with a commercially available point-of-care troponin T analysis: an observational prospective study. BMC research notes. 2015;8:210.
29. Marshall GA, Wijeratne NG, Thomas D. Should general practitioners order troponin tests? Med J Aust. 2014;201(3):155–7.
30. International Working Group on Chest Pain in Primary C. Aerts M, Minalu G, Bosner S, Buntinx F, Burnand B, et al. Pooled individual patient data from five countries were used to derive a clinical prediction rule for coronary artery disease in primary care. In: J Clin Epidemiol; 2016.
31. Gencer B, Vaucher P, Herzig L, Verdon F, Ruffieux C, Bosner S, et al. Ruling out coronary heart disease in primary care patients with chest pain: a clinical prediction score. BMC Med. 2010;8:9.
32. Nilsson S, Ortoft K, Molstad S. The accuracy of general practitioners' clinical assessment of chest pain patients. Eur J Gen Pract. 2008;14(2):50–5.
33. Mooney M, McKee G, Fealy G, O'Brien F, O'Donnell S, Moser D. A review of interventions aimed at reducing pre-hospital delay time in acute coronary syndrome: what has worked and why? Eur J Cardiovasc Nurs. 2012;11(4):445–53.
34. Bray JE, Stub D, Ngu P, Cartledge S, Straney L, Stewart M, Keech W, Patsamanis H, Shaw J, Finn J. Mass Media Campaigns' Influence on Prehospital Behavior for Acute Coronary Syndromes: An Evaluation of the Australian Heart Foundation's Warning Signs Campaign. J Am Heart Assoc. 2015;4(7). https://doi.org/10.1161/JAHA.115.001927.
35. Dracup K, McKinley S, Riegel B, Moser DK, Meischke H, Doering LV, et al. A randomized clinical trial to reduce patient prehospital delay to treatment in acute coronary syndrome. Circ Cardiovasc Qual Outcomes. 2009;2(6):524–32.
36. Albarqouni L, Smenes K, Meinertz T, Schunkert H, Fang X, Ronel J, et al. Patients' knowledge about symptoms and adequate behaviour during acute myocardial infarction and its impact on delay time: Findings from the multicentre MEDEA Study. Patient Educ Couns. 2016;99(11):1845–51.
37. World Medical Association. World Medical Association Declaration of Helsinki: ethical principles for medical research involving human subjects. JAMA. 2013;310(20):2191–4.

11

Changes in prescribed medicines in older patients with multimorbidity and polypharmacy in general practice

Fiona von Buedingen[1], Marc S. Hammer[1], Andreas D. Meid[2], Walter E. Müller[3], Ferdinand M. Gerlach[1] and Christiane Muth[1*]

Abstract

Background: Treatment complexity rises in line with the number of drugs, single doses, and administration methods, thereby threatening patient adherence. Patients with multimorbidity often need flexible, individualised treatment regimens, but alterations during the course of treatment may further increase complexity. The objective of our study was to explore medication changes in older patients with multimorbidity and polypharmacy in general practice.

Methods: We retrospectively analysed data from the cluster-randomised PRIMUM trial (PRIoritisation of MUltimedication in Multimorbidity) conducted in 72 general practices. We developed an algorithm for active pharmaceutical ingredients (API), strength, dosage, and administration method to assess changes in physician-reported medication data during two intervals (baseline to six-months: Δ_1; six- to nine-months: Δ_2), analysed them descriptively at prescription and patient levels, and checked for intervention effects.

Results: Of 502 patients (median age 72 years, 52% female), 464 completed the study. Changes occurred in 98.6% of patients (changes were 19% more likely in the intervention group): API changes during Δ_1 and Δ_2 occurred in 414 (82.5%) and 338 (67.3%) of patients, dosage alterations in 372 (74.1%) and 296 (59.2%), and changes in API strength in 158 (31.5%) and 138 (27.5%) respectively. Administration method changed in 79 (16%) of patients in both Δ_1 and Δ_2. Simvastatin, metformin and aspirin were most frequently subject to alterations.

Conclusion: Medication regimens in older patients with multimorbidity and polypharmacy changed frequently. These are mostly due to discontinuations and dosage alterations, followed by additions and restarts. These findings cast doubt on the effectiveness of cross-sectional assessments of medication and support longitudinal assessments where possible.

Keywords: Medication changes, Polypharmacy, Older adults, General practice, Multiple chronic conditions, Multimorbidity

* Correspondence: muth@allgemeinmedizin.uni-frankfurt.de
[1]Institute of General Practice, Johann Wolfgang Goethe University, Theodor-Stern-Kai 7, 60590 Frankfurt, Main, Germany
Full list of author information is available at the end of the article

Background

General practitioners (GPs) are confronted with older patients with multiple chronic diseases in up to 80% of their consultations, i.e. patients with multimorbidity [1, 2]. Multimorbidity is strongly associated with polypharmacy, most commonly defined as the regular use of five or more drugs [3]. Polypharmacy increases the risk of inappropriate prescriptions from drug misuse (e.g., drug-drug interactions, drug-disease interactions, and inappropriate dosages) and drug selection (overuse and underuse), and may result in hospitalisations, falls and related injuries, decreased quality of life, cognitive and physical dysfunction, loss of autonomy, and increased mortality as well as preventable health care spending [4–12]. The indiscriminate use of disease-specific treatment guidelines for patients suffering from multimorbidity and uncoordinated treatment by multiple physicians are drivers of polypharmacy and lead to complex medication regimens involving multiple drugs [13–15]. However, medication adherence in patients is inversely correlated with the number of drugs and the complexity of the medication regimen [16]. The higher the number of drugs and doses per day, pills per dosage, different administration methods and specific recommendations related to drug use, such as dietary recommendations, the greater is treatment complexity and burden, and the patient's inability to cope [14, 17, 18].

Medication changes over time may further increase treatment complexity because patients develop routines that enable them to manage their daily medication regimens, and adjusting them can be very troublesome for the chronically ill [19, 20]. On the other hand, medication changes often reflect patients' preferences, particularly when conditions are symptomatic. The assessment of patient priorities and shared decision making when evaluating and changing medication in older patients with multimorbidity have been identified as important [21–23]. From the physician's perspective, indications that an established drug regimen should be changed may be related to the development of new symptoms or worsening existing conditions, suspected medication-related adverse effects and because the treatment does not benefit the patient to the degree expected [24]. Particularly in patients with multimorbidity, evidence on effective treatment strategies is often lacking, and flexible and individualised pharmacotherapy is needed to meet their needs and preferences. As a result, GPs often rely on "hunches or best guesses" when deciding how to treat their patients [25]. Although, GPs frequently prefer to maintain the status quo once a patient appears to be stable [25], and are frequently reluctant to make changes to complex regimes, even if a potential problem has been identified [26, 27], their "hunches and best guesses" may lead to constant adaptation and frequent medication changes. Moreover, profound changes in a medication regimen are frequently made when patients are hospitalised and immediately thereafter. Newly introduced medication has not reached its steady state at discharge because inpatient care is frequently shorter than four to five half-lives of prescribed drugs, so that effectiveness and side-effects have not be properly assessed in hospital [28–30]. As variable discount contracts between pharmaceutical companies and statutory health insurers dictate the use of generic medicaments in Germany, changes may also be made in an attempt to reduce costs, rather than for medical reasons. Available consultation times apparently also influence prescribing behaviours. An average consultation time of less than seven minutes has been shown to be related to higher prescribing rates, whereas a consultation time of nine minutes or longer is associated with lower rates [31].

While all these determinants and consequences of prescribing behaviour and regimen complexity have been investigated in numerous cross-sectional studies, much less is known about how often medication regimens are changed over time, and what kind of changes older patients with multimorbidity and polypharmacy are faced with and have to manage. Improved insights into the number and nature of medication changes in this population may help strategies to be developed that avoid unnecessary medication changes. The goal of this study was therefore to explore changes in prescribed medication in older patients with multimorbidity and polypharmacy in primary care over a nine-month period.

Methods

Setting and population

We retrospectively assessed data from the pragmatic cluster-randomised controlled PRIMUM trial (PRIoritisation of MUltimedication in Multimorbidity) with the general practice as the unit of randomisation. The methods used in the PRIMUM trial are reported in detail elsewhere [32]. Briefly, the PRIMUM study evaluated the effectiveness of a complex intervention in improving medication appropriateness in comparison to usual care. The complex intervention consisted of four elements: the practice-based health care assistant (1) conducted a checklist-based interview with patients on medication-related problems and (2) reconciled their medications. (3) Assisted by a computerised decision-support system, the general practitioner optimised medication, and (4) discussed recommended changes with patients and adjusted medication regimens accordingly [32, 33]. Health care assistants in Germany receive less training than nurses, are comparable to certified medical assistants in the USA [34]. However, they have repeatedly and successfully carried out chronic care interventions that involve, for example, surveying patients by following protocols with fixed interview questions for conditions such as major depression, osteoarthritis and chronic heart failure, under the supervision of GPs [35–38].

Control practices continued with usual care. In usual care in Germany, patients regularly consult their GPs to discuss health problems, but, as GPs are not acting as 'gate keepers', may also contact ambulatory care specialists directly. Regular medication reviews were not conducted at the time of the study and health care for patients with chronic diseases has been characterized as fragmented and uncoordinated [39]. The presence of multiple conditions may have worsened the situation [40].

In total, 72 general practices located in the German state of Hesse participated in the PRIMUM trial. Of these practices, a random sample of 505 patients aged ≥60 years, with ≥3 chronic conditions for which they were treated with ≥5 drugs with systemic effects was included in the study. Patients were also required to be able to participate in telephone interviews, complete written questionnaires and provide written informed consent. Patients with cognitive impairment (Mini Mental State Exam < 26) and a life expectancy under 12 months were excluded. Patients' degree of multimorbidity was assessed at baseline using the Cumulative Illness Rating Scale (CIRS) [41, 42].

Measurement of medication changes

We assessed the number of changes to drugs, dosages and administration methods over a nine-month follow-up period. Data on prescribed medicines (active pharmaceutical ingredient (API) or trade name, dosage, and dosage form) were reported at baseline (T0), as well as six (T1), and nine (T2) months later. The first interval (Δ_1) was between baseline and the 6-month follow-up and the second interval (Δ_2) between the 6- and 9-month follow-ups.

At study visits, the attending health care assistant at the practice entered data on each participating patient into a paper-based case report form (CRF) and the GP checked the documentation before the CRF was sent to the study centre. At the study centre, a study assistant entered CRF data into an Access™ database where it was checked by another assistant. Based on an online database ("Gelbe Liste™"), an assistant coded the drugs according to API, strength, dosage form and a standardised package size of "N2" (generally containing the quantity of the drug required for 30 days of treatment) using the National Drug Code (PZN). PZN codes were converted into ATC codes, APIs, strengths, and dosage form automatically. Converted information was cross-checked against reported information for validation.

To explore medication changes in terms of medication usage, we adapted the algorithm suggested by Lam and co-workers [20]. We differentiated between changes (1) relating to API, (2) the strength of the API (amount of API per application unit e.g. tablet) (3) the dosage (the number of application units that make up the medication regimen) and (4) the administration method, reflecting the four main dimensions of a drug prescription (see Fig. 1).

API changes included the addition and discontinuation of drugs, restarts and intraclass-substitutions. Additions were medications that were present at one of the follow-up visits but were not reported before. Discontinuations referred to drugs that were mentioned previously but not reported at a later study visit. Restarts were drugs, which were discontinued between T0 and T1 but re-prescribed during the second interval (Δ_2). Intraclass substitutions were substitutions of a medicine by another drug of the same drug class, as reflected in the five-digit ATC-code. The strength of the API was changed if a higher or lower amount of the same API per unit of the medication was reported at one study visit compared to a previous one. The dosage was changed if the total daily dose (the amount of API per day) was increased or decreased, the application interval prolonged or shortened, and/or the application time altered between visits. The dosage was additionally modified when tablet splitting started or stopped. We measured changes to the administration method in accordance with the Medication Regimen Complexity Index (MRCI) [17]. CM assigned each of the 299 pharmaceutical dosage forms defined by the European Directorate for the Quality of Medicines & Health Care (EDQM) that were on the market at the time of the study to one of the 14 dosage forms used in the MRCI (immediate and extended release tablets, capsules, dragées, drops, liquids, effervescent tablets, sprays, ointments, plasters, metered-dose inhalers, syringes, suppositories, others). The classification was cross-checked by the clinical pharmacologist.

For medications with more than one active ingredient (combination drugs), we concentrated on changes in the active ingredient for the main indication of the drug. The main indication is represented by the three-digit ATC code describing the main therapeutic group for the particular medication. Changes in other active ingredients of combination drugs were not taken into consideration. FvB reviewed the medication changes of study participants. The algorithm was then applied electronically by MSH. Any disagreement was checked and corrected and the algorithm was refined where necessary.

Statistical analysis

Data were analysed descriptively on a patient level and on the level of prescriptions using STATA version SE 13. For this purpose, we collected prescription data on each patient from the physicians at each one of the three study visits (T0, T1, T2). Changes from one study visit to the next were assessed for both intervals (Δ_1, and Δ_2). A longitudinal prescription trajectory was developed for the prescriptions and study visits, with the patient's first

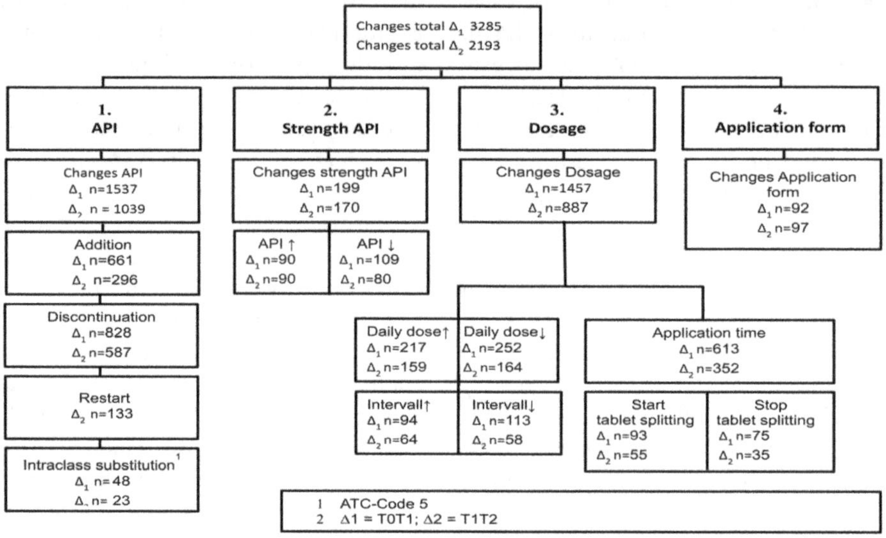

Fig. 1 Medication Changes at Prescribing Level. API: active pharmaceutical ingredient. [1]ATC-Code 5 digits. ATC: anatomical therapeutic chemical classification system. Interval Δ_1: baseline to six-month follow-up; interval Δ_2: six- to nine-month follow-ups

specific drug prescription as the reference (called *reference prescriptions* in the remainder of the article). The results are presented in absolute and relative numbers (percentages), means and standard deviations, or median and interquartile ranges (IQR).

The test for equal proportions was used to analyse changes and derive rate ratios between intervention and control groups. The Spearman correlation coefficient was used to analyse the relationship between the absolute numbers of medication changes in both time intervals.

The R software/environment version 3.3.2 (R Foundation for Statistical Computing, Vienna, Austria, 2016) was used for multivariate analyses and, in particular, to estimate and control for the intervention effect. Accounting for the clustering structure within GPs, a generalised linear mixed model was applied by the package *glmmADMB* [43]. Following an exploratory assessment of multi-collinearity and missing data patterns, the model was parameterised according to the independent variables *intervention status, age, sex* and respective changes in *number of previous hospital visits* at baseline, and the *Cumulative Illness Rating Scale (CIRS) summary score* between the follow-up visit and baseline. When modelling *total prescription* changes between study visits (T0, T1, T2), a negative binomial distribution provided the best fit to appropriately address overdispersion. Intra-cluster correlation (ICC) was obtained from the model in accordance with Aly and co-workers [44]. All tests were two-tailed. 95% confidence intervals (CI) were calculated, and P values < 0.05 were considered statistically significant.

Results

Of the 72 participating GP's, 41 worked in single-handed practices, and 31 in group practices. Their median age was 50 years (IQR 46.5–56), the majority was male (56.9%) and they had on average 23.5 years clinical experience (IQR 15.75–29).

We included 502 patients in our analyses (three had to be removed from the PRIMUM study population because they were younger than 60 at baseline), of whom 464 completed the study (see additional file 1). Their median age was 72 years (IQR 67–77), 52% of them were female (for patient' characteristics in intervention and control group, see Table 1). At baseline and the two follow-up visits, the sum of all prescriptions was 11,719 and the total number of reference prescriptions was 4999. The most commonly prescribed therapeutic subgroups were agents acting on the renin-angiotensin system (ATC code C09: $n = 514$ prescriptions accounting for 10% of reference prescriptions), drugs used in diabetes (A10: $n = 468$, 9%), antithrombotic agents (B01: $n = 409$, 8%), drugs acting on the lipid metabolism (C10: $n = 355$, 7%) and beta blocking agents (C07: 352, 7%). See also Table 2.

Medication changes at patient level

Cumulatively, 99% of patients showed at least one medication change over the nine-month period with a median of 9.5 (IQR 6–15) changes per patient. The maximum of medication changes was 21 (in one patient) during the six months of Δ_1 and 20 (in two patients) during the three months in Δ_2. The mean number of changes per patient was 6.5 (STD 4.3) in Δ_1 and 4.4 (STD 3.9) in Δ_2. The total number of drugs per patient

Table 1 Baseline characteristics of patients

Characteristics (median, IQR)[a]	Intervention group (*n* = 252)	Control group (*n* = 250)	Total (*N* = 502)
Age	72 (69–77)	72 (66–77)	72 (67–77)
Female sex (n, %)	133 (53%)	129 (52%)	262 (52%)
CIRS sum score	7 (5–11)	7 (4–10)	7 (4–11)
Number of prescriptions	8 (6–10)	8 (6–9)	8 (6–9)
MRCI	24 (17–36)	24 (18–33)	24 (18–34)

CIRS cumulative illness rating scale, *MRCI* medication regimen complexity index
[a]if not stated otherwise

remained relatively constant (the median number of prescriptions was 8 at all study visits, while the IQR was 6 to 9 at T0 and T1 and 6 to 10 at T2). (See Fig. 2).

The most frequent changes occurred in the active ingredient, the subcategories of which were addition, discontinuation, intraclass substitution and restart (Δ_2 only). The API was changed in 414 (83%) of the patients during Δ_1 and 338 (67%) during Δ_2 (in Δ_1 and Δ_2, the mean number of API changes per patient were 3.1 and 2.1 respectively). We observed up to eight additions per patient in both periods. The mean number of added drugs per patient was 1.3 (STD 1.5) during Δ_1 and 0.6 (STD 1.0) during Δ_2. Patients had discontinued up to 15 drugs in Δ_1 and 16 in Δ_2, with a mean number of de-prescribed drugs per patient of 1.6 (STD 1.9) in Δ_1 and 1.7 (STD 2.0) in Δ_2.

Changes in the strength of the API occurred in 158 (32%) patients in Δ_1 and 138 (28%) patients in Δ_2 (in Δ_1 and Δ_2, mean change per patient was 0.4 (STD 0.65) and 0.3 (STD 0.61) respectively). Dosages were altered in 372 (74%) patients in Δ_1 and in 296 (59.2%) patients in Δ_2. The mean number of dosage changes per patient was 2.9 (STD 2.87) and 1.8 (STD 2.21) respectively (Table 3).

There was no statistical correlation between medication changes in Δ_1 and Δ_2 with correlation coefficients indicating weak relationships, if any (Spearman correlation coefficient for overall medication changes between Δ_1 and Δ_2 was 0.321 and 0.005 between discontinuations in Δ_1 and any changes in Δ_2). The multivariate model showed that more medication changes occurred in the intervention group. We compared both groups and found 19% more medication changes in the intervention group (95% CI [0.3%; 41%], $P = 0.0046$), which was the only significant factor in the multiple regression model. It is noteworthy that an ICC of 0.146 was observed. Univariate analyses showed that the reduction in the dosage was slightly greater but significantly so in the intervention group compared to the control group but no further significant differences in the various types of medication changes were found between both groups (Table 3).

Table 2 Most commonly prescribed medicines

Chemical subgroup[b] / Most prevalent active pharmaceutical ingredient (API)[c]	Absolute and relative frequency of prescriptions[a] (n, %)
Platelet aggregation inhibitors excl. Heparin (B01AC):	323 (6.5%)
Acetylsalicylic acid (B01AC06)	261 (5.2%)
Beta blocking agents, selective (C07AB):	297 (5.9%)
Bisoprolol (C07AB07)	135 (2.7%)
Metoprolol (C07AB02)	128 (2.6%)
HMG CoA reductase inhibitors (C10AA)	297 (5.9%)
Simvastatin (C01AA01)	256 (5.1%)
Proton pump inhibitors (A02BC)	231 (4.6%)
Omeprazole (A02BC01)	126 (2.5%)
Pantoprazole (A02BC02)	93 (1.9%)
ACE inhibitors, plain (C09AA)	218 (4.4%)
Ramipril (C09AA05)	139 (2.8%)
Dihydropyridine derivatives (C08CA)	208 (4.2%)
Amlodipine (C08CA01)	148 (3.0%)
Sulfonamides, plain (C03CA)	176 (3.5%)
Torasemide (C03CA04)	133 (2.7%)
Thyroid hormones (H03AA)	159 (3.2%)
Levothyroxine (H03AA01)	119 (2.4%)
Biguanides (A10BA)	131 (2.6%)
Metformin (A10BA02)	131 (2.6%)
Preparations inhibiting uric acid production (M04AA)	123 (2.5%)
Allopurinol (M04AA01)	120 (2.4%)
Angiotensin II antagonists, plain (C09CA)	117 (2.3%)
Candesartan (C09CA06)	40 (0.8%)
Low-Ceiling Diuretics, Thiazides, plain (C03AA)	97 (1.9%)
Hydrochlorothiazide (C03AA03)	97 (1.9%)
Selective beta-2-adrenoreceptor agonists (R03AC)	95 (1.9%)
Salbutamol (R03AC02)	46 (0.9%)

[a]Relative frequency: absolute numbers of prescriptions with regard to the total number of reference prescriptions (*N* = 4999)
[b]according to the 4th level, chemical subgroup (5-digit ATC code)
[c]according to the 5th level, chemical substance (7-digit ATC code)

Medication changes at prescribing level

The analysis of the medication included $N = 4999$ reference prescriptions. In total, we detected $N = 5478$ cumulative changes in these reference prescriptions during the nine-month follow-up. Figure 1 shows the distribution of changes in reference prescriptions, as determined using our algorithm. The mean number of changes per reference prescription was 1.09 (STD 1.2). The most frequently changed drugs in our older study population with multimorbidity

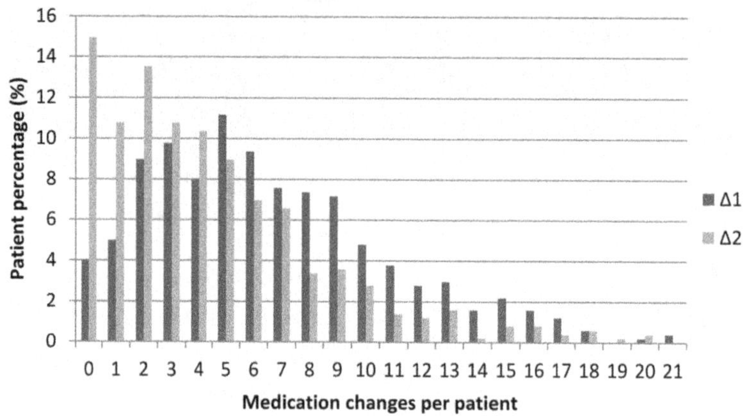

Fig. 2 Medication Changes at Patient Level. Interval Δ1: baseline to six-month follow-up; interval Δ2: six- to nine-month follow-ups

were simvastatin (mostly, a change in the strength of API, an increase or decrease of dosage, a change in the application time and starting or stopping tablet splitting), low dose aspirin (addition, discontinuation and restart as well as changes in time of application), metformin (application interval and time, and decrease in dosage), omeprazole (intraclass substitution of pantoprazole or esomeprazole) and ramipril (strength of API and application interval; see Table 4). Most of the restarts (after previous discontinuation) were seen in low dose aspirin, metoprolol, HCT, ramipril and diclofenac.

Discussion

Key findings

In our study population of older patients with multimorbidity and polypharmacy, more than three quarters of prescriptions was modified within six months (Δ_1) and another half in the three months thereafter (Δ_2). According to our algorithm, changes occurred in all categories, with changes in API (83%) the most common, and changes in administration method (16%) the least. The API was most often changed through discontinuation (in more than two thirds of the patients at least one drug was stopped during Δ_1 and in almost half the patients during Δ_2). However, our data also showed that at least one third of previously discontinued drugs were restarted (we could only measure restarts in the second period, Δ_2). Furthermore, the number of dosage alterations was high and observed in 82% of patients. Despite such high levels of prescribing and de-prescribing, the total number of medications per patient remained remarkably constant. This finding supports the general view that drug numbers barely reflect prescription appropriateness [45, 46]. In order to optimise a patient's medication, it can be warranted both to stop (i.e., de-prescribe) unnecessary drugs and to start taking indicated drugs [47].

On a prescription level, our research revealed that the most frequent modifications occurred in simvastatin and low-dose aspirin, which are both drugs that should be prescribed in relatively fixed doses in the treatment (or prevention) of chronic conditions. Changes in dosage were the most frequently observed modifications in both drugs. In the case of simvastatin, presumed or actual common side effects (myalgia) [48] may have encouraged the treating physician to replace the statin with an intermittent or pulsed dosing regimen [49], or to slowly increase doses in highly intolerant patients [50]. Restarts of metoprolol, ramipril, diuretics or diclofenac may have been decided when underlying health problems exacerbated and precluded a discontinuation or withdrawal symptoms occurred [51]. The intraclass substitution of pantoprazole for omeprazole may reflect the reduced likelihood of drug-drug interactions in pantoprazole [52]. Other frequent modifications, such as discontinuation or dosage alterations in diuretics or anti-diabetics are easier to interpret, but the reasons behind changes were not documented in our study.

Comparison with literature

The basic pattern of medication changes in our study was consistent with a previous observation study on older patients with multimorbidity and polypharmacy which also identified frequent starting, stopping and dosage changes [20]. However, the proportion of patients whose medication regimen was modified was higher in our study than in the previous one, in which additions were observed in 61%, discontinuations in 58%, dose changes in 51% and restarts in 21% of patients [20]. The differences may reflect different study designs and data collection methods. While we collected primary data from GPs in a polypharmacy study on medication optimisation, Lam et al. analysed claims data [20]. In our analysis, the intervention slightly increased the rate at which changes were made in the intervention group. In de-prescribing trials in community-dwelling elderly patients, 47% [53] and 48% [54] of patients reported at

Table 3 Medication changes at patient level

	Δ1 (baseline to 6-month follow-up)				Δ2 (6-month follow-up to 9-month follow-up)			
	Intervention group (IG) (n = 252)	Control group (CG) (n = 250)	Total (N = 502)	Proportion difference IG vs. CG (95% CI)	Intervention group (IG) (n = 252)	Control group (CG) (n = 250)	Total (N = 502)	Proportion difference IG vs. CG (95% CI)
API								
Addition	160 (63%)	153 (61%)	313 (62%)	0.02 (−0.07;0.11) *P* = 0.661	93 (37%)	88 (35%)	181 (36%)	0.02 (− 0.07;0.11) *P* = 0.761
Discontinuation	176 (70%)	161 (64%)	337 (67%)	0.05 (− 0.03;0.14) *P* = 0.229	119 (47%)	129 (52%)	248 (49%)	−0.04 (− 0.14;0.05) *P* = 0.373
Intraclass substitution	23 (9%)	18 (7%)	41 (8.2%)	0.02 (− 0.03;0.07) *P* = 0.532	14 (6%)	7 (3%)	21 (4%)	0.03 (− 0.01;0.07), *P* = 0.187
Restart of previously discontinued drugs	–	–	–	n.a.	51/176 (29%)	53/161 (30%)	104/337 (31%)	− 0.01 (− 0.08;0.07), *P* = 0.876
Strength of the API								
Increase	46 (18%)	36 (14%)	82 (16%)	0.04 (− 0.03;0.11) *P* = 0.295	45 (18%)	35 (14%)	80 (16%)	0.04 (−0.03;0.11), *P* = 0.29
Decrease	44 (17%)	49 (20%)	93 (19%)	−0.02 (− 0.09;0.05), *P* = 0.616	31 (12%)	37 (15%)	70 (14%)	− 0.02 (− 0.09;0.04), *P* = 0.492
Dosage								
Daily dosage increase	91 (36%)	80 (32%)	171 (34%)	0.04 (− 0.05;0.13), *P* = 0.38	67 (27%)	61 (24%)	128 (26%)	0.02 (−0.06;0.1), *P* = 0.646
Daily dosage decrease	106 (42%)	79 (32%)	185 (37%)	*0.1 (0.02;0.19), P = 0.019**	72 (29%)	58 (23%)	130 (26%)	0.05 (− 0.03;0.13), *P* = 0.203
Application interval shortened	55 (22%)	42 (17%)	97 (19%)	0.05 (− 0.02;0.12), *P* = 0.189	32 (13%)	20 (8%)	52 (10%)	0.05 (− 0.01;0.1), *P* = 0.114
Application interval prolonged	48 (19%)	35 (14%)	83 (17%)	0.05 (− 0.02;0.12), *P* = 0.161	28 (11%)	26 (10%)	54 (11%)	0.01 (−0.05;0.07), *P* = 0.91
Change in application time point	145 (58%)	155 (62%)	300 (60%)	− 0.04 (− 0.13;0.05), *P* = 0.353	98 (39%)	118 (47%)	216 (45%)	− 0.08 (− 0.17;0.01), *P* = 0.073
Pill splitting started	43 (17%)	35 (14%)	78 (16%)	0.03 (−0.04;0.1), *P* = 0.41	23 (9%)	19 (8%)	42 (8%)	0.02 (− 0.04;0.07), *P* = 0.648
Pill splitting stopped	30 (12%)	35 (14%)	65 (13%)	−0.02 (− 0.08;0.04), *P* = 0.571	13 (5%)	18 (7%)	31 (6%)	− 0.02 (− 0.07;0.03), *P* = 0.445
Administration method								
Change in administration method	47 (19%)	32 (13%)	79 (16%)	0.06 (− 0.01;0.13), *P* = 0.093	37 (15%)	42 (17%)	79 (16%)	−0.02 (− 0.09;0.05), *P* = 0.597

API active pharmaceutical ingredient
*Difference between intervention group and control group was statistically significant

Table 4 Most frequently changed drugs

Interval Δ_1 (baseline to 6 month follow-up)				Interval Δ_2 (6-month follow-up to 9-month follow-up)			
Intervention group		Control group		Intervention group		Control group	
Drug	Changes in Δ_1 / total prescriptions at T0[a] (n / N, %)	Drug	Changes in Δ_1 / total prescriptions at T0[a] (n / N, %)	Drug	Changes in Δ_2 / total prescriptions at T1[a] (n / N, %)	Drug	Changes in Δ_2 / total prescriptions at T1[a] (n / N, %)
Simvastatin	75 / 104 (72%)	Simvastatin	90 / 128 (70%)	Aspirin*	40 / 108 (37%)	Simvastatin	72 / 121 (60%)
Ramipril	70 / 67 (104%)	Aspirin*	58 / 126 (46%)	Omeprazole	39 / 48 (81%)	Aspirin*	50 / 122 (41%)
Metformin	63 / 61 (103%)	Metformin	49 / 57 (86%)	Simvastatin	38 / 107 (35%)	Metformin	39 / 50 (78%)
Amlodipine	63 / 76 (83%)	Allopurinol	43 / 47 (91%)	Ramipril	37 / 64 (56%)	Omeprazole	34 / 52 (65%)
Metoprolol*	59 / 69 (85%)	Amlodipine	40 / 57 (70%)	Metformin	34 / 60 (57%)	Torasemide	33 / 50 (66%)
Bisoprolol	58 / 62 (93%)	Pantoprazole	39 / 33 (118%)	Torasemide	34 / 57 (60%)	Metoprolol*	31 / 49 (63%)
Omeprazole	54 / 55 (98%)	Bisoprolol	39 / 65 (60%)	Pantoprazole	29 / 31 (93%)	Ramipril	29 / 58 (50%)
Aspirin*	53 / 105 (50%)	Metoprolol*	38 / 54 (70%)	Allopurinol	28 / 44 (64%)	Pantoprazole	28 / 29 (96%)
Torasemide	45 / 52 (87%)	Ramipril	38 / 54 (70%)	Metoprolol*	27 / 67 (40%)	Amlodipine	25 / 53 (47%)
Allopurinol	45 / 53 (85%)	Omeprazole	37 / 50 (74%)	Amlodipine	25 / 70 (36%)	Bisoprolol	24 / 62 (39%)
Levothyroxine	40 / 55 (73%)	Torasemide	37 / 55 (67%)	Bisoprolol	18 / 63 (29%)	Allopurinol	23 / 44 (52%)
Pantoprazole	37 / 30 (123%)	HCT	24 / 40 (60%)	Diclofenac	17 / 34 (50%)	Diclofenac	22 / 12 (183%)
Diclofenac	33 / 36 (92%)	Levothyroxine	23 / 55 (42%)	Ca + D3	16 / 14 (114%)	HCT	20 / 37 (54%)

[†]number of changed prescriptions during the interval per number of prescriptions at the begin of the interval, percentages > 100% indicate prescriptions with more than one change during the interval under investigation. API – active pharmaceutical ingredient, Aspirin* - low dose aspirin, Ca + D3 – combination of calcium and cholecalciferol (vitamin D3), HCT – hydrochlorothiazide, Metoprolol* - metoprolol-succinate

least one discontinuation and the average was 4.2 per patient [53]. In studies conducted in nursing homes, drugs were withdrawn in 59% [55] and 63% [56] of patients (on average 4.4 and 2.8 per patient respectively). However, no other medication changes were reported in these studies.

Strengths & Limitations

The robust design of the pragmatic cluster-randomised controlled PRIMUM trial was a major strength. This is particularly reflected in the random sample of patients per practice, the collection of primary data, the quality assurance and validation of medication data, the stepwise development and forward-backward validation of the algorithm to explore medication changes and its application by two independent researchers. This allowed a rich exploratory approach to the number and pattern of medication changes in older patients with multimorbidity and polypharmacy and the extension of the algorithm provided by Lam et al. to include the patient's perspective [20]. However, the study design was also a limitation because the intention of the intervention was to identify and change inappropriate medication regimens. The vast majority of patients included in the PRIMUM study received appropriate prescriptions according to the Medication Appropriateness Index (MAI) [57] and reported good quality of life and functional status. The intervention had no effect on primary and secondary outcomes [32], but medication changes did slightly increase (according to the multivariate model, 19% more frequently in the intervention group, with slightly more dosage reductions). The MAI does not reliably detect underuse [58] and our ratings may have missed also inappropriateness. Furthermore, the PRIMUM study included three measuring points over a period of nine months, which resulted in a series of cross-sectional measurements rather than continuous documentation, so we may have missed a number of medication changes between study visits and our results may therefore be rather conservative.

Implication

Our results illustrate that medication regimens in older patients with multimorbidity and polypharmacy are relatively unstable, and this has major implications. Firstly, future analyses should seek to discriminate appropriate from inappropriate, planned vs. ad hoc changes and examine changes in high-risk drugs, as these are more likely to be clinically significant for patients [59]. For clinicians and patients, it is of interest whether frequent medication changes increase longitudinal complexity and whether this affects patient adherence and health care costs in developing strategies to avoid unnecessary alterations in medication regimens in elderly, chronically ill patients with multimorbidity. Secondly, our findings pose fundamental methodological questions with respect to polypharmacy studies (no matter whether observational or interventional): how reliable are cross-sectional measurements of medication in this population, and what are suitable measurement intervals? Future studies should assess longitudinal changes so that researchers in the field can select appropriate study intervals.

Conclusion

Medication regimens in older patients with multimorbidity and polypharmacy change frequently. Most of the changes are discontinuations and dosage alterations followed by additional prescriptions and restarts. Modifications also include drugs, such as statins and low-dose aspirins, that are intended for prescription in relatively fixed dosages in the treatment of chronic conditions. These findings cast doubt on the effectiveness of cross-sectional assessments of medication (appropriateness) and support longitudinal assessments where possible. Dedicated future studies should longitudinally assess changes in medication regimens and seek to explain them. They should also study their effect on patient adherence.

Abbreviations

API: Active pharmaceutical ingredient; ATC: Anatomical therapeutic chemical classification system; CIRS: Cumulative illness rating scale; CRF: Case report form; EDQM: European Directorate for the Quality of Medicines & Health Care; GP: General practitioner; IQR: Interquartile range; MRCI: Medication regimen complexity index; PRIMUM: PRIoritisation of MUltimedication in Multimorbidity; PZN: National Drug Code; STD: Standard deviation

Acknowledgements

The authors would like to thank Sandra Heller and Zeycan Hezer-Albay for assistance and help with data processing.

Funding

Funding was provided by the German Federal Ministry of Education and Research, BMBF, grant numbers 01GK0702 and 01GY1320B. The funder had no role in study design, data collection and analysis, decision to publish, or preparation of the manuscript. The views expressed in this paper are those of the authors and not necessarily those of the funders.

Authors' contributions

FvB, WEM, FMG and CM designed the study. FvB, MSH, ADM and CM analysed the data. All authors contributed to the interpretation of the data. FvB and CM drafted the manuscript and all authors revised it critically for important intellectual content. All authors approved the version to be submitted for publication. FvB and CM had full access to all data and are responsible for the integrity and the accuracy of the data analysis.

Consent for publication

Not applicable.

Competing interests

FMG and CM report grants from German Federal Ministry of Education and Research, BMBF, grant no. 01GK0702, during the conduct of the PRIMUM study. ADM report grants from German Federal Ministry of Education and Research, BMBF, grant no. 01GY1320B, during the conduct of the PRIMUM study. FvB, MSH and WEM declared no conflicts of interest.

Author details

[1]Institute of General Practice, Johann Wolfgang Goethe University, Theodor-Stern-Kai 7, 60590 Frankfurt, Main, Germany. [2]Department of Clinical Pharmacology and Pharmacoepidemiology, University of Heidelberg, Im Neuenheimer Feld 410, 69120 Heidelberg, Germany. [3]Pharmacological Institute for Natural Scientists, Johann Wolfgang Goethe University, Max-von-Laue-Str. 9, 60438 Frankfurt am Main, Germany.

References

1. Salisbury C, Johnson L, Purdy S, Valderas JM, Montgomery AA. Epidemiology and impact of multimorbidity in primary care: a retrospective cohort study. Br J Gen Pract. 2011;61(582):e12–21.
2. van den Akker M, Buntinx F, Knottnerus J. Comorbidity or multimorbidity: what's in a name. A review of literature. Eur J Gen Pract. 1996;2:65–70.
3. Masnoon N, Shakib S, Kalisch-Ellett L, Caughey GE. What is polypharmacy? A systematic review of definitions. BMC Geriatr. 2017;17(1):230.
4. Campbell SE, Seymour DG, Primrose WR, Lynch JE, Dunstan E, Espallargues M, Lamura G, Lawson P, Philp I, Mestheneos E, et al. A multi-Centre European study of factors affecting the discharge destination of older people admitted to hospital: analysis of in-hospital data from the ACMEplus project. Age Ageing. 2005;34(5):467–75.
5. Davies EC, Green CF, Taylor S, Williamson PR, Mottram DR, Pirmohamed M. Adverse drug reactions in hospital in-patients: a prospective analysis of 3695 patient-episodes. PLoS One. 2009;4(2):e4439.
6. Deandrea S, Lucenteforte E, Bravi F, Foschi R, La VC, Negri E. Risk factors for falls in community-dwelling older people: a systematic review and meta-analysis. Epidemiology. 2010;21(5):658–68.
7. Grimmsmann T, Himmel W. Polypharmacy in primary care practices: an analysis using a large health insurance database. Pharmacoepidemiol Drug Saf. 2009;18(12):1206–13.
8. Hakkarainen KM, Gyllensten H, Jonsson AK, Andersson SK, Petzold M, Hagg S. Prevalence, nature and potential preventability of adverse drug events - a population-based medical record study of 4970 adults. Br J Clin Pharmacol. 2014;78(1):170–83.
9. Meid AD, Quinzler R, Groll A, Wild B, Saum KU, Schottker B, Heider D, Konig HH, Brenner H, Haefeli WE. Longitudinal evaluation of medication underuse in older outpatients and its association with quality of life. Eur J Clin Pharmacol. 2016;72(7):877–85.
10. Pirmohamed M, James S, Meakin S, Green C, Scott AK, Walley TJ, Farrar K, Park BK, Breckenridge AM. Adverse drug reactions as cause of admission to hospital: prospective analysis of 18 820 patients. BMJ. 2004;329(7456):15–9.
11. Thomson LA, Winterstein AG, Sondergaard B, Haugbolle LS, Melander A. Systematic review of the incidence and characteristics of preventable adverse drug events in ambulatory care. Ann Pharmacother. 2007;41(9):1411–26.
12. Viktil KK, Blix HS, Moger TA, Reikvam A. Polypharmacy as commonly defined is an indicator of limited value in the assessment of drug-related problems. Br J Clin Pharmacol. 2007;63(2):187–95.
13. Boyd CM, Darer J, Boult C, Fried LP, Boult L, Wu AW. Clinical practice guidelines and quality of care for older patients with multiple comorbid diseases: implications for pay for performance. JAMA. 2005;294(6):716–24.
14. Muir AJ, Sanders LL, Wilkinson WE, Schmader K. Reducing medication regimen complexity: a controlled trial. J Gen Intern Med. 2001;16(2):77–82.
15. Rambhade S, Chakarborty A, Shrivastava A, Patil UK, Rambhade A. A survey on polypharmacy and use of inappropriate medications. Toxicol Int. 2012; 19(1):68–73.
16. Horne R, Weinman J, Barber N, Elliott R, Morgan M, Cribb A, I K: Concordance, adherence and compliance in medicine taking. *National Coordinating Centre for the Service Delivery and Organisation (NCCSDO)* 2005. URL: http://www.netscc.ac.uk/hsdr/files/project/SDO_FR_08-1412-076_V01.pdf; Accessed: 08/07/2018.
17. George J, Phun YT, Bailey MJ, Kong DC, Stewart K. Development and validation of the medication regimen complexity index. Ann Pharmacother. 2004;38(9):1369–76.
18. Stone VE, Hogan JW, Schuman P, Rompalo AM, Howard AA, Korkontzelou C, Smith DK. Antiretroviral regimen complexity, self-reported adherence, and HIV patients' understanding of their regimens: survey of women in the her study. J Acquir Immune Defic Syndr. 2001;28(2):124–31.
19. Haslbeck JW, Schaeffer D. Routines in medication management: the perspective of people with chronic conditions. Chronic Illn. 2009;5(3):184–96.

20. Lam KD, Miao Y, Steinman MA. Cumulative changes in the use of long-term medications: a measure of prescribing complexity. JAMA Intern Med. 2013; 173(16):1546–7.
21. Muth C, van den Akker M, Blom JW, Mallen CD, Rochon J, Schellevis FG, Becker A, Beyer M, Gensichen J, Kirchner H, et al. The Ariadne principles: how to handle multimorbidity in primary care consultations. BMC Med. 2014;12:223.
22. NICE: Multimorbidity: clinical assessment and management. Multimorbidity: assessment, prioritisation and management of care for people with commonly occurring multimorbidity. NICE guideline NG56. National Institute for Health and Care Excellence. 2016. URL: https://www.nice.org.uk/guidance/ng56/evidence; Accessed: 08/07/2018.
23. Spinewine A, Schmader KE, Barber N, Hughes C, Lapane KL, Swine C, Hanlon JT. Appropriate prescribing in elderly people: how well can it be measured and optimised? Lancet. 2007;370(9582):173–84.
24. Bain KT, Holmes HM, Beers MH, Maio V, Handler SM, Pauker SG. Discontinuing medications: a novel approach for revising the prescribing stage of the medication-use process. J Am Geriatr Soc. 2008;56(10):1946–52.
25. Sinnott C, Hugh SM, Boyce MB, Bradley CP. What to give the patient who has everything? A qualitative study of prescribing for multimorbidity in primary care. Br J Gen Pract. 2015;65(632):e184–91.
26. Anderson K, Stowasser D, Freeman C, Scott I. Prescriber barriers and enablers to minimising potentially inappropriate medications in adults: a systematic review and thematic synthesis. BMJ Open. 2014;4(12):e006544.
27. Sinnott C, McHugh S, Browne J, Bradley C. GPs' perspectives on the management of patients with multimorbidity: systematic review and synthesis of qualitative research. BMJ Open. 2013;3(9):e003610.
28. Bergert FW, Braun M, Ehrenthal K, Fessler J, Gross J, Huttner U, Kluthe B, Liesenfeld A, Seffrin J, Vetter G, et al. Recommendations for treating adult and geriatric patients on multimedication. Int J Clin Pharmacol Ther. 2014; 52(Suppl 1):1–64.
29. Grimmsmann T, Schwabe U, Himmel W. The influence of hospitalisation on drug prescription in primary care--a large-scale follow-up study. Eur J Clin Pharmacol. 2007;63(8):783–90.
30. Larsen MD, Rosholm JU, Hallas J. The influence of comprehensive geriatric assessment on drug therapy in elderly patients. Eur J Clin Pharmacol. 2014; 70(2):233–9.
31. Wilson A, Childs S. The relationship between consultation length, process and outcomes in general practice: a systematic review. Br J Gen Pract. 2002; 52(485):1012–20.
32. Muth C, Uhlmann L, Haefeli WE, Rochon J, van den AM PR, Guthlin C, Beyer M, Oswald F, Valderas JM, et al. effectiveness of a complex intervention on Prioritising multimedication in multimorbidity (PRIMUM) in primary care: results of a pragmatic cluster randomised controlled trial. BMJ Open. 2018; 8(2):e017740.
33. Muth C, Harder S, Uhlmann L, Rochon J, Fullerton B, Guthlin C, Erler A, Beyer M, van den AM PR, et al. pilot study to test the feasibility of a trial design and complex intervention on PRIoritising MUltimedication in multimorbidity in general practices (PRIMUMpilot). BMJ Open. 2016; 6(7):e011613.
34. Bosley S, Dale J. Healthcare assistants in general practice: practical and conceptual issues of skill-mix change. *Br J Gen Pract*. 2008;58(547):118–24.
35. Gensichen J, von Korff M, Peitz M, Muth C, Beyer M, Guthlin C, Torge M, Petersen JJ, Rosemann T, Konig J, et al. Case management for depression by health care assistants in small primary care practices: a cluster randomized trial. Ann Intern Med. 2009;151(6):369–78.
36. Peters-Klimm F, Muller-Tasch T, Schellberg D, Gensichen J, Muth C, Herzog W, Szecsenyi J. Rationale, design and conduct of a randomised controlled trial evaluating a primary care-based complex intervention to improve the quality of life of heart failure patients: HICMan (Heidelberg integrated case management). BMC Cardiovasc Disord. 2007;7:25.
37. Rosemann T, Joos S, Laux G, Gensichen J, Szecsenyi J. Case management of arthritis patients in primary care: a cluster-randomized controlled trial. Arthritis Rheum. 2007;57(8):1390–7.
38. Rosemann T, Korner T, Wensing M, Gensichen J, Muth C, Joos S, Szecsenyi J. Rationale, design and conduct of a comprehensive evaluation of a primary care based intervention to improve the quality of life of osteoarthritis patients. The PraxArt-project: a cluster randomized controlled trial [ISRCTN87252339]. BMC Public Health. 2005;5:77.
39. Gensichen J, Muth C, Butzlaff M, Rosemann T, Raspe H, de Cornejo GM, Beyer M, Harter M, Muller UA, Angermann CE, et al. the future is chronic: German primary care and the chronic care model--the comprehensive principles in the proactive treatment of the chronically ill. Z Arztl Fortbild Qualitatssich. 2006;100(5):365–74.
40. Beyer M, Otterbach I, Erler A, Muth C, Gensichen J, Gerlach FM. Multimorbidität in der Allgemeinpraxis. Teil 1: Pragmatische definition, Epidemiologie und Versorgungsprämissen. [multimorbidity in general practice. Part I: a pragmatic definition, epidemiology, prerequisites of care.]. Z Allgemeinmed. 2007;83(8):310–5.
41. Hudon C, Fortin M, Soubhi H. Abbreviated guidelines for scoring the cumulative illness rating scale (CIRS) in family practice. J Clin Epidemiol. 2007;60(2):212.
42. Linn BS, Linn MW, Gurel L. Cumulative illness rating scale. J Am Geriatr Soc. 1968;16(5):622–6.
43. Fournier DA, Skaug HJ, Ancheta J, Ianelli J, Magnusson A, Maunder MN, Nielsen A, Sibert J. AD model builder: using automatic differentiation for statistical inference of highly parameterized complex nonlinear models. Optim Methods Softw. 2012;27(2):233–49.
44. Aly SS, Zhao J, Li B, Jiang J. Reliability of environmental sampling culture results using the negative binomial intraclass correlation coefficient. Springerplus. 2014;3:40.
45. Cadogan CA, Ryan C, Hughes CM. Appropriate polypharmacy and medicine safety: when many is not too many. Drug Saf. 2016;39(2):109–16.
46. Cooper JA, Cadogan CA, Patterson SM, Kerse N, Bradley MC, Ryan C, Hughes CM. Interventions to improve the appropriate use of polypharmacy in older people: a Cochrane systematic review. BMJ Open. 2015;5(12):e009235.
47. Meid AD, Haefeli WE. Age-dependent impact of medication underuse and strategies for improvement. Gerontology. 2016;62(5):491–9.
48. Rossello X, Pocock SJ, Julian DG. Long-term use of cardiovascular drugs: challenges for research and for patient care. J Am Coll Cardiol. 2015; 66(11):1273–85.
49. Backes JM, Ruisinger JF, Gibson CA, Moriarty PM. Statin-associated muscle symptoms-managing the highly intolerant. J Clin Lipidol. 2017;11(1):24–33.
50. Stulc T, Ceska R, Gotto AM Jr. Statin intolerance: the Clinician's perspective. Curr Atheroscler Rep. 2015;17(12):69.
51. Scott IA, Gray LC, Martin JH, Pillans PI, Mitchell CA. Deciding when to stop: towards evidence-based deprescribing of drugs in older populations. Evid Based Med. 2013;18(4):121–4.
52. Furtado RH, Giugliano RP, Strunz CM, Filho CC, Ramires JA, Filho RK, Neto PA, Pereira AC, Rocha TR, Freire BT, et al. Drug interaction between Clopidogrel and ranitidine or omeprazole in stable coronary artery disease: a double-blind, double dummy, Randomized Study. *Am J Cardiovasc Drugs*. 2016;16(4):275–84.
53. Garfinkel D, Mangin D. Feasibility study of a systematic approach for discontinuation of multiple medications in older adults: addressing polypharmacy. Arch Intern Med. 2010;170(18):1648–54.
54. van der Velde N, Stricker BH, Pols HA, van der Cammen TJ. Risk of falls after withdrawal of fall-risk-increasing drugs: a prospective cohort study. Br J Clin Pharmacol. 2007;63(2):232–7.
55. Potter K, Flicker L, Page A, Etherton-Beer C. Deprescribing in frail older people: a randomised controlled trial. PLoS One. 2016;11(3):e0149984.
56. Garfinkel D, Zur-Gil S, Ben-Israel J. The war against polypharmacy: a new cost-effective geriatric-palliative approach for improving drug therapy in disabled elderly people. Isr Med Assoc J. 2007;9(6):430–4.
57. Hanlon JT, Schmader KE, Samsa GP, Weinberger M, Uttech KM, Lewis IK, Cohen HJ, Feussner JR. A method for assessing drug therapy appropriateness. J Clin Epidemiol. 1992;45(10):1045–51.
58. Hanlon JT, Schmader KE. The medication appropriateness index at 20: where it started, where it has been, and where it may be going. Drugs Aging. 2013;30(11):893–900.
59. Howard RL, Avery AJ, Slavenburg S, Royal S, Pipe G, Lucassen P, Pirmohamed M. Which drugs cause preventable admissions to hospital? A systematic review. Br J Clin Pharmacol. 2007;63(2):136–47.

Access to primary and specialized somatic health care for persons with severe mental illness: a qualitative study of perceived barriers and facilitators in Swedish health care

Elisabeth Björk Brämberg[1,2*], Jarl Torgerson[3], Anna Norman Kjellström[4], Peder Welin[5] and Marie Rusner[6,7]

Abstract

Background: Persons with severe mental illness (e.g. schizophrenia, bipolar disorder) have a high prevalence of somatic conditions compared to the general population. Mortality data in the Nordic countries reveal that these persons die 15–20 years earlier than the general population. Some factors explaining this high prevalence may be related to the individuals in question; others arise from the health care system's difficulty in offering somatic health care to these patient groups. The aim of the present study was therefore to explore the experiences and views of patients, relatives and clinicians regarding individual and organizational factors which facilitate or hinder access to somatic health care for persons with severe mental illness.

Methods: Flexible qualitative design. Data was collected by means of semi-structured individual interviews with patients with severe mental illness, relatives and clinicians representing primary and specialized health care. In all, 50 participants participated.

Results: The main barrier to accessing somatic care is the gap between the organization of the health care system and the patients' individual health care needs. This is observed at both individual and organizational level. The health care system seems unable to support patients with severe mental illness and their psychiatric-somatic comorbidity. The main facilitators are the links between severe mental illness patients and medical departments. These links take the form of functions (i.e. systems which ensure that patients receive regular reminders), or persons (i.e. professional contacts who facilitate patients' access the health care).

Conclusions: Health care services for patients with severe mental illness need reorganization. Organizational structures and systems that facilitate cooperation between different departments must be put in place, along with training for health care professionals about somatic disease among psychiatric patients. The links between individual and organizational levels could be strengthened by introducing professional contacts, such as liaison physicians and case managers. This is also important to reduce stress and responsibility among relatives.

Keywords: Barriers and facilitators, Health services accessibility, Qualitative research, Semi-structured interviews, Severe mental illness

* Correspondence: Elisabeth.bjork.bramberg@ki.se
[1]Unit of Intervention and Implementation Research for Worker Health, Institute of Environmental Medicine, Karolinska institutet, 171 77 Stockholm, Sweden
[2]Närhälsan Eriksberg Primary Health Care Centre, Sjöporten 4, 417 64 Göteborg, Sweden
Full list of author information is available at the end of the article

Background

Persons with severe mental illness (SMI), defined as schizophrenia, bipolar disorder and psychosis, have a high prevalence of somatic medical conditions compared to the general population [1]. Mortality data for persons with SMI in the Nordic countries (Denmark, Finland, Sweden) reveal that these persons die 15–20 years earlier compared to the general population [2], mainly because of cardiovascular disease and cancer [3]. Persons with SMI experience a high number of risk factors that increase the prevalence of cardiovascular diseases and diabetes mellitus [4]. This is related to the side effects of prescribed antipsychotic medications [5], suboptimal lifestyle, lack of physical activity [3], poor diet and high rates of smoking [6–8]. A recent report from the Västra Götaland region of Sweden confirms the international data on mortality rates and the prevalence of somatic diseases within this patient group [9].

Other factors that explain the high prevalence of somatic diseases among persons with SMI are related to the health care system's difficulty in providing somatic health care which is appropriate to these persons' health care needs. Previous studies have explored factors which are barriers to and facilitators of access to health care for persons with psychiatric-somatic comorbidity [10–12]. Barriers at an organizational level were lack of communication and poor coordination between mental health and somatic care [11]. Lack of resources and productivity pressure, untrained staff, insufficient clinical support for staff, lack of established routines for referral of patients and lack of inter-agency collaboration were also seen as barriers [10, 12, 13]. Patient-related barriers were mental health stigma [14], along with socioeconomic barriers such as poverty, insecure housing and lack of transportation [15]. Difficulty in establishing and maintaining contact with a general practitioner also hindered access to health care [15]. Organization-related facilitators of access to health care were interdisciplinary, collaborative models of primary health care provision, which kept patients in regular contact with a primary health care clinician [15].

A limitation of previous research into barriers and facilitators is that it mostly uses data collected in countries other than Sweden, with different health care systems and treatment strategies for patients with SMI. These studies often lack a theoretical basis for identifying barriers and facilitators. We have therefore conducted a qualitative study of SMI patients, their relatives and clinicians working in primary and specialized health care. The study evaluates the factors which according to SMI patients, their relatives and clinicians, influence patient access to somatic health care. We aim to identify factors that may either hinder or facilitate implementation. To this end we will use the consolidated framework for implementation research (CFIR) [16], which will form the theoretical basis for the present study. According to CFIR, barriers or facilitators can be influenced by factors related to the following domains: intervention characteristics; characteristics of individuals; and inner and outer settings. Given the magnitude of the individual and societal costs related to the psychiatric-somatic comorbidity and disease burden, we need to gain a deeper understanding of the barriers and facilitators which affect patient access to health care in Sweden.

Aim

The aim was to explore the experiences and views of patients, relatives and clinicians regarding individual and organizational factors which facilitate or hinder access to somatic health care for persons with SMI.

Methods

Design

The present study applies a flexible, qualitative design. Qualitative data was collected by means of semi-structured individual interviews with patients with SMI, relatives and clinicians representing primary and specialized (somatic in-patient and psychiatric out-patient) health care. The qualitative interviews are based on the assumption that the interaction between the interviewer and the participant is an interplay between the interviewer's awareness of what and how the participant presents his/her answers and the participant's ability to explore and clarify his/her individual experiences and thoughts [17]. The method is reported in line with Tong A, Sainsbury P and Craig J [18].

Setting and participants

In Sweden, responsibility for health care is shared by national government, 20 county councils and 290 municipalities. The system is mainly tax funded. The government sets the political agenda and the principles and guidelines for the health care system by means of national legislation and/or agreements with the county councils and municipalities. Health care (primary as well as specialized care) is provided and funded chiefly by the county councils. The municipalities are responsible for the care and social security of people with psychiatric disorders [19]. As a consequence of this division of responsibilities, patients with SMI may have several health care contacts and providers.

The present study was conducted in a region of western Sweden. The selection of participants for the interviews was guided by strategic sampling in order to get a variation in participant experience of the questions under study. The study population consisted of persons suffering from SMI (hereafter called patients), relatives and clinicians. The recruitment of patients was based on psychiatric diagnosis, age, gender, and whether they lived in an urban or rural area. The inclusion criteria were: ongoing contact with psychiatric out-patient care; psychiatric diagnosis of bipolar disorder type I or II, psychosis or schizophrenia (ICD-10 codes: F2, F30.2, F31.2, F31.5, F32.3, F33.3); contact during the previous 12 months with primary or specialized health care for a somatic disease, such as type 2 diabetes mellitus, heart failure, hypertension or cancer. Exclusion criteria were: in-patient psychiatric care during the previous 12 months; ongoing investigation of patient's complaints by the patients' advisory committee. The selection of relatives was based on type of relationship (i.e. parent, adult child, sibling, spouse, co-habitant); the patient's psychiatric diagnosis and the patient's somatic diagnosis. The clinicians were chosen to represent different fields of primary and specialized health care (primary, somatic in-patient care, psychiatric out-patient care).

We presented the aims of the study to five managers representing five psychiatric out-patient units, 23 managers representing 23 units in primary and specialized care and six advocacy groups working with bipolar disorder or schizophrenia. All received oral and written information. The managers were asked to recruit clinicians and patients (primary and specialized health care). The representatives of the advocacy groups were asked to recruit relatives of SMI patients.

Four psychiatric out-patient units, 10 primary and specialized health care units and six of the advocacy groups helped to recruit patients, clinicians and relatives. The recruitment process was performed by unit managers (who recruited clinicians and patients) and representatives of advocacy groups (who recruited relatives). They received oral and written information about the recruitment process from the research group. The process resulted in 18 patients, 17 relatives and 21 clinicians agreeing to participate. Because the recruitment was performed by persons outside the research group, we cannot give an exact number for how many persons were invited to participate. Of those who initially agreed to participate, four of the patients and two of the relatives withdrew later for personal reasons. None of the clinicians withdrew from the study. Thus, interviews were conducted with 14 patients, 15 relatives and 21 clinicians. All participants received written information regarding the study's aim and content. They were given the choice of having the interview in their home town or nearby, at a time they found convenient.

Data collection

The interviews were held between May and September 2016. All interviews were semi-structured, i.e. three interview guides comprising a pre-determined set of open-ended questions were used. The interview guides were constructed for patients, relatives and clinicians and are further described below. All the interview guides were reviewed by the research group and pilot-tested at the first interview. Only small changes were made, such as a minor rephrasing of questions or changing the order of the questions. All interviews were conducted at face-to-face meetings, with no one other than the interviewer and the participant present. All except one were digitally recorded and transcribed verbatim. In the case of the latter interview, the patient did not allow the interview to be recorded and therefore notes were taken. No repeat interviews were carried out. A description of the participants is presented in Table 1.

The interview guides were developed for this study with inspiration from the CFIR guide http://www.cfirguide.org/. The following domains and their constructs

Table 1 Description of participants

Patients $N = 14$		
Female/male	10/4	
Age, years (mean)	35–77 (54)	
Psychiatric diagnosis (self-reported)		
Bipolar disorder	8	
Schizophrenia/psychosis	6	
Relatives $N = 15$		
Female/male	13/2	
Age, years (mean)	33–80 (55)	
Type of relationship		
Adult child	1	
Married	3	
Parent	6	
Sibling	5	
Psychiatric diagnosis (self-reported by the relatives)		
Bipolar disorder	4	
Schizophrenia/psychosis	11	
Clinicians $N = 21$		
Female/male	17/4	
Profession		Workplace
Assistant nurse	3	3 Psychiatric out-patient care
Behavioral scientist	2	2 Psychiatric out-patient care
Physician	7	3 Primary health care 1 Psychiatric out-patient care 3 Somatic in-patient care
Physiotherapist	1	1 Psychiatric out-patient care
Registered nurse	8	4 Primary health care 2 Psychiatric out-patient care 2 Somatic in-patient care

were addressed: outer setting (patient needs and resources); inner setting (structural characteristics, access to knowledge and information, leadership engagement); individual characteristics (knowledge and beliefs). The guide for patients consisted of eight questions, starting with "Can you tell me about when you had to contact the health services because of a physical illness?". The guide for the relatives consisted of seven questions and started with: "Can you tell me about a situation in which your relative with SMI had to contact the health services because of a physical illness?". The guide developed for clinicians contained 14 questions and started with: "Can you tell me about how your unit meets the somatic health care needs of patients with SMI?". The interview guides are presented in the Additional file 1. Follow-up questions (for example "Could you please tell me more about that situation?") were asked in all interviews when necessary.

Fourteen patients were interviewed in face-to-face meetings by the first author (EBB). She has a PhD, is an assistant professor and has broad experience of and training in qualitative methodology. The interviews lasted between 30 and 90 min and took place in public places (such as libraries or cafés) or in the interviewee's home. The patients had sought help from the primary or specialized care services for asthma, diabetes, various types of cancer, hypertension, myocardial infarction, renal insufficiency and non-specific musculoskeletal pain. All patients reported having more than one somatic diagnosis. Diabetes was the most common diagnosis. Fifteen relatives were interviewed in face-to-face meetings by a research assistant (SE). The interviews lasted between 15 and 50 min and were conducted in the interviewee's home, at the advocacy group or in a public place. Twenty-one clinicians were interviewed in face-to-face meetings by a research assistant (AJ). The interviews lasted between 10 and 45 min and were conducted at the clinicians' workplaces. Both research assistants were women and trained nurses. One has a PhD and the other a MSc. Both had prior training in qualitative methods and interview techniques.

Data analysis

The data (recordings and transcripts) were cross-checked for accuracy by ANK and JT. The data was analyzed by means of qualitative content analysis [20]. The analysis was performed according to the following steps: 1) The transcribed interviews were read through several times to gain an overall insight into the content. 2) All transcripts were explored by open coding, by marking sentences and/or paragraphs related to the study's aim and then condensed into meaning units, i.e. the marked text was summarized. 3) The meaning units were labeled with codes, which reflected different aspects of the content. 4) All meaning units and codes were transferred from the text to coding sheets in a MS Word document. 5) The codes were compared in order to identify similarities and differences. 6) Codes with similar content were classified as one category. 7) All codes and categories were compared with the interviews to ensure that they were appropriately linked to each other. 8) The categories were designated as barriers or facilitators according to their content. 9) Themes describing main barriers and facilitators were derived from the respective categories. Examples of the data analysis process are given in Table 2. Throughout the analysis procedure, the authors went back and forth between the transcripts, meaning units, codes and categories to make sure that the results

Table 2 Description of the analysis process

Meaning unit	Code	Category	Barrier/facilitator at individual or organizational level	Theme
When I finally did go to emergency department for help, my blood sugar levels were so high that I really shouldn't have been able to stay upright. What I mean is, the reason why I waited so long before getting help was that I'm afraid they're going to tell me you've got these problems because of your bipolar illness and the side effects of your drugs. You're afraid to go to the doctor's because that's the last thing you want is to be told.	Afraid of not being taken seriously	Self-stigmatization	Individual-level barrier	Main barrier: the gap between the organization of the health care system and patients' health care needs.
When our patients seek treatment for their somatic conditions it's usually got quite advanced. They don't seek help for the early symptoms and they often aren't already registered at a health centre. If you need help, it's very difficult for them to make a phone call, wait in a telephone queue, wait to be phoned back. Which means that I, as the person who is treating them, often make the phone calls for my patients to make things easier.	Making it easier for patients to get in touch with the health services.	Access to a professional contact	Organizational-level facilitator	The main facilitators: the links between the patients with SMI and the health care departments.

had been conceptually created and developed from the data by the analysts and did not lose their content in relation to the context described in the interviews. EBB had chief responsibility for the analysis in close collaboration with MR. In the latter phase of the analysis, the authors jointly discussed the analysis and agreed on the results. Short quotations from the data were used to illustrate the link between the data and the analysis.

Results

For an overview of the results, see Table 3.

Barriers

The main barrier is the gap between the organization of the health care system and the patients' health care needs. This is observed at both individual and organizational levels. In particular, the somatic health care system seems unable to support SMI patients with psychiatric-somatic comorbidity. The data indicates that the system relies on the individual's ability to initiate contact with health care providers, which is a problem for these patients. Another barrier is the lack of contact between different health care sectors.

Individual-level barriers

The results indicate that patients' self-stigmatization and cognitive disabilities together with clinicians' lack of knowledge of SMI are individual factors which constitute barriers to obtaining somatic health care.

All patients reported **self-stigmatization** as a barrier to accessing health care. They described previous experience of not being believed and not being taken seriously. This, in combination with their own thoughts about psychiatric disease, sometimes made the patient doubt whether the somatic symptoms were "for real". Previous experience of seeking help had left patients with the impression that mental illness was used as a framework for interpreting their somatic symptoms. The perceived tendency of clinicians to see the psychiatric diagnosis first and foremost was a major concern for the patients and seemed to increase their self-stigmatization.

When I came in they couldn't even do tests at the emergency clinic. So it was a real emergency. But what I mean, what I want to get to, is that the reason I just hung around at home so long is that I'm scared they're going to say "You've got these problems because of your bipolar diagnosis and the side effects of your medication." You're scared of ever going to the doctor's, because that's absolutely not what you want thrown at you. (Patient 2).

It's a lot like you're imagining things. Because you think... you've got this terrible thing, and it becomes a kind of self-condemnation. That it's something bad. And then you kind of end up at the back of the queue. You think you're being discriminated against all the time. And maybe that's not how things are in reality always. But you think, as soon as they get to know about this (the psychiatric diagnosis, author's note) I'll get worse treatment. Because I'm not worth as much in society. If you don't pay tax and are ill. It's terrible. (Patient 13).

Relatives and clinicians reported that a **patient's cognitive disabilities** were barriers to accessing health care. Relatives had first-hand experience of how patients' disabilities could affect medical visits, with clinicians interpreting symptoms as resulting from the psychiatric condition rather than as symptoms of a somatic disease. As one parent said at the interview:

Now, I haven't been with her every time, but when she talks about it she feels that they just... That they've

Table 3 Overview of the findings

	Individual-level	Organizational-level	Themes
Barriers	Self-stigmatization[a]	The fragmentation of the previously comprehensive county council primary care system[a, b, c]	The main barrier is the gap between the organization of the health care system and the patients' health care needs
	The patient's cognitive disability[b, c]	The lack of cooperation between different parts of the health care system[a, b, c]	
	The clinician's lack of knowledge of mental illness[c]	Lack of psychiatric expertise[b, c]	
		Single-disease paradigm[b, c]	
Facilitators	The relative as a spokesperson[b]	Access to a professional contact person[a, b, c]	The main facilitators are the links between the patients with SMI and the health care departments
	The clinician's own interest in developing a better understanding[c]	Continuity among clinicians[a, b, c]	
		Annual reminders[a, c]	

[a]Barrier/facilitator reported by patients
[b]Barrier/facilitator reported by relatives
[c]Barrier/facilitator reported by clinicians

> *largely neglected her, and that's how I see it too, even when I phone and talk to them I feel that... it's as if she's been labelled. She does behave a bit differently. She has a different way of talking, it might be that kind of thing that makes people not believe her. (Relative 10)*

This barrier was also mentioned by the clinicians working in somatic health care. They sometimes found it hard to understand psychotic patients' descriptions of the symptoms they were experiencing. As a consequence, the clinicians struggled to get the patient's medical history, sometimes with the help of other persons such as family members. The clinicians themselves suspected that they often underestimated patients' symptoms because of the difficulty of establishing the medical history.

> *I can see extra needs, these particular patients can be more difficult to assess and in some cases can be dissimulating, that they don't express the morbidity they may have in the same way other people do. There's a risk that you don't take their complaints as seriously, I think, there's a risk of making light of them in some way. I worked in psychiatric care for a while before I became a doctor. That's why I'm extra cautious in a way. (Clinician 1 somatic in-patient care).*

The clinicians' lack of knowledge of mental illness was a barrier reported by the clinicians working in somatic health care (primary and specialized in-patient care). Their medical training had included psychiatry, but this was perceived as insufficient. The clinicians also recognized that they had difficulty in dealing with non-adherence to medication and/or treatment in this patient group. They identified the need for training and cooperation to address these problems.

> *Maybe you don't have good enough specialist knowledge about these groups (author: patients) and the problems they can have, what we do in principle is treat them like any other patient. Then you usually get, can get problems with communication, or compliance, and then we usually get help from a psychiatric consultant. (Clinician 15 somatic in-patient care).*

Organizational-level barriers

The results indicate that, according to the interviewed patients, relatives and clinicians, there are a number of organizational factors that negatively impact the patients' ability to access health care.

The fragmentation of the previously comprehensive county council primary care system was described as a barrier by patients, relatives and clinicians. Since 2009 patients have had the right to choose their primary care provider. Private care providers and free-market competition between these providers was also introduced. The clinicians in the present study regarded this system as a hindrance because it does not give priority to clinical continuity and gives no incentives for clinicians at different units to cooperate with each other.

> *Previously (author: before the introduction of the right to choose) you never talked about medical priorities in relation to what the diagnosis was and what you got money for. But today everything is steered by which patients and diagnoses are registered at the health centre. You should really... If you haven't got enough time for everything, you should remove what you don't get money for. We don't actually say that, but that's the reality. (Clinician 17 primary health care).*

The lack of cooperation between different parts of the health care system, i.e. between primary and specialized care, within specialized institutions and between the county council's health services and municipal care, was seen as a barrier by patients, relatives and clinicians. The patients felt that, in one way, the lack of cooperation protected their integrity, such as when the health care institutions did not exchange patient-related information. On the other hand, this put the onus on the patients themselves to obtain information and decide what the next step should be.

> *So I go to the bipolar clinic, you know that, and then I get sent to the emergency unit, and at the emergency unit they say no, you're heart's beating slowly because of your medication. So I go back to the bipolar clinic and "No, I don't think so because the dose is so low". Ok. You can never get the whole picture, it's always just bits like this, so you just have to try to piece it together yourself. (Patient 10).*

The lack of cooperation was seen by the clinicians and relatives as reflecting the way in which specialized care focuses on a **single-disease paradigm**. This paradigm was seen as a facilitator for highly specialized care, but also as a barrier for persons with psychiatric-somatic multi-morbidity with regard to cooperation between different care sectors such as psychiatry and medicine, and primary and specialized care.

Almost all of the clinicians and relatives highlighted the **lack of psychiatric expertise** (i.e. clinicians such as physicians, psychiatrists, registered nurses with a specialization in psychiatry) as a barrier to accessing somatic health care. The clinicians felt they had limited opportunities to cooperate, refer patients and discuss issues related to the patient group. This barrier was also related to the perceived uncertainty about which health care institution (and therefore which clinician) had chief responsibility for the patient. Two of the clinicians said:

If a patient has had Alvedon for pain, for example, there's absolutely no communication that this is what we prescribe, this is what we do, this is our bit. It's only psychiatric. And primary care can take the other bit. And they think just the same, that no, psychiatry can prescribe that medication. So there's absolutely no communication. And no one has main responsibility for the patient. If you've got a pain problem and are in touch with another clinic at the hospital there's no contact between the doctors. (Clinician 4, psychiatric out-patient care).

The barriers are the shortage of doctors and lack of time with the doctor. Long waiting times, sometimes much too long so they have to go to the psychiatric emergency department instead. (Clinician 12 primary health care).

Facilitators

The results show that the main facilitators of access to somatic health care are the links between the patients with SMI and the medical departments. These take the form of functions (e.g. systems which ensure that patients receive regular reminders) or persons (e.g. professional contacts who facilitate patients' access to health care). Other facilitators are clinical continuity and better knowledge about SMI patients.

Individual-level facilitators

The individual-level facilitators of access to healthcare are the relatives who act as spokespersons for the patients and the clinicians' own interest in improving their knowledge about the patient group and SMI.

The relatives perceived **themselves as spokespersons** who facilitated patients' access to health care by accompanying them to appointments, asking questions and helping them with information about treatments, etc. The relatives described the spokesperson role in a positive way. However, those relatives who were parents of a son or daughter with SMI also discussed their worries about the future and who would support their child when they were no longer able to help. As one parent said:

She doesn't really understand that this (symptom, author's note) isn't good. That's when we have to push as parents. And she's got an appointment next week and then we can do our bit as parents... So of course we'll go with her. But I think about if we haven't got the strength or if we weren't around, who would go with her then? Then there wouldn't be any appointment. That's when there would be consequences (Relative 12).

The clinicians regarded their **own interest in developing a better understanding** of patients with SMI as a facilitating factor. A greater awareness of patients' needs facilitated access to health care. Some of the clinicians had previous experience of psychiatric in-patient care and could therefore draw in this experience when caring for patients with SMI in primary or specialized care. However, bridging the knowledge gap was the responsibility of the individual clinician. Some of them reported that they, for example, searched for information on the Internet about patients' symptoms and how to meet the needs of this patient group in an appropriate way.

Organizational-level facilitators

The organizational-level factors which facilitated access to health care were seen to be: having a professional health-care contact; continuity among clinicians; and patients being contacted annually.

The patient's **professional contact,** i.e. a nurse or assistant nurse at a psychiatric out-patient unit, was described by patients, relatives and clinicians as facilitating access to health care. The professional contact facilitated access by coordinating communication between the patient and the various health care units about such issues as medication, referrals and visits outside the psychiatric sector. Having a well-functioning professional contact was also seen as enhancing the patient's trust in the health care system. One positive consequence of this was better adherence to referrals. As one patient commented:

So, even though I do want them to know, in one way I also don't want them to know. Because it's a bit embarrassing. And I don't know if they'll get it, if they find out. It's, for example, at my psychiatric clinic, they wanted me to start collecting my medication at the health centre instead. They wondered if I would be prepared to do it. No, I'm not going to get that medication there, I don't want to because they don't know anything about this kind of thing. And if I've got any questions or if I maybe refuse to take the medication... they won't be able to help me with it. (Patient 2).

Continuity among clinicians was reported to be an organizational-level facilitator of access to health care. Continuity facilitated exchange of knowledge between clinicians as well as continuity for the patients. Both patients and clinicians described continuity as an opportunity to build a patient-clinician relationship based on a trusting alliance. They described this as a vital factor in helping to prevent difficulties arising in patient contacts.

Continuity of staff is vital, it's absolutely vital. And especially for the weaker members of society, continuity is incredibly important for them. It's more important than anything else, actually, and the health centre which has had the same staff for a long time, where there's good continuity, well it obviously works much better, and when the doctor has known the patients since way back, then there'll be fewer problems, so continuity is incredibly important. (Clinician 14).

Both patients and clinicians regarded **annual reminders** about primary health care and psychiatric out-patient appointments as an organizational-level facilitator. The clinicians reported that the annual health surveys for patients in psychiatric care helped them to be better informed and facilitated contact.

Discussion

The study's aim was to explore the experiences and views of patients, relatives and clinicians about individual and organizational factors which either facilitate or hinder access to somatic health care for persons suffering from SMI. The results reveal the main barrier to be the gap between the organization of the health care system and the patients' health care needs. Thus, the health care system is unable to meet the needs of patients with SMI. In addition, all patients reported self-stigma as a barrier to accessing health care. The main facilitators are the various links between SMI patients and the medical departments involved in their care. These facilitators can be functions, persons or factors such as clinical continuity and understanding of the SMI patients.

Primary care and general practitioners constitute the basic level of the Swedish health care system, both for somatic and psychiatric disorders. Patients with SMI are cared for by specialized psychiatric care services. Psychiatric out-patient units are mainly community based. They are thus located far from hospitals and seldom close to primary care centers. There is thus a geographical gap within the health care system that can be difficult to bridge for patients with SMI. There is also a knowledge gap within the system, in the sense that psychiatrists seldom know how to treat somatic disorders and vice versa. This is a consequence of the single-disease paradigm [21]. Specialist physicians in somatic health are often experts in a relatively small number of diseases, which means that a psychiatric patient with, for instance, type 1 diabetes and congestive heart failure, will need two somatic physicians as well as their psychiatrist. Patients with SMI and somatic comorbidities will thus be in contact with a number of medical departments. This can be a problem for any patient but is especially so for patients with impaired cognitive function and possibly also delusions. This is also the case for other patients with multi-morbidity such as the elderly [22]. It is therefore important for somatic clinicians to learn how to interact with SMI patients. As discussed below, physicians trained to provide somatic care in psychiatric settings might help to close or bridge this gap. We believe that this knowledge gap problem is an issue concerning all health care professionals.

Self-stigmatization was identified as an individual-level barrier for access to health care and was reported by all patients included in the study. This is in line with previous research [23–25]. Self-stigmatization is defined as a process in which the individual endorses stereotypes, avoids social interaction and regards him-/herself as a devalued member of society [23, 26]. Previous research has shown that self-stigma is negatively correlated with hope, self-esteem, empowerment and adherence to treatment [24, 25]. Self-stigmatization must be taken into account when developing interventions aimed at increasing access to health care for patients with SMI.

There is limited evidence about the effectiveness of interventions which aim to increase access to somatic health care for patients with psychiatric-somatic multi-morbidity [27]. A recent British report from the Royal College of Psychiatrists looks at the increased somatic disease burden among patients with SMI. The report suggests that a new specialist medical field of liaison physicians should be introduced [28]. One of the reasons for this is the geographical separation of somatic and psychiatric care that seems to be the rule in modern health care. As a consequence it is generally difficult for psychiatrists and their patients to consult physicians from somatic specialist disciplines. Patients tend instead to be referred to hospitals or primary care centers. This is often a problem for patients with cognitive impairments and leads to unnecessary delays or cancelled appointments, and ultimately impaired somatic health. A liaison physician is a general practitioner or specialist in internal medicine trained in the somatic comorbidities of severe mental illness. The liaison physician supports psychiatric departments and out-patient units both at individual patient level and at organizational level, for example treating patients for somatic comorbidities and teaching psychiatric staff about somatic diseases. The liaison physician could help to bridge the gap between somatic and psychiatric care, thus making it easier to meet the medical needs of psychiatric patients (cf. [27]). This recommendation is well in line with the results of the present study, which suggest that there should be professional contact personnel to act as links between SMI patients and the somatic health care services.

The present study highlights the potential of relatives and professional contact personnel to liaise between patients with SMI and the somatic health care services. This would help SMI patients to attend somatic medical appointments, overcome mistrust and maintain communication. However, the use of relatives and/or professional contacts has both advantages and disadvantages. On the one hand, our results showed that relatives regarded themselves as helping to empower patients to participate more actively in their own health care needs. This is in line with one systematic review, which demonstrated that knowledge provision and the patient's perceived capacity are two key factors for successful shared decision-making [29]. On the other hand, the presence of relatives and professional contacts resulted in transparency between the persons involved, which in turn suggests a paternalistic perspective which may interfere with the patient's legal right to autonomy. This was highlighted by the SMI patients in the present study. We therefore need to understand whether and in what way, the need for access to somatic healthcare for SMI patients may justify increased transparency.

One way to balance paternalism and the patient's right to autonomy is to empower patients to share decision-making [29]. When this is the case, increased transparency can be seen as an empowering factor for patients with SMI. A study of conditions that help to create a good life for people with bipolar disorder demonstrates that professional and reliable private relationships can help individuals to carry out their wishes at times when they are not able to do so on their own [30]. Voluntary chosen dependency of this kind contributes to the quality of life of persons with bipolar disorder, while at the same time enhancing their power and control.

Methodological considerations

The strength of the present study is that the data reflects a variety of perspectives (i.e. those of patients, relatives and clinicians). The participants (patients, relatives and clinicians) interviewed for the present study were strategically chosen to produce a wide variety of participants' experiences. Of the 23 clinics which were invited to take part (primary and specialized somatic in-patient care), 13 declined due to heavy work load and limited time, even if their managers were willing to allow their clinicians to participate during working hours. We sought to include patients with a wide range of psychiatric diagnoses because patients with SMI are not a homogeneous group. Four of the patients who had agreed to participate withdrew their consent before the start of the interviews without giving any specific reason. The interview topics could have been perceived as violating personal integrity or recalling memories of feeling discriminated against. Two of the relatives withdrew from the study; none of the clinicians withdrew.

Another strength of the study was that the data collection was based on questions recommended by CFIR, aimed at identifying factors that hinder or facilitate access to health care for SMI patients. To ensure the integrity of the qualitative analysis and the results, the meaning units and codes were kept close to the interview data. Throughout the analysis process the researchers went back and forth between the interviews, meaning units and codes in several steps. In addition, the analysis was conceptually created and developed based on the data, and the results were continuously discussed in the inter-professional research group in order to improve rigour [18]. With regards to thematic saturation, we suggest that the data facilitated the categorization and abstraction of the results. Thus, saturation of the analysis was achieved [31].

The recruitment of patients by health care managers in primary and specialized health care may have affected the patients' willingness to participate. However, we considered it necessary to use the recruitment process described here in order to create a safe setting for this vulnerable group of patients. Recruitment via managers gave patients the opportunity to discuss the interviews with their health care professionals. Because managers outside the research team were in charge of the recruitment process, it is not possible to give the exact number of non-participants. A relative limitation of the study is the small number of men it contains. In all other ways the strategic sampling was satisfactory.

Conclusions

We conclude that health care services for SMI patients would benefit from reorganization. We recommend that structures and systems that facilitate cooperation between medical departments are established at organizational level. This might include economic incentives for cooperation and clinical continuity. Furthermore, we see the need for the ongoing education of professionals about SMI patients and somatic diseases which would include both medical knowledge and how to interact with SMI patients. We suggest that the links between individual and organizational level should be strengthened by the introduction of professional contact personnel in the form of liaison physicians and case managers who have a good knowledge of somatic conditions. This can reduce the levels of stress and responsibility experienced by relatives. The present study has a qualitative design which reflects the health care system in Sweden. We conclude that our results could also be of interest in other countries (with comparable health care systems) which are seeking to facilitate SMI patients' access to somatic health care.

Abbreviations
CFIR: Consolidated framework for implementation research; SMI: Severe mental illness

Acknowledgements
The authors would like to acknowledge Susanne Erkell and Annika Jakobsson for their contribution to the data collection and Anna Dittrich for her administrative support.

Funding
This study was funded by the Centre for Equity in Health, Department of Data Management and Analysis, Head Office, and the Centre for Mental Health, Region Västra Götaland, Sweden.

Authors' contributions
MR had main responsibility for the project. EBB, JT, ANK, PW and MR designed the study. EBB and MR drafted and wrote the manuscript. EBB developed the interview guides. EBB collected the data with the support of two research assistants. EBB and MR analyzed the data and conceptualized the results with continuing support from JT, ANK and PW. All authors read and approved the final version of the manuscript.

Authors' information
Not applicable.

Ethics approval and consent to participate
The Regional Ethics Review Board in Gothenburg approved the study (Reg. no. 276–16). Before the interviews all participants were informed that participation in the study was voluntary, that they could withdraw at any time without giving any reason and that it would not be possible to identify the participants when the results were reported. Written informed consent was obtained from all participants.
In the present study we have included patients suffering severe mental illness. In order to ensure that the patients were able to provide consent to their participation, managers in primary and specialized health care were engaged in the recruitment of patients. The managers received information from the project group regarding the study's inclusion and exclusion criteria. Thereafter, they started the recruitment. Furthermore, we have also assured that all patients who took part in the study had an ongoing contact with out-patient psychiatric care.

Consent for publication
All participants (patients, relatives, clinicians) consented to publication of their anonymous quotes.

Competing interests
The authors declare that they have no competing interests.

Author details
[1]Unit of Intervention and Implementation Research for Worker Health, Institute of Environmental Medicine, Karolinska institutet, 171 77 Stockholm, Sweden. [2]Närhälsan Eriksberg Primary Health Care Centre, Sjöporten 4, 417 64 Göteborg, Sweden. [3]Department of Psychosis, Sahlgrenska University Hospital, 431 80 Mölndal, Sweden. [4]Department of Data Management and Analysis, Head Office, Region Västra Götaland, 541 80 Skövde, Sweden. [5]Centre for Equity in Health, Region Västra Götaland, Regionens Hus, 405 44 Göteborg, Sweden. [6]Department of Research, Södra Älvsborgs Hospital, Brämhultsvägen 52, 501 82 Borås, Sweden. [7]Institute of Health and Care Sciences, Sahlgrenska Academy, University of Gothenburg, 405 30 Gothenburg, Sweden.

References
1. Janssen EM, McGinty EE, Azrin ST, Juliano-Bult D, Daumit GL. Review of the evidence: prevalence of medical conditions in the United States population with serious mental illness. Gen Hosp Psychiatry. 2015;37:199–222.
2. Vancampfort D, Wampers M, Mitchell AJ, Correll CU, De Herdt A, Probst M, De Hert M. A meta-analysis of cardio-metabolic abnormalities in drug naive, first-episode and multi-episode patients with schizophrenia versus general population controls. World Psychiatry. 2013;12:240–50.
3. Scott D, Happell B. The high prevalence of poor physical health and unhealthy lifestyle behaviours in individuals with severe mental illness. Issues Ment Health Nurs. 2011;32:589–97.
4. Druss BG, Zhao L, Von Esenwein S, Morrato EH, Marcus SC. Understanding excess mortality in persons with mental illness: 17-year follow up of a nationally representative US survey. Med Care. 2011;49:599–604.
5. Vancampfort D, Stubbs B, Mitchell AJ, De Hert M, Wampers M, Ward PB, Rosenbaum S, Correll CU. Risk of metabolic syndrome and its components in people with schizophrenia and related psychotic disorders, bipolar disorder and major depressive disorder: a systematic review and meta-analysis. World Psychiatry. 2015;14:339–47.
6. Henderson DC, Vincenzi B, Andrea NV, Ulloa M, Copeland PM. Pathophysiological mechanisms of increased cardiometabolic risk in people with schizophrenia and other severe mental illnesses. Lancet Psychiatry. 2015;2:452–64.
7. Smith DJ, Langan J, McLean G, et al. Schizophrenia is associated with excess multiple physical-health comorbidities but low levels of recorded cardiovascular disease in primary care: cross-sectional study. BMJ Open. 2013;3:e002808. doi:https://doi.org/10.1136/bmjopen-2013-002808.
8. Smith DJ, Martin D, McLean G, Langan J, Guthrie B, Mercer SW. Multimorbidity in bipolar disorder and undertreatment of cardiovascular disease: a cross sectional study. BMC Med. 2013;11:263.
9. Torgerson J, Kjellström A, Overgaard K, Dimberg Jonson H: Vårdbehov i Västra Götaland. Somatisk vård och hälsoutfall vid samtidig psykisk sjukdom (In Swedish with a summary in English) http://analys.vgregion.se/contentassets/4ecc73f2879543bbb2b258b04836c292/somatisk-vard-och-halsoutfall-vid-samtidig-psykisk-sjukdom.pdf. 2016.
10. Groenkjaer M, de Crespigny C, Liu D, Moss J, Cairney I, Lee D, Procter N, Galletly C. "The chicken or the egg": barriers and facilitators to collaborative Care for People with Comorbidity in a metropolitan region of South Australia. Issues Ment Health Nurs. 2016;38(1):18–24.
11. Levinson Miller C, Druss BG, Dombrowski EA, Rosenheck RA. Barriers to primary medical care among patients at a community mental health center. Psychiatr Serv. 2003;54:1158–60.
12. Loeb DF, Bayliss EA, Candrian C, deGruy FV, Binswanger IA. Primary care providers' experiences caring for complex patients in primary care: a qualitative study. BMC Fam Pract. 2016;17:34.
13. De Hert M, Cohen D, Bobes J, Cetkovich-Bakmas M, Leucht S, Ndetei DM, Newcomer JW, Uwakwe R, Asai I, Moller HJ, et al. Physical illness in patients with severe mental disorders. II. Barriers to care, monitoring and treatment guidelines, plus recommendations at the system and individual level. World Psychiatry. 2011;10:138–51.
14. Happell B, Scott D, Platania-Phung C. Perceptions of barriers to physical health care for people with serious mental illness: a review of the international literature. Issues Ment Health Nurs. 2012;33:752–61.
15. Ross LE, Vigod S, Wishart J, Waese M, Spence JD, Oliver J, Chambers J, Anderson S, Shields R. Barriers and facilitators to primary care for people with mental health and/or substance use issues: a qualitative study. BMC Fam Pract. 2015;16:135.
16. Damschroder LJ, Aron DC, Keith RE, Kirsh SR, Alexander JA, Lowery JC. Fostering implementation of health services research findings into practice: a consolidated framework for advancing implementation science. Implement Sci. 2009;4:50.
17. Kvale S. Interviews. Thousand Oaks: Sage; 1996.
18. Tong A, Sainsbury P, Craig J. Consolidated criteria for reporting qualitative research (COREQ): a 32-item checklist for interviews and focus groups. Int J Qual Health Care. 2007;19:349–57.
19. Health care in Sweden [https://sweden.se/society/health-care-in-sweden/]. Accessed 3 Aug 2017.
20. Graneheim UH, Lundman B. Qualitative content analysis in nursing research: concepts, procedures and measures to achieve trustworthiness. Nurse Educ Today. 2004;24:105–12.
21. Moffat K, Mercer SW. Challenges of managing people with multimorbidity in today's healthcare systems. BMC Fam Pract. 2015;16:129.

22. Farmer C, Fenu E, O'Flynn N, Guthrie B. Clinical assessment and management of multimorbidity: summary of NICE guidance. BMJ. 2016;354:i4843.
23. Picco L, Pang S, Lau YW, Jeyagurunathan A, Satghare P, Abdin E, Vaingankar JA, Lim S, Poh CL, Chong SA, Subramaniam M. Internalized stigma among psychiatric outpatients: associations with quality of life, functioning, hope and self-esteem. Psychiatry Res. 2016;246:500–6.
24. Livingston JD, Boyd JE. Correlates and consequences of internalized stigma for people living with mental illness: a systematic review and meta-analysis. Soc Sci Med. 2010;71:2150–61.
25. Lundberg B, Hansson L, Wentz E, Bjorkman T. Are stigma experiences among persons with mental illness, related to perceptions of self-esteem, empowerment and sense of coherence? J Psychiatr Ment Health Nurs. 2009; 16:516–22.
26. Corrigan PW, Watson AC. Understanding the impact of stigma on people with mental illness. World Psychiatry. 2002;1:16–20.
27. Coventry P, Lovell K, Dickens C, Bower P, Chew-Graham C, McElvenny D, Hann M, Cherrington A, Garrett C, Gibbons CJ, et al. Integrated primary care for patients with mental and physical multimorbidity: cluster randomised controlled trial of collaborative care for patients with depression comorbid with diabetes or cardiovascular disease. BMJ. 2015;350:h638.
28. Royal College of Psychiatrists: Improving the physical health of adults with severe mental illness: essential actions Working Group for Improving the Physical Health of People with SMI; 2016.
29. Joseph-Williams N, Elwyn G, Edwards A. Knowledge is not power for patients: a systematic review and thematic synthesis of patient-reported barriers and facilitators to shared decision making. Patient Educ Couns. 2014;94:291–309.
30. Rusner M, Carlsson G, Brunt D, Nystrom M. A dependence that empowers: the meaning of the conditions that enable a good life with bipolar disorder. Int J Qual Stud Health Well-being. 2010;5
31. Creswell JW. Research design: qualitative, quantitative, and mixed methods approaches. Sage cop: Thousand Oaks; 2009.

13

Experiences and needs of carers of Aboriginal children with a disability

Michelle DiGiacomo[1], Anna Green[1], Patricia Delaney[1], John Delaney[1], Patrick Patradoon-Ho[2,4], Patricia Mary Davidson[1,3] and Penelope Abbott[4*]

Abstract

Background: Australian parents/carers of a person with a disability experience higher rates of depression, more financial stress, and are twice as likely to be in poor physical health than the general population. Aboriginal and Torres Strait Islander peoples experience worse health, social and economic outcomes than other Australians, and those with a disability face 'double disadvantage'. This study aimed to better understand the experiences and needs of parents/carers/families of Aboriginal children with a disability.

Methods: Semi-structured in-depth interviews were conducted with parents or primary carers of Aboriginal children aged zero-eight with disability. Interviews were analysed using thematic analysis.

Results: Nineteen women (sixteen mothers and three grandmothers) were interviewed. More than half were lone carers (without a partner or spouse). Participants described their experiences, including challenges and facilitators, to providing and accessing care, impacts on their health and wellbeing, and associated economic and non-economic costs of caregiving. Financial strain and social isolation was particularly prominent for lone carers.

Conclusions: Tailoring services to the needs of carers of Aboriginal children with a disability means supporting kinship caregiving, facilitating engagement with other Aboriginal families, and streamlining services and systems to mitigate costs. The experiences described by our participants depict an intersection of race, socio-economic status, gender, disability, and caregiving. Services and funding initiatives should incorporate such intersecting determinants in planning and delivery of holistic care.

Keywords: Caregivers, Childhood disability, Aboriginal and Torres Strait islander, Indigenous, Qualitative

Background

Increasingly, family carers of people with a disability are subsuming greater responsibilities while caring for people at home [1, 2]. They are often required to fill in the gaps in fragmented service and support systems through their caregiving [2]. Consequences of caregiving responsibilities for parents/carers include adverse health and social outcomes related to high levels of stress experienced in dealing with challenges of caring and juggling the demands of daily life [3, 4]. Parents/carers of a person with a disability have been found to experience higher rates of depression, stress, including financial stress, and are twice as likely to be in poor physical health compared to the general population [2, 3, 5]. Family relationships can also be strained as high stress in carers and concern for other household members are prominent reasons for decisions to place children in out-of-home-care (OOHC) [1, 3, 6].

Influence of specific contexts on the caregiving experience

While similar impacts of caring for a person with a disability have been reported across populations, contextual differences highlight the need to explore the experiences of parents/carers/families within priority populations, or those who experience health inequities, as they may face unique and additional challenges [7]. Experiences of

* Correspondence: P.Abbott@westernsydney.edu.au
[4]Western Sydney University, Locked Bag 1797, Penrith, NSW 1797, Australia
Full list of author information is available at the end of the article

stigma towards disability, different conceptualisations of disability, personal factors including resilience, cultural variations in support-seeking behaviours, and variations in access to available support services and resources can impact caring [4, 7, 8]. Obtaining a better understanding of the caring experience in priority populations, is particularly important in facilitating access to supports [9].

The Aboriginal context of caregiving

Aboriginal and Torres Strait Islander peoples are one such priority population who experience worse health, social and economic outcomes than other Australians [2]. Government policies of dispossession and racism have contributed to Aboriginal people being one of the most disadvantaged socio-economic groups in Australia. Chronic illnesses are much more prevalent among the Aboriginal population and they impact at younger ages. They are more likely than other Australians to experience poverty [10, 11], unemployment [12], make less money, and live in rented homes and homes that are overcrowded (National Aboriginal and Torres Strait Islander Social Survey [12]. These disparities are also apparent in disability throughout the life course. Aboriginal children aged 0–14 years are more than twice as likely as non-Indigenous children to have a disability. High educational attainment and employment is less likely in Aboriginal and Torres Strait Islander people with disability compared to non-Indigenous people with disability [13].

These disparities likewise affect Aboriginal and Torres Strait Islander carers who are more likely to be an unpaid carer for a person with a disability than non-Indigenous Australians [14]. The impact of caring is more pronounced for Aboriginal and Torres Strait Islander carers and their communities due to the high levels of socioeconomic and health disadvantage [15]. Furthermore, conceptualisations of caregiving are different in Aboriginal families where family obligation is part of the culture. Connotations of family extend to all relatives who are nurtured within a community context, as in a kinship system, and it is appropriate for families and communities to look after one another [16]. For example, many Aboriginal carers rely on the extended family to give them a break from caring rather than approaching formal (paid) services for respite [15]. Kinship care is currently the most common form of out-of-home-care (OOHC) for Aboriginal children [17]; this has specific implications on the impact of caregiving for Aboriginal kinship carers of a child with a disability. Also, the term 'carer' may not resonate with Aboriginal carers who perceive it as reflecting formal care workers; thus, Aboriginal carers may not identify as carers despite significant care responsibilities.

In addition to this culture of shared caring within families and communities, Aboriginal carers may not access formalised external supports for other reasons. Historical mistrust of government institutions and a lack of culturally acceptable services and resources mean that parents/carers may only seek help when there is a crisis [18]. Lack of cultural awareness and sensitivity in mainstream service providers can result in misunderstandings and fractured trust and relationships. Aboriginal carers may also be unaware or have little knowledge of services and supports, their eligibility requirements, and how to access them. Low income and lack of transport are additional barriers to services for carers.

Despite the disparity and the significant role played by carers, little attention has focused on the needs of Aboriginal parents/carers of a person with a disability. It is necessary to facilitate timely access of children with a disability and their families to appropriate health services, social support services, and treatment because addressing problems early is crucial in reducing long-term negative impacts on health, education and employment outcomes [19–21].

Aim

We conducted this study to better understand the experiences and needs of parents/carers/families of Aboriginal children with a disability. Understanding the experiences and impact of caring on Aboriginal parents/carers/families is critical in establishing a baseline to inform improvement of services.

Methods

This study was informed by a socio-ecological framework situating carers' experiences at the macro- (government), exo- (organizational), meso- (provider), and micro (family/child) system levels in recognition of the inter-dependence of these factors. The carer, child, and family are positioned at the centre of the framework. This micro-level experience is the focus of this paper. Findings related to navigating systems external to the family and additional methodological detail are reported elsewhere [22]. We used a qualitative approach using thematic analysis underpinned by phenomenology to facilitate understanding experiences of carers for Aboriginal children with a disability. [23].The sampling frame consisted of participants who were parents or primary carers (hereafter, carers) of Aboriginal children aged zero to eight years who attended a developmental clinic at an Aboriginal health service in a suburban area near a capital city in eastern Australia. The clinic, run by a team of visiting paediatricians, Aboriginal Health Workers, nurses, and midwives, catered to children with developmental problems aged from birth to sixteen years. Problems managed in this clinic are similar to those seen in other developmental clinics, although it catered specifically to Aboriginal and Torres Strait Islander children. Recruitment was facilitated by clinic staff who verbally informed potential participants about the study and supplied written information to interested parties upon presentation to the clinic for scheduled appointments or during home visits. Sampling was purposive in that recruitment targeted carers of children attending the clinic. We used an inclusive definition of disability to intercept experiences relating to mild, moderate and severe, physical, intellectual, or developmental conditions. Recruitment continued until no new issues emerged during interviews.

Data collection

Between April 2013 and June 2015, in-depth semi-structured interviews were conducted on two occasions within twelve months with each participant to capture a range of experiences and perspectives of caring for a child with a disability. Initial interviews were conducted at the health facility in private clinic rooms, were audio recorded, and ranged in duration from 20 to 60 min. Participants were reimbursed for travel and child care expenses incurred as a result of participation. Interview topics were derived from a literature review [24] and the social determinants of health and social capital frameworks [25–27]. Within the interviews, we explored participants' meanings and interpretations of their experiences with the child's disability, the 'patient/family journey' enacted to access services and support, and participants' perceptions of the effects of the child's disability and 'journey' on the carer and family.

Follow-up interviews were conducted with participants, in-person or via telephone, to document activities related to the carer's experience since the first interview twelve months prior. For example, some participants described attending ongoing medical appointments or changes in living arrangements since the first interview and how they made sense of these experiences. This second interview was also an opportunity to summarise thematic content of the first interview to seek confirmation of its validity with participants [28]. Any noted discrepancies were discussed, clarified, and resolved to the satisfaction of the participant.

Research team

The research team was co-led by Aboriginal and non-Aboriginal team members, who frequently met to discuss research processes and debrief about ongoing data collection. The core research team comprised four female researchers supported by a male Aboriginal elder (JD) who provided cultural mentorship to the team. One member of the research team was an Aboriginal woman from the local community with experience in health service delivery, Aboriginal health, and childhood disability (PD). Both these team members worked in the Aboriginal health service in health promotion roles. One of the researchers (MD) who conducted interviews and analysis was a qualitative researcher based at a university and had qualifications in psychology. She had had an 8-year relationship at the study site wherein she worked with staff on health promotion and secondary prevention program research, but was unknown to participants. Another interviewer and analyst (PA) was a general practitioner (GP) employed at the service and was a university-based academic. While she had met some of the participants in the context of primary care consultations, she was not involved directly in the child's healthcare, and ensured that participants were aware that her role in the research was separate to her role as a GP at the service.

Analysis

Thematic analysis began with development of a contact summary sheet for each interview with key demographic information and emergent issues noted [29]. Thematic analysis was used because our aim was to understand carers' experiences and perceptions, yet we focused more on patterned meaning across the data-set [23], rather than prioritising the idiographic focus, as in interpretive phenomenological analysis. One researcher (MD) undertook preliminary analysis wherein she read transcripts to familiarise herself with the data, added notes to each document, including analytic observations for individual transcripts and as well as the entire set, and developed a coding system with semantic and latent codes to elucidate categories. Data relevant to each code was collated individually for each transcript and at the end of the coding process. To facilitate rigor, a second researcher (BA) independently coded unmarked transcripts. The full research team met regularly to discuss code development throughout the data collection and preliminary analysis stages; differences in coding scheme were discussed until consensus was reached. The interview transcripts were then coded according to the developed scheme with consideration of emerging categories. Categories were then collapsed into themes. Emerging themes were discussed with the full research team before analysis was finalised. To further enhance trustworthiness, a stakeholder check was undertaken, whereby preliminary analysis of findings was presented to clinic staff, some of whom were also Aboriginal carers of a child with a disability, for their feedback. Feedback was incorporated into theme development.

Ethical considerations

Ethical approval was granted by the Aboriginal Health and Medical Research Council (AH&MRC) (762/10) and

University Human Research Ethics Committee (UTS HREC 2011-417R). The study adhered to key principles for research with Aboriginal and Torres Strait Islander peoples as espoused by the AH&MRC [30]. Participants were made aware that all identifiable information would remain confidential and that they could withdraw from the study at any time and that this would not affect any relationship they may have with the health service or researchers. Permission to audio record interviews was obtained from each participant. To preserve anonymity and confidentiality, names were replaced with pseudonyms and identifying information was removed following verbatim transcription of recordings.

Results

Participants were sixteen mothers and three grandmothers, of whom 53% ($n = 10$) were lone carers (without a partner), and were taking care of 60 children at home, half of whom were identified as having a disability or developmental delay (Table 1). Types of disabilities or disorders represented in the care recipients were predominantly developmental disabilities including intellectual disability, autistic spectrum disorder, ADHD, language and communication disorders and hearing impairment, as well as associated conditions such as epilepsy and genetic disorders.

Participants described their experiences in terms of caring for their child and family, challenges and facilitators of this caring, carer health and wellbeing, and associated financial expenses and non-economic costs. Our focus on costs of caring arose from the coding process. This led us to seek out a framework to assist in exploring and organising these economic and non-economic consequences of caring [31]. The data reflecting explicit content are thus presented in tabular form (Table 2) to provide specific examples of how participants experienced each consequence in the framework and are summarised narratively below. Following the discussion of economic and non-economic costs incurred by informal caregivers, factors that influence these costs are presented.

Table 1 Demographic details of carers ($N = 19$)

Characteristic	N (%)
Female	19 (100)
Sole carer	10 (52.6)
Relationship to child:	
Mother	16 (84.2)
Grandmother	3 (15.8)
# of children with a disability/developmental disorder they care for	30
Average age of child with a disability/ developmental disorder	6.4 years (Range: 5 months – 13 years)
Other children in their care	30

Costs incurred by caregivers

Economic costs

We organised findings reflecting economic and non-economic costs incurred by family caregivers using the taxonomies developed by Keating et al. [32] and Lero et al. [31](discussed below). Keating's taxonomy depicts economic costs as employment consequences, out-of-pocket expenses, and caregiving labour, or time spent on caregiving and related activities. Excerpts reflecting each domain appear in Table 2 because they illustrate manifest content regarding caregiving costs. Caregivers referred to limiting or rearranging paid working hours or resigning from employment to accommodate their children's needs. Inability to juggle demands of employment and attending multiple appointments, providing care on non-school days, and managing behaviour resulted in exiting the workforce. Out-of-pocket expenses involved purchasing supplies, accessing health services, and transport costs. Despite the context of universal health care coverage, accessing specialist or private health providers required a financial outlay considered significant in light of other household expenditures. Parking fees and meals were indirect costs of care-seeking. Financial pressure was unabated in carers receiving government subsidies. Conditions that were undiagnosed or not recognised as subsidiary-worthy translated to an increase in out-of-pocket costs for carers. Financial strain was particularly prominent for lone carers with only a single income. Related to both out-of-pocket expenses and caregiver burden were costs associated with traveling to and from multiple appointments and distant schools.

Non-economic costs

Lero's three non-economic cost domains are physical, psychological, and social health and wellbeing [31]. Participants discussed the ways in which their physical and psychological health and wellbeing had been affected over the course of their caring role, from the period prior to diagnosis through ongoing management as the child aged. Stress reported by carers often centred around their child's behavioural problems. Ongoing aggressive behaviour, even by very young children, challenged caregiving and caused injury to carers and siblings. The impact of concurrent stressful life events, such as the loss of a partner, further amplified the emotional impact of caring. In addition to sleep deprivation, worry, frustration, anger, and grief were described by participants. Carers' other roles and relationships suffered as did self-management of their own health care needs. Family relationships were affected by the strains of caregiving and needs of the child with a disability in the family home. There were several examples of the

Table 2 Economic and non-economic costs incurred by informal caregivers

Economic Costs	Employment Consequences	Labour force exit/ preclusion	Well I was working. But I have stopped…Yeah, the amount of time that I have off. It was my decision, it's the school, a handful of weeks like every day. But she has at least one day off here or, like, five days off. She had had two weeks off, you know like. (Nadia)
			when we got the one that was 13 weeks, (my husband) gave up his job and stayed with him. Virtually raised the third one. The first two we stayed at work and tried to cope, and then with the bad behaviour and that it just got a bit too much. And yeah, so I only work two days a week now, and my husband doesn't work, he had got a carer's pension for the children. (Bree)
		Restricted work hours/absences	It is hard with the boys. I work three days a week at the moment, because both the boys do speech therapy every week, and it is hard, but such is life. We've always done it. (Barbara)
	Out of Pocket Expenses	Purchases for Care Recipient: supplies	money is a big issue for me too. Like, for me to have a house, raise my daughter and buy her medical needs, her clothing, her food, like, just anything in general, with the house, electricity and that, I'm pretty much looking at nothing at the end of when I get paid. Like, it's not enough. I'm on a single parenting payment and I get the carer's allowance. Not enough at all. (Samantha)
			…they ended up getting me an authority script for the [over-the-counter pharmaceutical] because it's, like, $18 a box, but I was buying three boxes a week. And it's got very expensive. Basically my husband works overtime to pay off our credit cards that pay for when I have been in hospital and you know we have to eat at the hospital, parking at the hospital, I am not entitled to anything. So, I don't have a disabled sticker, I don't have anything. (Nadia)
			Well, the problem is there is Centrelink won't accept that she has a problem. I have been to them and [her condition] is not considered, so therefore I am eligible for nothing. So yeah, it's quite frustrating…they tell me that they are looking into a healthcare card, but nothing else. She is not going to get – I am not going to get carers [support], I am not going to get support or anything like that because they don't see it, they don't recognise her problem as a problem. So that was the next thing Dr. X was sort of saying when we have the biopsy done maybe he can try again, but I try until I am blue in the face to tell them she has a problem, but it's not on their list, so it's not recognised. (Nadia)
		Purchases for Care Recipient: health services	So then I became a single mum, done this. Now I live in my own place where you've got to pay rent, it's baby food, and – not baby food, nappies, food and all – I end up being broke. (Tabitha)
			Because you're putting so much effort into getting them to different places, especially if you've got to pay privately as well, it really does hit the hip pocket. Um, sometimes it can make you go without your petrol because you've either got to weigh it up what is more important. (Rita)
			the therapy stuff was a lot – it's a lot harder to access than – even with children that have very clear diagnoses and very clear needs, I mean unless you've got money to, sort of, get the private stuff. (Ainslee)
			I mean it's – it's significant because, especially, um, we did OT for a while through the kids' hospital and the private one there, um, I mean the initial, the very first visit and it was literally half an hour, it cost – it was, like, $180… and you only got, like, $40 back. Like, it was really small… And then it was – I mean every subsequent half hour was, like, 50 bucks and you got $25 back, or something, so – but it's that initial, sort of, um, cost - and plus travel and plus with young kids, you know…a lot of it was just play therapy and, you know, stuff that we do at home anyway, and I just thought, you know, it was such a waste of time and money. (Ainslee)
			he was seeing another paediatrician and I just could not afford to send him when he needed to go because it was like a hundred and something dollars. I know that you get money back but its $100 that you have to fork out to pay for it up front. (Grace)
			Cause it's expensive. If they didn't have a free service like this, what would they do?...You know, and living expenses – living. I – I get broke you know what I mean? But that's with the circumstances of taking a pay cut and them sorts of things. (Laura)
		Transportation/travel	Costs me about a hundred and two dollars to fill up my car. And that means if I go to (hospital) more than four times a week I have to fill up again. (Lesley)

Table 2 Economic and non-economic costs incurred by informal caregivers *(Continued)*

			There's no way, I would never afford the petrol; it's right out [distant suburb]. Then you're stuck in traffic, you may as well wait out there at the gate [laughs], take a pillow. (Melanie)
	Caregiving labour	Time spent getting to services	You don't pick the school they actually go to. Um, when they've got a certain level of disability where they need to be at a special school, um, you don't get to pick…they decide where she fits best and where there's space… Because there's not very many specialist schools in Sydney…it's an hour each way for us, basically…it makes it hard, and I think people just, sort of, take that stuff for granted that you just can't send her to the school next door… you have to send her to the place that they think is going to give her what she needs…I mean it's a really good school, and stuff. It was just the distance, and it's not feasible for us to move closer 'cause it's more expensive to live close to there. (Ainslee)
			…when they have got appointments and they are all bang, bang, bang, and that's a bit challenging because I have also got my own appointments and so I try and work around so it all fits in. (Stacey)
Non-economic costs	Physical Health and Wellbeing	Injuries/Physical Stress/Fatigue	they didn't put [the child] on drugs, they put me on drugs … because she was so bad before I got here, um, I had a broken nose from her… I couldn't touch her without her attacking me, yeah, really violent. (Jocelyn)
			It's tiring and especially when I work nights… It's tiring to, um, drag the kids around and – yeah…I mean it is - it's very tiring, emotionally and physically. (Ainslee)
	Mental Health/ Emotional Wellbeing	Depression, Anxiety/ Psychological strain	And then, yeah, when she got diagnosed with it – it's hard…I stress a lot, I cry a lot. (Rachel)
			It's become very stressful, yeah. At the doctor's today, before I was going to the hospital, I am on edge and I am, like, fighting doesn't get it done, but I can't just sit back and agree anymore and say, 'Yeah don't worry, you know it's okay. We will see.' (Nadia)
			I feel a little bit, you know, like last night, oh, my chest started getting a bit tight, you know…She takes out a lot of frustrations out on me and, well, I've got nobody to take mine out on, so I need my time out. I'll lock myself out in the backyard if I have to. Lock myself in the toilet [laughs]. It's only five minutes, but that five minutes is all you need to calm down. (Jocelyn)
			It is – it was very hard after I lost her dad. But I found it very – I'm finding it very hard to cope some days, and find it easy other days…[She was] shaking, and the eyes rolling back in her head, and all that. Yeah…I just wish that – it's just like living in a nightmare. (Susan)
	Social Wellbeing	Activity engagement/ Social Participation/ Isolation	Yeah, I don't take her anywhere anymore. I don't take her food shopping. I don't take her – like my aunt's wedding was on the weekend… I don't take her anywhere with me anymore because she's just too full on and I can't – it stresses me out at the shops when I'm trying to do shopping and I can't – I can't think what I need to get. (Rachel)
			I've moved down here [three years ago][to have better access to health services], I have been out bush for 20 years, so I've got no friends down here… (Jocelyn)
			I don't have no support…I do everything on my own…Sit in the hospital all day by myself… I don't get people coming to the hospital bringing me meals…I wish I just had a little bit more support, you know. Like, a little bit more. It's depressing sitting in the house by yourself and having no-one to talk to. (Susan)
		Relationships	It's affected it big time. Um, because I can't go to see my grandkids anymore. Um, I worked, you know, and you have got to move around things looking after these two girls (Stacey)
			With my daughter, it was hard until I got her into a boarding school. She started Year 7 this year, and she's over at [Sydney suburb]. So she just comes home on the holidays.(Barbara)
			My youngest daughter, she doesn't live with me, she lives with my auntie because at the time I – like, I'm still a single mother but I can't raise a child with a disability and a newborn on my own. It was way too much. My auntie, she can give, like, she can give my daughter a life I never could. (Samantha)
			You're too ashamed to be able to tell family. Some think 'oh, that's just gammon, the ADHD...he's just mucking up...just give them a hiding.' (Laura)

physical separation, whereby the child with a disability or their sibling(s) were sent to live with other family members or to boarding schools to facilitate educational and social growth.

Lone carers, or those without a partner or spouse, were especially vulnerable to social isolation. The lack of emotional support was prominent in their narratives and it impacted on carers' ability to cope with strain. Relocating to be closer to service networks sometimes hindered beneficial social support networks. Yet, feelings of isolation despite proximity of family sometimes surfaced due to lack of acknowledgement and understanding of the carers' experiences.

Factors that influence the impact of costs of caregiving

Lero et al.'s [31] framework for caregiving suggests that characteristics of the caregiver, care recipient, the relationship of the dyad, and the context and nature of care influence costs of caregiving and thereby challenge or facilitate resilience. Findings depicting the context and nature of care reflected latent content as they reported concepts underpinning the data.

Balancing needs of differently-abled children

Diverse needs related to learning, psychosocial support and development, healthcare, and safety all need to be balanced by carers of children with and without disability. Siblings and the family unit sometimes bore the brunt of the accommodations required. Concerns ranged from developmental, behavioural, and learning-related to the physical safety of siblings.

Younger siblings of a child with a disability occasionally modelled behaviours of the older brother or sister. For example, Ainslee was challenged by regressed speech and toileting behaviours in her son who does not have a disability or delay, unlike his older sister:

> *"Certain things he's very regressed in because he's modelling himself from her and because she, sort of - toilet training's a big issue for her - so it's a big issue for him...And speech is an issue for him because he's, sort of, learning speech from her ... we try really hard not to treat our kids any different. I know there's nothing wrong with him, he's far more ahead than Sally was, but I worry that he's going to learn bad habits and he's going to not be able to stop." (Ainslee).*

Managing multiple children's diverse needs could tax a carer's resources, particularly a lone carer, and lead to choices about who missed medical care or school:

> *"For the first two months of the baby's life, it was a bit hard...So there were two months there where my kids didn't get the services they needed." (Barbara)*

> *"Even if one of the kids has to go to the doctor, I have to get them all out of school." (Helen)*

In several other cases, parents referred to their children without disabilities as missing out on attention:

> *"...the other ones feel it. So you've got to make sure you make that time for them as well...And say, 'No, no. We're talking. Your time is later.'...But yeah. It's so much attention around him." (Laura)*

Some participants reported aggression perpetuated by their child with a disability either towards the carer or siblings. These violent interactions were described as frightening, disrupting family harmony, and shifting household dynamics:

> *"He is now starting to slap [his sister] across her face, pulling her hair, and I'm trying to explain to him that is naughty. So now she's got a big bruise on her face where he's bit her." (Tabitha)*

Physical aggression between siblings could jeopardize safety of family members and consequences reportedly included physical separation via changed living circumstances in some situations.

Family resources support the disability journey

Although caring for child with a disability impacts on the family, family also impacts on the caregiving and disability journey. The resources within families were used to provide respite, access services, afford instrumental and emotional support, and facilitate empowerment of carers.

For many families, respite is a family matter and using respite service rather than a family member or friend was perceived as unacceptable. They would not feel confident that an unknown respite provider would understand their child's needs:

> *"She can't get minded by a lot of people because they don't know what to do with her." (Lesley)*

Many carers were fortunate to have family members willing to act in an informal respite capacity. However, planning for informal respite was difficult given multiple competing demands and at times, several children who need looking after.

> *"We had family to help to look after the other ones while we have to do things for her, but, that's still difficult depending on what times of the day and I work nights, so it definitely has a big impact." (Ainslee)*

Even brief periods of care provided by trusted others afford the carer time to rest and restore.

> *"I have a lot of support from my mother-in-law, like she's really good... 'cause I don't get a break really from her and the only time I do is when my mother-in-law does take her for the night or something like that. She plays up for her, but my partner's mum is very strict and won't put up with it." (Rachel)*

> *"My sister goes, 'Go outside, get a bit of fresh air, and come in when you are ready.'" (Tabitha)*

Examples of kinship care arrangements helping to keep separated families together were described. Despite the pain of family separation, one lone carer explained that she takes solace in having a family member act as her newborn's primary carer:

> *"My auntie, she can give my daughter a life I never could. She can give her anything she wants. She'll never need for nothing, so that's enough for me." (Samantha)*

In this carer's case, she maintains a healthy relationship with her auntie and this arrangement means that both of the girls are cared for within the family, albeit only one child remains in her home. Likewise, other carers, some of whom were grandparents, explained that they assumed the primary carer role to keep the children within the family.

> *"Our daughter had a drug and alcohol problem and her older two children were removed by [social services], and we didn't want them to go into foster care, so we took them. Then she seemed to get her act together for a while and had the third child, and then ended up relapsing and they removed him. And the same story with the younger one." (Bree)*

Indeed, family support was discussed as a critical element of coping with having a child with a disability. In some cases, carers moved from distant areas to obtain more support from health services as well as to be closer to family.

In addition to providing emotional and instrumental support in the form of respite and caregiving, several family members were able to leverage their employment and social networks to facilitate access to schools, housing, and non-government organisation resources. In one example, a carer moved to a capital city to be closer to her mother and grandmother who were able to obtain support and advocacy from various organisations.

> *"(My Nan) is very highly respected in the community, so she knows a lot of people. So, yeah, it's not about what you know, it's pretty much who you know these days...The [caseworker] was one of my Nan's best friends, so she come and picked me up, picked my nan up, took me to Housing and then we sat down with the Department of Housing and they got the manager out and we told them my situation. The manager was like, 'alright, I'll ring you back in a week,' and they ended up offering me a house." (Samantha)*

In her perspective, this carer's experiences highlighted the role of her influential, well-networked family member and caseworker friend as facilitating an unfettered path to housing. Conversely, there were several other examples of participants who did not have such resourceful networks. As previously described, some carers experienced social isolation after having moved away from family to have better service access closer to a metropolitan area or were estranged from family (Table 2). Also described were family members acting to validate concerns and difficulties or prompt to seek care. One carer explained that her mother-in-law recognized the need to seek care based on previous personal and professional experience:

> *"Cause I had a lot of problems with (my daughter) beforehand, but I was kind of in denial and didn't want people to say that she had problems. But, [my partner's] mother had told me to come here to see a paediatrician because she knew (there was a problem)." (Rachel)*

Another woman discussed social support as the main influence on her ability to cope. Barbara described the support she received from her brother, friends, and work colleagues as integral to her coping.

> *"I was lucky I had my brother. My brother's always been with me... So I think if I didn't have him I would have lost the plot." (Barbara)*

These examples exemplify the influential role of the familial context in mitigating or intensifying the costs of caregiving.

Discussion

Our data show that carers bear the costs, both economic and non-economic, of fragmented systems and complex pathways to care. Aboriginal carers' ability to draw on family resources to care for their children with disability, despite these high costs demonstrates strength and resilience.

Bearing the costs

In spite of the Australian context of universal health care and specific policy initiatives aimed to reduce costs of healthcare for Aboriginal and Torres Strait Islander peoples, such as Closing the Gap [25], carers in this study reported that financial costs incurred as part of their caring roles strained resources and exceeded their capacity. While financial stress previously has been reported in literature on caregiving for people with a disability [2], we have contributed the experiences and perspectives of costs and resources associated with caring for an Aboriginal and Torres Strait Islander child with a disability. Lone carers or single parents are recognised as some of the most economically disadvantaged groups in Australian society and there is a higher prevalence of lone-parenthood in Indigenous women than others [11, 33]. Our participants were all women, mostly mothers and some grandmothers, half of whom were lone carers for one or more child with a disability. Previous research has reported that single mothers with a child with a disability are less likely to be in the labour force than single mothers of a young child without a disability [34], thereby constraining income. Even small out-of-pocket expenses can contribute to financial strain in carers, particularly those whom are financially disadvantaged [35, 36]. Providers should consider the financial outlays characteristic of many care pathways and forewarn carers of service costs and caveats [22]. Concerted efforts to streamline services and systems may mitigate these costs. The experiences described by our participants depict an intersection of race, socio-economic status, gender, disability, and caregiving. Services and funding initiatives should incorporate such intersecting determinants in planning and delivery of holistic care.

In most instances, living within a context of a multiple child household challenged the lone carers' ability to meet needs of all household members. Research on siblings of children with disability has identified siblings may witness or experience physical violence perpetrated by their sibling with a disability that makes them feel unsafe and anxious at home [37]. As in the present study, long-term alternate accommodations were sometimes sought for the non-disabled sibling to enable them educational opportunities and physical safety that were not necessarily available living at home because of the high level needs and behavioural problems of their sibling. While in some families, the child with a disability is accommodated elsewhere which enables other members of the family to have quality time spent together, in other families, the child(ren) with a disability remained at home and siblings were accommodated elsewhere.

One option for accommodation of children outside their parental home is kinship care, a formal or informal arrangement when care is provided within the family or friendship network [38]. This arrangement has been associated with greater psychological benefit [39], stability of care, more contact with parents and other family members, less trauma being separated from parents, and less stigma [40]. These are beneficial outcomes for children, but the kinship carers may not fare as well. A study of Indigenous and non-Indigenous kinship carers from urban and rural areas of New South Wales, Australia, revealed extensive and complex support needs. This was particularly the case for older carers, often grandparents, who were resuming previous caregiving roles [39]. Indigenous kinship carers were more likely to have poor health, financial hardship, and have multiple caregiving roles [39], yet were less likely to seek help from statutory agencies [41]. The Kinship Care Family Research Report concluded that needs of kinship carers included increased financial and non-financial support to caregivers of Aboriginal children, recognition of Aboriginal caregivers as more likely being older, single, have poorer health, and caring for and supporting multiple children [38]. Financial and support services may be particularly beneficial for such carers to mitigate the negative impact on health and wellbeing [42]. Despite these concerns, however, grandparent and other kinship caregivers are reported to be extremely resilient, thus demonstrating the importance of developing mechanisms to support resilience [42].

The social capital of family

Family is a cornerstone of Aboriginal culture and includes nuclear and kinship or extended family as well as others within the community who are considered to be family, and who will potentially provide support for children throughout their lives [43]. Family functioning can influence the adverse effect of disadvantage on health and wellbeing in Aboriginal culture [44]. Good family functioning is associated with improved mental and physical health of parents/carers of a person with a disability [3] and as such, should be supported. A key finding of this study was the important role of family as a resource to enact respite, provide instrumental and emotional support, and facilitate service access and empowerment of carers. Use of social and familial networks to obtain resources and facilitate access is a universal behaviour, yet it should be appreciated that some carers may not be networked and thus are vulnerable to isolation and obstacles to needed support.

Our findings indicate that respite is perceived as a family matter. Participants reported that they did not trust 'outsiders' with providing the same level of care that the family can provide. It is therefore particularly important that family kinship systems be supported in their roles as respite providers for carers [1]. For carers who are un-networked and vulnerable, provision of support mechanisms should be specifically targeted to their needs to facilitate resilience [45].

Facilitating networks

Formal and informal social support is beneficial to being able to cope as well as mitigate stress and some of the negative health impacts from caring for a child with a disability. Several participants voiced their desire for opportunities to speak, share experiences, and garner strength from linking with other Aboriginal family carers of children with a disability. Participants in support groups can gain emotional and practical information, experiential knowledge, and empathy via reciprocity of peer support [46]. Such groups can provide a sense of community, unconditional acceptance and information, and help to facilitate relationships with family and friends [4]. There is a dearth of information on how Aboriginal carers of children with a disability can best be supported through their disability journey by culturally-appropriate groups and whether this might be one way of overcoming the challenges and disparities faced by Aboriginal Australians.

Limitations

The small self-selected sample preclude generalisation to other Aboriginal and Torres Strait Islander populations or to indigenous populations more widely. Yet, these information-rich narratives were elicited from participants who were purposively recruited from a developmental clinic sample, and as such, the findings may be transferable to individuals in that type of setting. Clinic staff enacted a type of gatekeeping role during recruitment by alerting the researcher to eligible participants who were attending the fortnightly clinic. Being recruited from this clinic may mean that participants were more likely to be receiving care for their child and their access challenges were different because of the increased support or other circumstances related to being a patient of the health service. For example, some participants used the transport service provided by the facility to attend the clinic appointment. Interviews were conducted at an Aboriginal health service, by individuals with organisational affiliations which may have inhibited disclosure of information regarding experiences with that service. Only women carers' perspectives were represented, so future research should seek out male carer perspectives.

Conclusions

Addressing the needs of carers of Aboriginal and Torres Strait Islander children with a disability is vital in the shift to providing community-based care for people and families living with disability. Tailoring services to these carers' needs means supporting kinship caregiving, engaging with other Aboriginal families, and the needs of Aboriginal women who are lone carers and especially vulnerable to financial strain and social isolation. Family resources can mitigate the costs associated with caring for a child with a disability in Aboriginal families and facilitate resilience.

Abbreviations

AH&MRC: Aboriginal Health and Medical Research Council; GP: General practitioner; OOHC: Out-of-home care

Acknowledgements

The research team appreciate the recruitment support and consultation provided by the staff of the Aboriginal health service.

Funding

This work was supported by an Australian Research Council Linkage Project [LP120200484]. AG is a PhD student supported by LP120200484.

Author's contributions

MD contributed to study conceptualization and design, data acquisition and analysis, and drafting the manuscript. AG contributed to data collection, analysis, and manuscript development. PA contributed to study conceptualization, data collection and analysis, and manuscript revision. PMD contributed to study conceptualization and design and manuscript revision. PPH contributed to study conceptualization, data collection, and manuscript review. PD and JD contributed to study conceptualization, data collection and analysis, manuscript revision, and cultural mentorship. All authors read and approved the final manuscript.

Consent for publication

Not applicable

Competing interests

The authors declare that they have no competing interests.

Author details

[1]University of Technology Sydney, Faculty of Health, PO Box 123, Broadway, Sydney, NSW 2007, Australia. [2]Blacktown and Mt Druitt Hospitals, Western Sydney Local Health District, Blacktown Road, Blacktown, NSW 2148, Australia. [3]Johns Hopkins University, School of Nursing, 525 N. Wolfe Street, Baltimore, MD 21205, USA. [4]Western Sydney University, Locked Bag 1797, Penrith, NSW 1797, Australia.

References

1. Llewellyn G, et al. Family factors influencing out-of-home placement decisions. J Intellect Disabil Res. 1999;43(3):219–33.
2. National People with Disabilities and Carer Council, SHUT OUT: The Experience of People with Disabilities and their Families in Australia. 2009, Australian Government: Canberra.
3. Edwards B, et al. The nature and impact of caring for family members with a disability in Australia. Research Report No. 16. Canberra: Australian Institute of Family Studies; 2008.
4. Llewellyn G, et al. Health status and coping strategies among older parent-carers of adults with intellectual disabilities in an Australian sample. Res Dev Disabil. 2010;31:1176–86.
5. Breen C, Burns L. Improving services to families affected by FASD. Final report prepared for the Foundation of Alcohol Research and Education. In: National Drug and Alcohol Research Centre. Sydney: University of New South Wales; 2012.
6. Brown JD, Moraes S, Mayhew J. Service needs of Foster families with children who have disabilities. J Child Fam Stud. 2005;14(3):417–29.
7. Azar M, Kurdahi Badr L. Predictors of coping in parents of children with an intellectual disability: comparison between Lebanese mothers and fathers. J Pediatr Nurs. 2010;25:46–56.
8. McCubbin HI, et al. Culture, ethnicity, and the family: critical factors in childhood chronic illnesses and disabilities. Pediatrics. 1993;91(5):1063–70.

9. Schofield HL, et al. Family carers: women and men, adult offspring, partners, and parents. J Fam Stud. 1997;3(2):149–68.
10. Steering Committee for the Review of Government Service Provision, Overcoming Indigenous Disadvantage: Key Indicators 2014. 2014, Productivity Commission: Canberra.
11. Melbourne Institute of Applied Economic and Social Research, 2014 Household, Income and Labour Dynamics in Australia (HILDA) survey, in Families, Incomes and Jobs, R. Wilkins, Editor. 2014, University of Melbourne: Melbourne.
12. Statistics, A.B.o., National Aboriginal and Torres Strait Islander Social Survey, 2014–15. 2016, Australian Bureau of Statistics: Canberra.
13. Statistics, A.B.o., Aboriginal and Torres Strait Islander People with a Disability, 2012. 2017, Australian Bureau of Statistics.
14. Hunter, B., M. Gray, and H. Crawford, Who cares and does it matter for the labour market? A longitudinal analysis of the labour force status of Indigenous and non-Indigenous carers, in CAEPR WORKING PAPER NO. 105/ 2016. 2016, Centre for Aboriginal Economic Policy Research: Australia National University.
15. Services, N.S.W.D.o.C., Working with Aboriginal People and Communities, a practice resource. 2009, New South Wales Department of Community Services: Ashfield.
16. Hepburn R. Be with us feel with us act with us: counselling and support for indigenous carers. Carers Victoria: Footscray; 2005.
17. Boetto H. Kinship care. Family Matters. 2010;85:60–7.
18. Aboriginal Disability Network New South Wales, Telling it like it is: a report on community consultations with Aboriginal people with disability and their associates throughout NSW, 2004-2005. 2007, Aboriginal Disability Network NSW: Sydney.
19. Australian Institute of Health and Welfare, The health and welfare of Australia's Aboriginal and Torres Strait Islander people: an overview. 2011, Australian Institute of Health and Welfare: Canberra.
20. Morris PS, et al. Otitis media in young aboriginal children from remote communities in northern and Central Australia: a cross-sectional survey. BMC Pediatr. 2005;5(1):27.
21. Williams CJ, Jacobs AM. The impact of otitis media on cognitive and educational outcomes. Med J Aust. 2009;191(9):S69–72.
22. Green A, et al. Navigating the journey of Aboriginal childhood disability: a qualitative study of carers' interface with services. BMC Health Services Research. 2016;16:680.
23. Braun V, Clarke V. Using thematic analysis in psychology. Qual Res Psychol. 2006;3(2):77–101.
24. DiGiacomo M, et al. Childhood disability in Aboriginal and Torres Strait Islander peoples: a literature review. International Journal for Equity in Health. 2013;12:7.
25. Commission on Social Determinants of Health, Closing the gap in a generation: health equity through action on the social determinants of health. Final Report of the Commission on Social Determinants of Health. 2008, World Health Organization: Geneva.
26. Kawachi I, Subramanian SV, Kim D. Social capital and health: a decade of progress and beyond, in Social capital and health. In: Kawachi I, Subramanian SV, Kim D, editors. . New York: Springer; 2008.
27. Loppie Reading C and Wien F, Health Inequalities and Social Determinants of Aboriginal Peoples' Health. 2009, National Collaborating Centre for Aboriginal Health: British Columbia.
28. Mays N, Pope C. Qualitative research in health care: assessing quality in qualitative research. BMJ. 2000;320(7226)
29. Minichiello V, et al. In-depth interviewing: principles, techniques, analysis 2nd ed. Cheshire: Longman; 1995.
30. AH&MRC Ethics Committee, AH&MRC Guidelines for Research into Aboriginal Health: Key Principles. 2013, Aboriginal Health & Medical Research Council of New South Wales: Sydney.
31. Lero DS, et al. The interplay of risk factors associated with negative outcomes among family caregivers: a synthesis of the literature. University of Guelph & University of Alberta: Canada; 2007.
32. Keating N, et al. A framework and literature review on the economic costs of care. University of Guelph & University of Alberta: Canada; 2013.
33. (DEECD), D.o.E.a.E.C.D., The state of Victoria's children 2008. 2009, Department of Education and Early Childhood Development (DEECD): Melbourne.
34. Porterfield SL. Work choices of mothers in families with children with disabilities. J Marriage Fam. 2002;64:972–81.
35. Johnston C, Mash EJ. Families of children with attention-deficit/hyperactivity disorder: review and recommendations for future research. Clin Child Fam Psychol Rev. 2001;4(3):183–207.
36. Lukemeyer A, Meyers MK, Smeeding T. Expensive children in poor families: out-of-pocket expenditures for the care of disabled and chronically ill children in welfare families. J Marriage Fam. 2000;62(2):399–415.
37. Benderix Y, Sivberg B. Siblings' experiences of having a brother or sister with autism and mental retardation: a case study of 14 siblings from five families. J Pediatr Nurs. 2007;22(5):410–8.
38. Kiraly M and Humphreys C, 'It is the story of all of us.' Learning from Aboriginal communities about supporting family connection. Report 2 Family Links: Kinship Care and Family Contact Series. 2011, Child Safety Commissioner: Melbourne.
39. Spence N. Kinship care in Australia. Child Abuse Rev. 2004;13(4):263–76.
40. Cuddleback G. Kinship family foster care: a methodological and substantive synthesis of research. Child Youth Serv Rev. 2004;26:623–39.
41. Powell Sears K. Improving cultural competence education: the utility of an intersectional framework. Med Educ. 2012;46(6)
42. Fuller-Thomson E. Canadian first nations grandparents raising grandchildren: a portrait in resilience. Int J Aging Hum Dev. 2005;60(4):331–42.
43. Secretariat of National Aboriginal and Islander Child Care (SNAICC). Connection to Family. Available from: www.supportingcarers.snaicc.org.au/connecting-to-culture/connection-to-family/.
44. Walker R, Shepherd C. Strengthening aboriginal family functioning: what works and why? Australian Institute of Family Studies: Canberra; 2008.
45. Hassall R, Rose J, McDonald J. Parenting stress in mothers of children with an intellectual disability: the effects of parental cognitions in relation to child characteristics and family support. J Intellect Disabil Res. 2005;49(6): 405–18.
46. Munn-Giddings C, McVicar A. Self-help groups as mutual support: what do carers value? Health & Social Care in the Community. 2007;15(1):26–34.

14

Prevalence of anal symptoms in general practice

Géraldine Tournu[1*], Laurent Abramowitz[2], Camille Couffignal[3,4,5], Frédéric Juguet[6], Agnès Sénéjoux[7], Stéphane Berger[8], Anne-Laure Wiart[9], Marc Bernard[10], Françoise Provost[11], Hélène Pillant-Le Moult[12], Dominique Bouchard[13], Jean-Pierre Aubert[14], for the GREP study group and for the MG-PREVAPROCT study group

Abstract

Background: Anal disorders are largely underestimated in general practice. Studies have shown patients conceal anal symptoms leading to late diagnosis and treatment. Management by general practitioners is poorly described. The aim of this study is to assess the prevalence of anal symptoms and their management in general practice.

Methods: In this prospective, observational, national study set in France, all adult patients consulting their general practitioner during 2 days of consultation were included. Anal symptoms, whether spontaneously revealed or not, were systematically collected and assessed. For symptomatic patients, the obstacles to anal examination were evaluated. The general practitioner's diagnosis was collected and a proctologist visit was systematically proposed in case of anal symptoms. If the proctologist was consulted, his or her diagnosis was collected.

Results: From October 2014 to April 2015, 1061 patients were included by 57 general practitioners. The prevalence of anal symptoms was 15.6% (95% CI: 14–18). However, 85% of these patients did not spontaneously share their symptoms with their doctors, despite a discomfort rating of 3 out of 10 (range 1–5). Although 65% of patients agreed to an anal examination, it was not proposed in 45% of cases with anal symptoms. Performing the examination was associated with a significantly higher diagnosis rate of 76% versus 20% ($p < 0.001$). Proctologist and general practitioner diagnoses were consistent in 14 out of 17 cases.

Conclusions: Patients' concealed anal symptoms are significant in general practice despite the impact on quality of life. Anal examination is seldom done. Improved training of general practitioners is required to break the taboo.

Keywords: General practice, Proctology, Anal, Examination, Epidemiology, Haemorrhoids

Background

General practitioners (GP) should be first in line to manage anal disorders, given their high prevalence in the general population and their simple medical treatment. However, epidemiological research concerning general practice is poor and difficult to obtain because of patients' reluctance to discuss symptoms and to agree to anal examination. Existing studies have evaluated anal symptoms only by questioning patients, without any anal examination. Therefore results of the prevalence of anal disorders vary, from 20% to 40.5% [1–3]. In 2014, Abramowitz et al. evaluated the prevalence of anal symptoms in general practice. Among 1079 patients who consulted their GP in France, 2% consulted spontaneously for an anal symptom. However, after systematic questioning of all patients, the prevalence was in fact 14.2% [4]. Patients do not freely discuss their symptoms, despite an effect on quality of life [5]. Furthermore, anal examination is seldom done by doctors [4], even though it is considered important [6]. A 1990 study assessed the practice of family doctors in England. Reasons for not performing a rectal examination included patients' reluctance, lack of time or repetition of the examination by a proctologist [7].

To pursue the research by Abramowitz et al. [4], we conducted this study to assess the prevalence of anal symptoms, this time by systematic questioning and clinical examination, and to evaluate their management in general practice, by assessing the diagnostic approach,

* Correspondence: gtournu@gmail.com
[1]General practice department, University Paris Diderot, F-75018 Paris, France
Full list of author information is available at the end of the article

the clinical examination proposal rate, the diagnosis rate and the frequency of referral to a proctologist.

Methods

GP recruitment

This observational prospective study was conducted in 5 cities in France: Beausoleil, Bordeaux, Nîmes, Paris and Rennes. Eight referent proctologists were recruited by the French group for proctological research (GREP). Secondly, each proctologist provided a list of his or her usual contact GPs, who were recruited: two hundred and fifty one GPs were contacted by telephone. Eight centres were organised around the 8 proctologists and their contact GPs (1 centre in Beausoleil, 3 centres in Bordeaux, 1 centre in Nîmes, 2 centres in Paris and 1 centre in Rennes). Prior to the study, an optional 2 h medical lecture on anal disorders was proposed to all GPs.

Patient recruitment

All patients were included over 1 to 2 days of consultation. Each GP was first given the option of choosing 1 day within a predefined week for inclusion, but due to lack of GP participation, an additional day was proposed. GPs proposed participation to all consecutive adult patients. Home visit patients were excluded. Data on the reason for refusal to participate was also documented.

Data collection

The presence of anal symptoms, at the time or over the past month, was assessed using a self-administered survey, completed in the waiting room by the patient just before consultation. Patients could choose among a list of symptoms: bleeding, anal pruritus, anal pain, anal swelling, anal discharge and uncontrolled anal leakage. They specified if the anal symptom was the reason for consultation and assessed the level of discomfort and pain on a 0 to 10 numeric rating scale. For each patient included, GPs completed an electronic Case Report Form during consultation. They identified the presence of constipation and diarrhoea. GPs then proposed an anal examination to all symptomatic patients. If they did not propose the examination, the reason of refusal was documented.. Proctologic diagnoses and prescription were also recorded. Additionally, GPs estimated the time dedicated to the proctological issue during the consultation, from patient questioning to prescription.

Proctologist consultation

Patients with anal symptoms were offered a consultation with a proctologist, which would take place within 3 days after the GP visit. If the patient refused, the cause was documented by the GP during consultation.

Statistical methods

Statistical analysis was made for all patients with complete data. Patients with missing data from the self-administered survey were excluded. Continuous variables were expressed as median and range and categorical variables as counts and percentages. To compare the distribution of quantitative variables, the Wilcoxon rank sum test was used. To compare the distribution of qualitative variables, the chi-square test was used.

The concordance rate between the GP and the proctologist diagnoses were measured by the Kappa coefficient. All analyses were performed using SAS software (SAS Institute, Cary, NC). Statistical significance level was defined by $p < 0.05$.

A sample size of 1920 participants would allow an accuracy of 3% for an expected prevalence of 14% as shown in the previous study by Abramowitz et al. [4]. For each of the 8 referent proctologists, 15 GPs were to be contacted. Considering an average of 20 patients seen each day in each GP office in France and an estimated refusal rate of 20%, this would lead to an estimated inclusion of 1920 participants. One centre in Paris was excluded before the beginning of the study due to the lack of GP participation.

Results

Population included

Among 251 doctors contacted, 80 accepted the study and 59 included at least 1 patient. The two main reasons for doctors' refusal to participate were lack of time or interest in the research. Doctors' average age was 50 years (range 42–57) and 52.6% were male. Two doctors who did not follow the research protocol during patient inclusion were excluded. Assessment took place from October 2014 to April 2015, and 1315 patients were screened by the 57 doctors. The median number of patients assessed by each doctor was 19 (range 15–29). Among the 1315 screened patients, 60 patients were excluded for missing age or sex, and 1061 (84.5%) accepted to participate in the study. The median age was 52 years (range 37–67), 414 were males (39%). Causes for refusal to participate are listed in Fig. 1.

Prevalence of anal symptoms

After targeted questioning, anal symptoms were found for 166 patients (15.6%; 95% CI: 14–18), of which only 25 (2.3%; median age: 43 years, range 32–54) declared it was the reason for consultation. One hundred forty-one patients (13.3%; median age: 49 years, range 38–61) had an anal symptom though this was not the reason for consultation (Table 1). No difference in distribution of anal symptoms was found between centres.

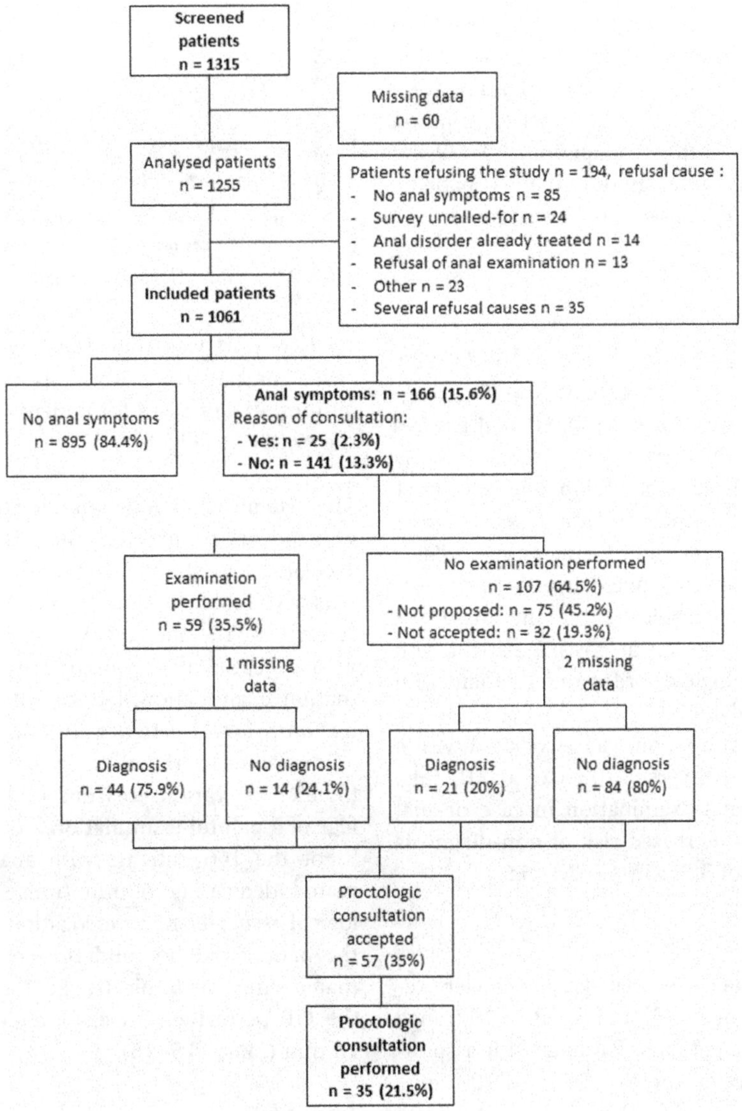

Fig. 1 Patient flow-chart

Table 1 Prevalence of anal symptoms and diagnosis approach

Anal symptom	Total anal symptoms (*n* = 166)	Reason for consultation (*n* = 25)	Revealed by questioning (*n* = 141)	*p* value[a]
Anal symptom				
Bleeding	77 (46.4%)	13 (52%)	64 (45.4%)	0.66
Anal pruritus	74 (44.6%)	11 (44%)	63 (44.7%)	1
Pain	57 (34.3%)	17 (68%)	40 (28.4%)	<0.001
Anal swelling	45 (27.1%)	12 (48%)	33 (23.4%)	0.01
Anal discharge	17 (10.2%)	1 (4%)	16 (11.3%)	0.47
Uncontrolled anal leakage	15 (9%)	3 (12%)	12 (8.5%)	0.70

[a]chi-square test *p*-value

Patients spontaneously consulting for an anal complaint in comparison with patients who revealed the symptoms after questioning

Anal symptom and constipation or diarrhoea

GPs assessed the presence of constipation or diarrhoea for patients with anal symptoms (Table 2). Constipation and a combination of diarrhoea and constipation were associated with the presence of an anal symptom. Among the 127 patients with constipation, 50 (39.4%) had anal symptoms. Likewise, among the 44 patients with a combination of diarrhoea and constipation, 22 (50%) had anal symptoms.

Proctological diagnoses

A diagnosis was made for 65 patients out of 165 (39.9%), and there was no diagnosis for 98 patients (60.1%). Diagnoses included: 42 haemorrhoids (25.8%), 10 anal fissures (6.1%), 3 dermatologic disorders (1.8%), 2 condyloma (1.2%), 2 anal abscesses, 2 marisca, 2 idiopathic pruritus, 1 mycosis, 1 lichen, 1 anal erythema, 1 anal excoriation, 1 anal incontinence after surgery and 2 unidentified disorders. Five patients had more than one diagnosis (2 patients were diagnosed with haemorrhoids and an anal fissure, 1 patient with haemorrhoids and a mycosis, 1 patient with an abscess and a dermatologic disorder and 1 patient with an anal fissure and a condyloma).

Performing an anal examination was associated with a higher diagnosis rate of 76% versus 20% ($p < 0.001$) (Fig. 2). Not performing an anal examination in case of anal symptoms resulted in an increased risk of non-diagnosis with a relative risk (RR) of 3.5; 95% CI: 2.1–5.6.

Pain and discomfort

Pain and discomfort induced by anal symptoms were respectively 2 out of 10 (range 0–5) and 3 out of 10 (range 2–6) for all symptomatic patients. Patients with a spontaneous anal complaint rated the pain 5 out of 10 (range 2–7) versus 1 out of 10 (range 0–4) for patients who did not consult for the symptom ($p = 0.001$). Likewise, discomfort was more important among patients with a spontaneous anal complaint, 5 out of 10 (range 3–8) versus 3 out of 10 (range 1–5) ($p = 0.006$) for patients who did not consult for the symptom.

Table 2 Prevalence of diarrhoea and constipation, depending on the presence of an anal symptom (n = 1061)

Intestinal transit disorders (n = 249)	Patients with anal symptoms (n = 166)	Patients without anal symptoms (n = 895)	p-value[a]
Diarrhoea (n = 78)	17 (10.2%)	61 (6.8%)	0.12
Constipation (n = 127)	50 (30.1%)	77 (8.6%)	< 0.001
Both (n = 44)	22 (13.3%)	22 (2.5%)	< 0.001

[a]chi-square test p-value

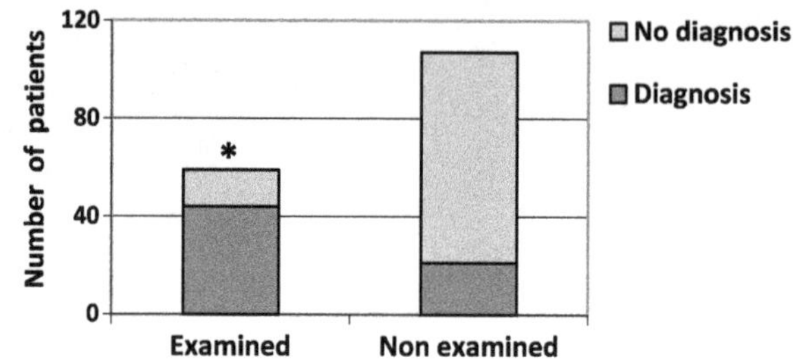

Fig. 2 Proportion of diagnoses depending on clinical examination

Discomfort was considered average or high in 43% of cases for patients with a spontaneous anal complaint and for 40% of cases for patients who did not consult for the symptom (Fig. 3).

Anal examination in general practice

GPs did not propose any anal examination for 75 out of 165 (45.2%) patients with anal symptoms, for different reasons (Table 3). None of the GPs declared being constrained by the anal examination. Among the 59 patients who accepted the examination, all underwent an anal margin examination, but digital rectal examination was not done for 24 patients (40.7%).

The anal examination was refused by 32 patients (35.2%) for various reasons (Table 3). None declared a fear of a painful examination.

For the 166 patients with anal symptoms, GPs estimated dedicating 6 min (range 5–10) to the proctological issue, from interrogation to prescription. When the patient did not undergo an anal examination, estimated time was 5 min (range 3–8). Comparatively, when the GP performed an examination, estimated time was 10 min (range 8.5–15).

Treatments

Haemorrhoids was the most frequent diagnosis. For those patients with this diagnosis, ointments were then most often prescribed (69%), followed by suppositories (45.2%), phlebotonic drugs (31%), laxatives (28.6%), oral anti-inflammatory drugs (21.4%) and oral analgesics (14.3%). Phlebotonic, also known as venoactive, drugs increase venous tone leading to an increase in capillary resistance, improvements in lymphatic flow and reduction in oedema.

Proctologist's follow-up consultation

Among the 166 patients with anal symptoms, fifty-seven (34.9% on 163 with complete data) accepted a consultation with the referent proctologist. Thirty-five (21.2%) patients were seen in consultation. Among them, 17 had a diagnosis from the GP, of which 14 were in concordance with the proctologist's diagnosis (Kappa = 0.66; 95% CI: 0.27–0.91).

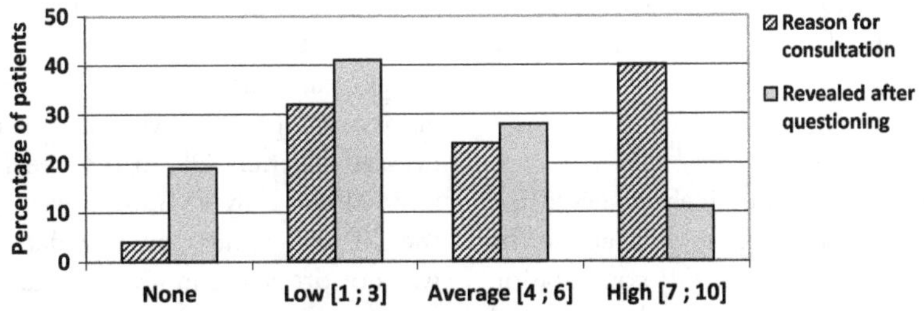

Fig. 3 Level of discomfort due to the anal symptom, when it was spontaneously declared or revealed after questioning

Medical lecture

Among the 57 participating GPs, 40% (n = 23) attended the lecture before screening. The lecture did not have any impact on their practice. The rate of anal symptoms found by patient questioning was no different. Furthermore, GPs who attended the lecture did not perform more anal examinations.

Discussion

Summary

For this study we assessed the diagnostic approach, the clinical examination proposal rate, the diagnosis rate and the frequency of referral to a proctologist.

Table 3 Anal examination in general practice

Reasons GPs did not propose an anal examination	Patients (n = 75)
Another predominant cause of consultation	n = 24 (32%)
Lack of time	n = 21 (28%)
Patient already under treatment	n = 19 (25%)
Fear of embarrassing the patient	n = 4 (5%)
Patient directly addressed the proctologist	n = 4 (5%)
Other	n = 9 (1%)
Reasons GPs did not perform a digital rectal examination	Patients (n = 24)
Fear of causing pain	n = 10 (42%)
Absence of indication	n = 5 (21%)
Patient's reluctance	n = 3 (12%)
Embarrassment	n = 2 (8%)
Lack of knowledge in proctology	n = 2 (8%)
Lack of time	n = 2 (8%)
Other	n = 5 (21%)
Reasons patients refused the anal examination	Patients (n = 32)
Discomfort	n = 11 (34%)
Anal symptoms considered of minor importance	n = 11 (34%)
Examination already performed for the symptom	n = 8 (25%)
Knowing the examination would be repeated by the specialist	n = 7 (22%)
Lack of time	n = 4 (12%)
Other	n = 2 (6%)

In our cohort of 1061 patients, 2.3% spontaneously consulted their GP for an anal symptom. However, after questioning all patients, the prevalence of anal symptoms was 15.6% (95% CI: 14–18). This not only reveals the high prevalence of anal symptoms in general practice but also highlights that they are under-reported by patients and underestimated by practitioners.

Furthermore, half the patients presenting a combination of diarrhoea and constipation had an anal symptom.

While the main diagnoses were haemorrhoids (25.8%) and anal fissures (6.1%), 60.1% of patients had no diagnosis. Only 54.8% of symptomatic patients were proposed an anal examination by their GP. Yet, our results show that performing an examination was associated with a higher diagnosis rate, of 76% versus 20% ($p < 0.001$). When the examination was not done, there was an increased risk of non-diagnosis. This highlights the importance of the examination in the diagnosis approach. GPs estimated devoting 5 min to the proctological issue when the examination was not done and 10 min when it was done.

We studied the management of anal disorders by GPs. Although anal examination was not proposed for 45.2% of patients, none of the GPs declared being constrained by it. They complained of lack of time, especially because of another reason of consultation. In other cases, they were afraid of embarrassing the patient or they directly addressed the patient to the proctologist.

Concerning patients, anal examination was accepted by the majority (64.8%) but still refused by a third. The principal reason was discomfort, followed by the fact that the anal symptoms were considered of minor importance. In other cases, patients refused, knowing the examination would be repeated by a specialist or because they were in a hurry. One of the factors influencing the patient's decision could be the doctor's confidence and motivation.

Finally, concerning treatments, first line treatment in haemorrhoids and anal fissures involves treating constipation and dyschesia [8–10]. Yet in our study, for haemorrhoids, laxatives were not prescribed in 28.6% of cases and no treatment was given in 14.3% of cases.

Likewise, for anal fissures, no treatment was given in 20% of cases and only half of patients were prescribed laxatives.

Strengths and limitations

This is the first study to have prospectively assessed the management of anal symptoms in general practice, by describing the patient's path from their GP consultation to the proctologist's follow-up visit. This observational study presents limits. First, due to low GP participation, it was necessary to increase inclusion per GP, by setting up an additional day of inclusion during consultation. This could have led to a recruitment bias, as the volunteering GPs could have been sensitized to anal diseases and their medical practice does not necessarily reflect the general practice. Inclusion rate was lower than intended, diminishing the study's strength. Yet our data show no difference between the 7 centres. Distribution was similar in different French cities, hence representing French medical practices. Secondly, anal symptoms were sought up to 1 month preceding consultation. Therefore patients could have no more symptoms at the time of the study, leading to a low rate of examination and a high rate of non-diagnosis in our study (60.1%). Finally, the referent proctologist saw few patients, meaning the GPs diagnoses were confirmed only for a few cases.

Comparison with existing literature

A study by Nelson et al. found a prevalence of anal symptoms of 20% in the general population, using a telephone survey with 102 adults in the Joliet, Illinois area [1]. Abramowitz et al. found similar results to our work: 14.2% of anal symptoms [4] in France but among a different population of GPs and in different areas of the country. The concealment of symptoms was already reported by Siproudhis et al. with 58.3% of patients suffering from proctological disorders who never consulted their GP [2]. In our study, 85% of patients revealed their symptoms only after questioning.

Concerning anal symptoms, our data was similar to those of a French study by Pigot et al. where 161 doctors recruited 831 patients consulting for a proctological complaint. Symptoms recorded using an information sheet were: pain (48%), bleeding (37%), anal swelling (26%) and anal pruritis (24%) [3]. In this study, the subjective impact of anal symptoms (none, little, important, enormous) on quality of life was assessed. It was considered important or enormous for 44% of patients who consulted for that symptom. In our work, on a numeric rating scale from 0 to 10, discomfort was considered average or high in 43% of cases. Our study is the first to evaluate the impact on patients who had not spontaneously revealed their symptoms. For these patients, discomfort was average or high in 40% of cases.

Regarding doctors' diagnosis approach, our survey confirms the low rate of anal examination, especially rectal examination. In a study by Springall and Todd, among 305 patients with anal or digestive symptoms addressed by their GP to the specialist, 31% were not examined and only 48% underwent a rectal examination by the GP [6], similar to our data where an examination was not proposed in 45.2% of cases.

Implications for practice

Patients don't spontaneously reveal anal symptoms, despite affecting quality of life. Patient discomfort towards anal examination could be a restraint. A systematic screening for anal disorders is already recommended for HIV (Human Immunodeficiency Virus) patients [11] and is common practice for pregnancy and postpartum patients [12]. Screening should also be systematic in case of constipation and/or diarrhoea, given the high rate of anal symptoms in these populations.

In parallel, informing patients about the frequency of anal disorders could help encourage patients to spontaneously share their symptoms, to avoid inadequate self-medication or aggravation of certain disorders. Similarly, medical training for students and practitioners could sensitize the medical profession, especially the importance of examination, which is seldom done and could lead to absence or error in diagnosis. Regarding anal fissures, late diagnosis can lead to chronic or infected fissures, which could put patients at risk of faecal incontinence due to surgery. As for haemorrhoids, simple medical or instrumental treatment is often sufficient, but late diagnosis could also lead to complications due to necessary surgery. Finally, there is the risk of overlooking an anal or rectal cancer.

Conclusion

2.3% of patients consult GPs spontaneously for an anal complaint. However, after targeted questioning of patients, 15.6% (95% CI = 14 to 18) of adult patients have an anal symptom. Despite the impact on quality of life, leading to discomfort and pain, these symptoms are seldom declared.

In 60.1% of cases, GPs do not diagnose for reported anal symptoms. It is of note that performing an anal examination is associated with a 3.8 times higher diagnosis rate. Yet examination is insufficiently proposed by GPs. When proposed, it is accepted by patients two thirds of the time. To break the taboo and improve management, better information concerning anal symptoms could be provided to both patients and practitioners.

Abbreviations

GP: General practitioner; HIV: Human Immundeficiency Virus

Acknowledgements
The authors wish to thank Caroline Barnes who contributed to the translation of the article.
Group authorship: the members of the MG-PREVAPROCT study group are: Cédric Laouénan, Sandrine Calonne, Sonia Corral, Philippe Uge, Thomas Tarjus, Raymond Wakim, Thierry Dubon, Pierre Fenouillet, Gregory Lovato, Alain Lovato, Valérie Berthelot-Calmels, Philippe Denoyelle, Gregory Moisset, Anne Youssefian, Valérie Douillard, Michel Geffrault, Marie-Pierre Bouchara, Mathieu Petit, Bertrand Leblanc, Claudine Brune Ropert, Emmanuel Fournier, Cécile Andreu, Isabel Ferraris, David Ferraris, Nora Gauffier, Ismaël Nureni Banafunzi, Claire Salanova, Michael Boyadjian, Joelle Desaize, Catherine Dubertret, Cornélis Floor, Catherine Majerholc, Ewa Rudnicka, Hélène Vitou, Hélène Carrez-Louys, Frédéric Dumas, Monique Horwitz-Guérin, Marina Lavigne, Valérie Lubert, Eric Penichou, Julien Pouyanne, Sophie Sauvage-Rigal, Igor Sozonoff, Sandrine Baux, Marianne Guern, Bruno Calmels, Jamila Jamil, Catherine Chaumie, Guy Millou, Bernard Foinant, Alain Frangeul, Pascal Roger, Garry Magendie, Didier Marion and Jean-François Toledo.
The members of the GREP study group are: Cécile Laclotte, Dominique De Faucal, Thierry Higuero, Guillaume Bonnaud, Vincent De Parades and Véronique Vitton.

Consent to participate
Not applicable.

Funding
This study was financed by a grant of BAYER laboratories. The study design, analysis, results and write up were performed independently to the BAYER laboratories.

Authors' contributions
GT designed the study, prepared data for inclusion in the manuscript and participated in manuscript writing. LA designed the study and oversaw writing. CC conducted statistical analyses, prepared data for inclusion in the manuscript and oversaw writing. FJ, AS, HPLM, DB oversaw the design, participated in data acquisition and oversaw writing. SB, ALW, MB, FP participated in data acquisition and oversaw writing. The GREP study group participated in data acquisition and oversaw design and writing, the MG-PREVAPROCT study group participated in data acquisition and oversaw writing. JPA designed the study and oversaw manuscript writing. All authors read and approved the final manuscript.

Competing interests
LA is a consultant for Bayer, Sanofi, Abbvie, Allergan, MEDAPharma and Coloplast. This study was financed by a grant of BAYER laboratories.

Author details
[1]General practice department, University Paris Diderot, F-75018 Paris, France. [2]AP-HP and GREP; Gastroenterology and proctology unit, Bichat University hospital, Paris, France. [3]INSERM, IAME, UMR 1137, F-75018 Paris, France. [4]University Paris Diderot, IAME, UMR 1137, Sorbonne Paris Cité, F-75018 Paris, France. [5]AP-HP, Bichat hospital, Biostatistics unit, F-75018 Paris, France. [6]Tivoli Ducos Clinic, Bordeaux, France. [7]Proctology unit, Private hospital, Saint Grégoire, France. [8]Montigny les Cormeilles, France. [9]Bordeaux, France. [10]Cadaujac, France. [11]Rennes, France. [12]Blomet Clinic, Paris, France. [13]Proctology unit, Bagatelle hospital, Talence, France. [14]Sorbonne Paris Cité, General practice department, University Paris Diderot, F-75018 Paris, France ; REMES, F-75018 Paris, France.

References

1. Nelson RL, Abcarian H, Davis FG, Persky V. Prevalence of benign anorectal disease in a randomly selected population. Dis Colon rectum. 1995;38:341–4.
2. Siproudhis L, Pigot F, Godeberge P, Damon H, Soudan D, Bigard MA. Defecation Disorders: a French Population Survey. Dis Colon rectum. 2006; 49:219–27.
3. Pigot F, Siproudhis L, Bigard M-A, Staumont G. Ano-rectal complaints in general practitioner visits: consumer point of view. Gastroentérologie Clin Biol. 2006;30:1371–4.
4. Abramowitz L, Benabderrahmane M, Pospait D, Philip J, Laouénan C. The prevalence of proctological symptoms amongst patients who see general practitioners in France. Eur J Gen Pract. 2014;20:301–6.
5. Damon H, Guye O, Seigneurin A, Long F, Sonko A, Faucheron J-L, et al. Prevalence of anal incontinence in adults and impact on quality-of-life. Gastroentérologie Clin Biol. 2006;30:37–43.
6. Springall RG, Todd IP. General practitioner referral of patients with lower gastrointestinal symptoms. J R Soc Med. 1988;81:87–8.
7. Hennigan TW, Franks PJ, Hocken DB, Allen-Mersh TG. Rectal examination in general practice. BMJ. 1990;301:478–80.
8. Perry WB, Dykes SL, Buie WD, Rafferty JF. Practice parameters for the Management of Anal Fissures (3rd revision). Dis Colon rectum. 2010;53: 1110–5.
9. Slim K, Siproudhis L. Fissure anale. Quel traitement de première intention ? Ann Chir. 2004;129:290–2.
10. Zeitoun J-D, de Parades V. Pathologie hémorroïdaire : de la physiopathologie à la clinique. Presse Med. 2011;40:920–6.
11. Morlat P. Prise en charge médicale des personnes vivant avec le VIH. Recommandations du groupe d'expert 2013;237. http://solidarites-sante.gouv.fr/IMG/pdf/Rapport_Morlat_2013_Mise_en_ligne-6.pdf.
12. Abramowitz L, Sobhani I, Benifla JL, Vuagnat A, Daraï E, Mignon M, et al. Anal fissure and thrombosed external hemorrhoids before and after delivery. Dis Colon rectum. 2002;45:650–5.

15

Health care provider experiences in primary care memory clinics: a phenomenological study

Linda Sheiban[1,2], Paul Stolee[1,3*], Carrie McAiney[4] and Veronique Boscart[1,2,3]

Abstract

Background: There is a growing need for community-based services for persons with Alzheimer's disease and related dementias (ADRD). Memory clinic (MC) teams in primary care settings have been established to provide care to people with ADRD. To consider wider adoption of these MC teams, insight is needed into the experiences of practitioners working in these models. The purpose of the current study is to explore the experiences of health care providers (HCPs) who work in primary care Memory Clinic (MC) teams to provide care to persons with Alzheimer's disease and related dementias (ADRD).

Methods: This study utilized a phenomenological methodology to explore experiences of 12 HCPs in two primary care MCs. Semi-structured interviews were completed with each HCP. Interviews were recorded and transcribed verbatim. Colaizzi's steps for analyzing phenomenological data was utilized by the authors.

Results: Three themes emerged from the analysis to describe HCP experiences: supporting patients and family members during ADRD diagnosis and treatment, working in a team setting, and personal and professional rewards of caring for people with ADRD and their family members.

Conclusions: Findings provide insight into current practices in primary care MCs and on the motivation of HCPs working with persons with ADRD.

Keywords: Alzheimer's disease, Dementia, Primary health care, Gerontology, Phenomenology, Qualitative methodology, Memory clinics

Background

As the prevalence of Alzheimer's disease and related dementias (ADRD) increases, there is a growing pressure on the healthcare system to provide care for individuals with dementia and their caregivers. Primary care is the first level of health care in which people with dementia seek and receive care (family physician clinic). However, there are concerns about the capacity of primary care [1] to address complex, chronic conditions [2]. Implementing collaborative care models for chronic conditions such as ADRD has been shown to improve quality of care, and is linked to positive health outcomes for patients [3, 4]. The diagnosis and management of patients with ADRD is a challenge in primary care [5]. A systematic review by Bradford and colleagues [6] found that ADRD is difficult to diagnose and manage in primary care settings due to several factors, including lack of proper training in distinguishing between the different types of dementia.

The Ontario College of Family Physicians developed a five-day training program to implement a primary care-based Memory Clinic (MC) model that supports multidisciplinary team approaches to diagnose and treat people with ADRD [5]. This specialized memory clinic model has been adapted to fit a primary care structure, training already-established primary care teams on adopting a memory clinic model within their current primary care practice setting [7]. Teams who have embedded this model hold MC days monthly to assess referred patients [5]. The memory clinic model in Ontario offers a multidisciplinary team training approach to better assist in the diagnosis and

* Correspondence: stolee@uwaterloo.ca
[1]School of Public and Health and Health Systems, University of Waterloo, Waterloo, Ontario, Canada
[3]Schlegel-UW Research Institute for Aging, Kitchener, Ontario, Canada
Full list of author information is available at the end of the article

treatment of ADRD among health teams [8]. Team members are trained to work in this clinic, and provide comprehensive, collaborative assessments to patients who present with memory issues [5]. These clinics offer an intermediate level of care between primary and specialist care for patients who present with symptoms of ADRD. Family Health Teams (FHTs) are the most common teams to embed this model, with various healthcare providers (such as nurses, physicians, social workers and pharmacists) collaborating [5].

The effectiveness of primary care MCs and their societal impact is not yet understood. Previous studies have examined experiences of those working with people with ADRD in acute care [9] and psychiatric care [10]. Lee and colleagues [5] showed that a MC decreased the number of unnecessary referrals to specialists and physicians believed that MCs improved the quality of care they provided. In order to consider wider adoption of primary care based models, insight is needed into the experiences of practitioners working in these models.

The purpose of this study was to explore the experiences of health care providers (HCPs) who work with people with ADRD and their families. Understanding the experiences of HCPs in MCs will assist in developing strategies to enhance primary care services [11]. This work could promote understanding of HCPs' responsibilities and practices and inform future policy.

Methods

A phenomenological approach was employed to explore the essence of the experience of HCPs working in primary care MC teams in Ontario when caring for people with ADRD. This approach aimed to obtain a deeper understanding of the nature of the shared experience of HCPs who care for patients with ADRD in primary care memory clinics [12, 13]. These HCPs share a common experience of working in an enhanced model of primary care (memory clinic) and in a team setting to provide care for patients with ADRD. The study received ethics clearance from the University of Waterloo Office of Research Ethics in Ontario, Canada (ORE # 19001).

Recruitment & interview protocol

Eligibility criteria for HCP participation included: 1) currently working in FHT-based primary care MC; and 2) English-speaking. Interested team members contacted the Principal Investigator (PI) to schedule an interview. Participants signed an informed consent prior to participation. Individual interviews took place in a private room within the work setting. The PI utilized a semi-structured interview guide, allowing for flexible probing of examples, thoughts and ideas.

Data analysis

Interviews were recorded and transcribed verbatim. The authors used Colaizzi's [14] steps to analyze the data. These steps included the following procedure. First, each participant's transcript was reviewed by the PI by reading what they stated during their interview. This step allowed the researcher to gain a sense of their experience. Next, phrases that pertained to the phenomenon were extracted [14]. The PI then "formulated meanings" by moving beyond each statement to determine its meaning, while keeping the original transcription in mind [14]. The meanings of statements were then organized into theme clusters. Two authors compared these themes to the transcripts, validating that emerging themes kept the essence of the original statements [14]. If authors revealed differences in opinions, they reflected on the purpose of the study and engaged in several discussions to ensure agreement on the final themes [15]. Themes were then used to construct a description of the topic under investigation. Member-checking ensured themes captured the true nature of experiences.

Results

Background of participants

A total of 12 HCPs from two MC teams participated in the study. Participants included four nurses, two primary care physicians, two social workers, two pharmacists, one physician assistant and one occupational therapist. Participants' experience ranged from 1 to 7 years in the MC and from 1 to 33 years in their HCP role. Interviews lasted 30 minutes. Data saturation was reached after six interviews as no new themes and ideas emerged [13]; however, the PI completed 12 interviews to ensure a full range of experiences were included. Four HCPs provided feedback as part of the member-check, assisting in validating the findings.

Themes

Three main themes emerged from the analysis (Table 1): 1) supporting patients and family members during ADRD diagnosis and treatment, 2) working in a team setting, and 3) personal and professional rewards of caring for people with ADRD and their family members.

Theme 1: Supporting patients and family members during ADRD diagnosis and treatment

HCPs in the MC felt they supported patients and their families through the course of the ADRD diagnosis and the care plan. They felt responsible for patients and families, and discussed the importance of supporting patients while maintaining their dignity.

Subtheme 1: Maintaining patient dignity Obtaining the health and social history of patients allows HCPs to understand the patient's identity, which assists

Table 1 Overview of themes and subthemes

Themes	Subthemes
Supporting patients and family members during ADRD diagnosis and treatment	*Maintaining patient dignity*
	Balancing emotional situations and responsibilities
Working in a team setting	*Feeling valued and connected to team members*
	Unique health care provider experiences
Personal and professional rewards of caring for people with ADRD and their family members	*Complexities*
	Ongoing learning opportunities
	Personal and professional fulfillment

them in maintaining a patient's dignity. One HCP described the MC as a "soft place to land" for patients, providing them and their family the opportunity to discuss challenges and solutions with the HCPs. The HCPs take the time to listen while demonstrating a caring attitude:

> "I like to think of it, like, we're a soft place to land. We can sort of help buffer whatever hell they're going through. So if they go away going 'wow, somebody cares' that makes it all worthwhile," [HCP11].

HCPs described how an ADRD diagnosis affects the emotional state of patients and families and how their role consists of seeing the person behind the diagnosis:

> "I think that the most challenging part would be, dancing around the dignity piece. Many people don't want to hear the word dementia. So it's being able to deliver the language or concerns with still maintaining who they are and the dignity behind that person," [HCP03].

Understanding the stigma associated with an ADRD diagnosis helps HCPs to recognize and respond to these feelings and was perceived as an important role of their work in the MC.

Subtheme 2: Balancing emotional situations and responsibilities One of the most difficult situations for HCPs in the MC was delivering the "bad news" of an ADRD diagnosis. When asked how one "breaks bad news", participants talked about empathic responses and the importance of observing patients' and families' reactions to the diagnosis. These emotions often directed how HCPs responded to the situation:

> "Sometimes, if they're really sad or upset, then I feel that too. I feel sad for them. But some patients, they understand. So I sort of react according to how the patient reacts. If they're OK with it, then I feel OK. If they're really upset and sad, then I feel really upset and sad too" [HCP06].

Once a diagnosis had been made, HCPs discussed feeling responsible to help patients and their families on this emotional journey. One responsibility of the HCPs at the MC is assessing the patient's ability to maintain their driver's license. When asked how revoking licenses made them feel, many HCPs described feelings of sadness. HCPs understand that driving is an important part of most peoples' lives so it is a difficult issue for them to discuss:

> "Reporting licenses? Huge, huge. Like the hardest thing you have to do. People hate you, scream at you, yell at you, walk out, storm out. It's really hard for people and you hate doing it." [HCP11].

HCPs discussed the importance of gaining all necessary information from patients and families in order to accurately diagnose ADRD. HCPs described how a limited understanding of the disease by patients and families could form a barrier to adherence, such as issues around adhering to prescribed medications and attending follow-up appointments. One HCP described the struggle of accepting decisions made by patients and families:

> "Once in a while, you get somebody who just says: "I don't want the pills. I don't want anything". And you know they have things really wrong with them that you could help with" [HCP09].

All HCPs described how they try to understand the journey of a patient and their family, and their role of helping people make decisions that could enhance quality of life. HCPs saw this as their main responsibility at the MC:

> "I just love the fact that so many people surround this family and form a safety net. So I think that's really rewarding and you can see the difference that it makes and how much people appreciate that kind of care" [HCP10].

HCPs aim to provide various levels of support to patients and families when giving difficult news. HCPs talked about using their expertise to guide people on the ADRD journey.

Theme 2: Working in a team setting

The second theme describes HCPs' experiences working as a team within the MC. HCPs spoke about their strong connection with their colleagues, feeling part of a "family". HCPs explained the unique experience of working at the MC versus other health teams, specifically other FHTs. Two subthemes describe *feeling valued and connected to team members* as well as having *unique HCP experiences.*

Subtheme 1: Feeling valued and connected to team members HCPs described the value of individual roles in the MC. They believed that having a variety of disciplines on the team enhanced opportunities for comprehensive and multi-faceted care:

> "The disciplines all bring their own lens and perspectives. Bringing that to the table and having a really open, fulsome discussion is a much richer, and fulsome assessment than any individual physician can have in their office visit" [HCP08].

HCPs discussed their professional experience and contributions to the team. One HCP described a situation where the team brought different perspectives and collaborated to develop an individualized care plan for a patient:

> "[the other HCPs are] quite respectful if I see something differently. There was a client with some behaviours. They were going to look at medication. I was trying to figure out why that behaviour was happening instead of just medicating the behaviour. And they were quite open to that" [HCP04].

Another HCP talked about being valued as a member of the team:

> "I don't think I want the team to go ahead without me. It's part of a family and you want to be involved... I feel like there is a significant role there for [me] and that without it, there would be something missing" [HCP02].

Many HCPs described their team as a "family," working together to care for patients with ADRD and families. HCPs felt comfortable stating their opinions during consultations. Yet, inviting different perspectives from the team could also lead to conflicting opinions. One HCP described:

> "I think you could call it a challenge, like someone thinks the complete opposite of what I'm thinking. I think that's what we're looking for, the different perspectives" [HCP05].

HCPs saw benefits in gaining different perspectives, expressing opinions, and, at times, disagreeing with each other. Perceiving the team as a family allowed HCPs to speak freely and share perspectives: "...We hear everybody's opinion, work it out and by the time everybody leaves the room [they've] all kind of come to an agreement" [HCP02].

A well-connected team brings advantages to caring for people with ADRD, as patients and families benefit from all HCPs' expertise, insights and opinions.

Subtheme 2: Unique health care provider experiences HCPs discussed the unique experience of working in the MC. The "tight-knit" team and the clinic set-up allowed for face-to-face consultations with team members:

> "[The MC is] truly a team whereas in a Family Health Team, we have different practitioners working side by side - often still in a bit of a silo in terms of doing our own thing." [HCP02].

HCPs described the MC team as a "little family within a big family" [HCP03]. HCPs explained how the MC set-up allows for different HCPs to see the patient during the same appointment:

> "I think [the MC is] a true team environment, whereas in all the other settings, you're kind of doing the dual role, but we're not actually a team—we're more kind of different cogs in a machine" [HCP06].

HCPs described that the time spent with the patient is unique in primary care. Having more time to consult with the patient and team members was seen as beneficial:

> "I just found it so hard in the regular structure of practice—that 10-minute office visit. With these seniors, 10 minutes are to deal with the most acute problem, and memory problems are not acute until they hit crisis. So that all just got pushed back and then, nothing would be done" [HCP08].

HCPs perceived extra time to assess the patient as necessary to provide an accurate ADRD diagnosis, and positively impacts care for patients and families:

> "I really like that we get to see patients consistently. When people are diagnosed with dementia, you're told and you never see that doctor again. I feel like that we are consistently seeing people at follow-up" [HCP07].

HCPs expressed that extra time provides patients and families with an opportunity to feel connected to and comfortable with the care team. Follow-up with patients is a benefit of the MC structure and supports HCPs to provide continuous care:

"We always get the same nurses to test each person over time and they have a really good sense if the person is declining. And sometimes, it's very subtle. There is just something about him that is not right. Even though his cognitive test scores seem the same. There's so many aspects to how a person functions. Those pieces of information will get lost if there wasn't this real time discussion" [HCP08].

The MC structure provides HCPs the opportunity to maintain care continuity with patients and families so they can notice changes over time. This structure also allows HCPs to connect with patients and families at different points in the ADRD journey:

"Working with the elderly, you're working at all parts of the system—right from primary care to long-term care. You meet [people] at this part, but you might meet them again at this end. So we are helping them get to the next place that they need to be..." [HCP01].

Although the MC structure allows HCPs to deliver resources to patients and families, navigating the healthcare system is a difficult task, even for HCPs. Connecting patients with the appropriate resources was challenging. One HCP explained the difficulty of finding resources for those whose drivers' licenses were revoked:

" [A challenge is] trying to figure what resources are available, and how we get those services in place. Specifically around driving. It's a huge cost to the family and there's nothing really local." [HCP05].

Another HCP described being frustrated with the waitlists for long-term care. "The waitlists for a lot of things - in long-term care, sometimes people have to be placed on waitlists for that, it's frustrating," [HCP11]. Contrastingly, HCPs described the benefit of linking with community partners to assist patients and family members:

"Those community partners that we've connected with—the day program, the Alzheimer's Society, and other community networks. There's been some amazing links" [HCP03].

The MC structure allowed HCPs within that "little family" to support the "bigger families." HCPs described the benefit this structure has for community physicians:

"We're actually there to support the physicians in our community. We can be someone that our FHT can lean on. I like that feeling" [HCP03].

HCPs in the MC worked within a larger realm of care to provide ongoing support to those with ADRD. Although navigating resources was challenging, community partners allowed HCPs to provide additional support and resources to patients.

Theme 3: Personal and professional rewards of caring for people with ADRD and their family members

The final theme describes how HCPs felt they have grown personally and professionally through their work on the MC team. HCPs emphasized how the complexity of ADRD creates learning opportunities, as "no two patients are the same" [HCP01]. HCPs explained how collaborating to diagnose and support patients was like solving a puzzle, with each team member adding pieces of information.

Subtheme 1: Complexities When asked about their motivations for working with the ADRD population, HCPs described finding complexities intriguing, and preferred to delve into patients' past and current medical and social conditions in order to better understand the patient and develop a treatment plan. One HCP described the unique aspects of older patients:

"What we do in geriatrics is so much more different than, what I call the, single disease state of 'whoa, we have your blood pressure at a great number' and that's easy to do, relatively speaking. That's why I love what I do, because it's much more complicated—a lot of other pieces to consider—and to try to figure them out in a way that makes sense for the patient." [HCP09].

Greater patient information was perceived as important for HCPs caring for those with ADRD. The MC allowed for more time to be spent with patients, so HCPs could collaboratively unravel the complexities and develop proper treatment strategies. One HCP described:

"...I have two new patients on Wednesday, they're two-hour appointments. And it's a long process. I think we live in a society where everything is quick and easy. This isn't fast... A lot of people [say]: 'I don't want to deal with that. I want pretty medicine', but they don't know what they're missing..." [HCP11].

Other HCPs described working in the MC as "solving a puzzle", as there are many complex components that must fit together in order to provide quality care. One HCP described the experience of solving a mystery in the game Clue™:

"It's like a game of Clue™. It's like we're all part of this detective game, we're all doing a piece to put in" [HCP01].

HCPs also discussed the importance of using a team approach to solve these "puzzles":

"We're truly kind of all coming together, putting everything together... like putting a puzzle together. We're all in the room with all the pieces, versus you all have a quarter of the puzzle... And you're in your own offices trying to put these pieces together, it doesn't work, unless you all come together in the same space" [HCP02].

HCPs relied on the team, patients and families to collect all necessary pieces of information, "a triangulation of evidence" [HCP08], to properly diagnose and support patients with ADRD. Working in the MC allowed HCPs to collaborate and develop innovative ways of supporting patients and families. A HCP described a team approach to managing one patient's hallucinations:

"He has Lewy Body, and he sees these creatures that come out of the wall at night. And we needed to help them ... We came up with, let's put a spot light in his room at night, and put it towards that part of the wall [where the creatures come though]. And let's add a fan, so the light goes on and the fan blows them [creatures] away. So he could sleep through the night. We come up with strategies and roles and supportive ideas..." [HCP11].

This HCP described helping patients with complexities and taking the time to solve the "puzzles" in collaboration with colleagues, patients and families.

Subtheme 2: Ongoing learning opportunities HCPs felt rewarded working with the ADRD population as it allowed for professional growth and enhanced knowledge in dementia and patient complexities. The MC was described as a setting with learning opportunities that other care environments may not offer:

"We've learned from each other. So when I'm in my office working solo, the things that I now think of, I wouldn't have thought of before..." [HCP02].

HCPs developed other care strategies through working within a MC team. Interprofessional collaboration allowed HCPs to understand how other disciplines respond to situations. HCPs described these unique opportunities:

"I learn something from every one of them, almost every week... about what they do, what their role is, or how they approach patients and families. Everybody has their own way of saying it or maybe an expression that they use to get them to understand." [HCP12].

The training for MCs increased HCP confidence in their knowledge and understanding of ADRD. One HCP described a previous experience regarding the challenges of a dementia diagnosis:

"...prior to working here, I probably did come across people with Alzheimer's, but I wouldn't have recognized that. I had zero training other than what we touched upon in school. I would just think: they're old or they're difficult. So it wasn't actually until I started working here that I even knew anything about it at all" [HCP12].

Subtheme 3: Personal and professional fulfillment Personal and professional fulfillment emerged as a distinctive part of HCPs' experiences working in the MC. One HCP described knowing they were "making a difference" was a major motivation to remain at the MC:

"...even though at the end of a memory clinic day, I'm utterly exhausted... we know we've done good work, we've made a difference. And, that's my motivation—knowing that we're making a difference for the good" [HCP03].

Another HCP provided an example of making a difference in the MC:

"We've had a patient who was psychotic and had hallucinations of infidelity... great deal of stress for everybody. So with a little bit of fiddling around with one medication, after a couple of weeks, day and night difference. It's one of those few things where you can just say 'wow you've made a difference.' And so it's always rewarding," [HCP09].

Other HCPs described the drive behind their motivation:

"If you didn't have a passion for what you were doing, I don't think you could do [it], because it's a really tough clinic. But the passion keeps me going. And there's such a need. These people need help and a lot of people don't want to help them, so that's what keeps me going." [HCP11].

HCPs explained that only those committed to this work find it meaningful. "Just knowing it's effective and good work" [HCP07] is a motivator for HCPs to keep them at the MC. In addition, receiving positive feedback from patients and families was rewarding.

When asked why they choose to provide care to seniors, HCPs often alluded to previous exposure to gerontology and a growing interest, and others discussed influential mentors. HCPs described mentors as individuals who understood the demanding, yet rewarding nature of working with patients with ADRD, and who assisted them in shaping their career path.

HCPs believed that their work was a "good fit" with their personality traits and professional backgrounds, and that working with the elderly takes a special kind of person: "I feel motivated to work with this population because it's something that takes a special person to work with the geriatric population..." [HCP05]. Another HCP stated:

> "I always say, "I'd do this for free if I had to". Because I love it - but why do I love it? I love it because it just suits the way I think" [HCP01].

HCPs are strongly motivated by the team, previous experiences, mentors, and positive feedback from patients and families.

Discussion

Findings of this study provide insight into HCPs' experiences supporting patients and families in MC teams. HCPs take pride in their work in MCs. HCPs described how their roles fit well within the clinic team, and the difference working in the FHT versus the "tight-knit" MC, particularly opportunities for strong assessments and rich professional experiences.

HCPs described themselves as a source of support for patients and families. Maintaining patients' dignity and identity is important for HCPs, which is consistent with other research [16, 17]. Organizations such as the Alzheimer Society of Canada stress the importance of respecting persons with ADRD by reaffirming their sense of self [18].

During MC appointments, patients are asked to bring a family member or friend. HCPs described these individuals as key players to absorb information that may be missed by MC patients. Strong relationships between patients and family members or friends enable better dementia care as families/friends may notice changes that clinicians may not [19]. Contrastingly, denial and misinformed families could prohibit an accurate ADRD diagnosis and treatment plan for patients [19]. This study confirms the essential role of families in ADRD care.

Negative reactions from patients and family during a diagnosis such as ADRD can sometimes evoke emotions among HCPs, such guilt and may lead to job stress and burnout [20]. In a systematic review by Wilkinson and colleagues [21] there was a negative relationship found between burnout and empathy amongst HCPs. Thus, obtaining necessary information in order to accurately diagnose ADRD is important to support HCPs' job quality. One of the challenges faced by HCPs in MCs was the responsibility of revoking driver licenses. It is important to recognize that a diagnosis of ADRD may pose risks to those who are driving [22]. This study found that not only did the physicians feel responsible for revoking licenses, but other team members felt they have an important role in ensuring patient safety. Goldman and colleagues [23] identify shared responsibility as an important aspect of efficient teamwork. Although HCPs stressed the provision of alternate resources for patients after revoking a license, they expressed frustrations with navigating the system.

HCPs felt they were connected and worked well together to support patients with ADRD. Constant connectedness, close working relationships and communication within teams enhance care provided [24]. A disconnect and lack of integration among team members can potentially impede care for patients [24]. Although HCPs acknowledged these potential issues, they valued each other's opinions, explaining that clear communication led to effective collaboration. Clear communication was the main theme in HCP interviews by Moore and colleagues [11], who investigated perspectives of physicians and nurses in a primary care program for seniors. Despite the unique context of the Ontario, Canadian funding of these primary care memory clinics, in the increase of dementia diagnosis, the importance of care team approaches can be found in European studies [25].

HCPs discussed their interest in geriatrics. Low interest in geriatrics may stem from the lack of exposure and acquired knowledge during education [26, 27]. HCPs in this study identified past experiences in gerontology as motivators to pursue their careers. HCPs preferred working in a team and discussed learning opportunities when addressing care complexities.

HCPs described the opportunity for personal and professional growth in the MC. Uncertainties in diagnosing ADRD are common among primary care physicians [19, 28]. In this study, HCPs feel comfortable with the diagnosis process, are motivated by their team, and see the importance and value of each role and the contributions they bring to the team. Goldman and colleagues [23] stressed the importance of understanding the responsibility of each role in effectively working in a health team setting. Moore and colleagues [11] found that lack of role clarity hindered effective communication between team members. HCPs in this study felt their role was clearly defined and valued by others.

Strengths and limitations

Several strengths and limitations should be discussed. Contacting the MC Directors may have created pressure for HCPs to participate; yet, HCP participation was voluntary and participation information was not shared with Directors. Furthermore, transferability of the findings may be limited, as participating teams may have been high-functioning. Though these teams have been collaborating for several years, experience varied among participants; however, this did not seem to affect participants' perspectives. Saturation was reached halfway through data collection, but 12 interviews were completed to ensure representative data. The researchers attempted to increase transferability by including one rural and one urban MC. In addition, participants may not have been comfortable enough to speak to the challenges of working in team settings to provide care for persons with ADRD. The PI attempted to lessen this bias by reminding participants of the confidentiality measures being taken. Lastly, interviews completed were shorter in length than typical phenomenological interviews [13], due to time constraints. However, interviews allowed the researchers to ask all questions and use probes to gain further insight.

Conclusions

This study provides insight into HCPs' experiences in primary care MCs. Understanding HCPs' motivations to work with complex populations may assist in motivating future HCPs. Knowledge of the complexity of ADRD is important to ensure proper care and services. The study also provides support for team-based approaches in primary care.

Abbreviations

ADRD: Alzheimer's disease and related dementias; HCP: Health care providers; MC: memory clinic

Acknowledgements

The authors are grateful to the healthcare providers who took the time to participate in the study.

Funding

This research was supported by funding from the Canadian Institutes of Health Research (ETG-92249 and KTB-114392).

Authors' contributions

LS was the primary writer of this manuscript and was involved in the conceptualization, study design, participant recruitment and analysis of the study. PS was involved in the conceptualization, analysis of the study and drafting of the manuscript. CM was involved in the conceptualization, interpretation and drafting of the manuscript. VB was involved in the conceptualization, analysis, and drafting of the manuscript. All authors read and approved the final version of the manuscript.

Consent for publication

Health care providers who participated in the study provided written informed consent to publish anonymous quotes within the manuscript.

Competing interests

The authors declare that they have no competing interests.

Author details

[1]School of Public and Health and Health Systems, University of Waterloo, Waterloo, Ontario, Canada. [2]Schlegel Centre for Advancing Seniors Care, Conestoga College, Kitchener, Ontario, Canada. [3]Schlegel-UW Research Institute for Aging, Kitchener, Ontario, Canada. [4]Department of Psychiatry and Behavioural Neurosciences, McMaster University, Hamilton, Ontario, Canada.

References

1. Mitchell AJ, Meader N, Pentzek M. Clinical recognition of dementia and cognitive impairment in primary care: a meta-analysis of physician accuracy. Acta Psychiatr Scand. 2011;124(3):165–83. https://doi.org/10.1111/j.1600-0447.2011.01730.x.
2. Dixon JA, editor. Proceedings from queens health policy change conference series: backgrounder: healthcare reform in Canada. Toronto: The Monieson Centre for Business Research in Healthcare; 2013.
3. Callahan CM, Boustani MA, Weiner M, Beck RA, Livin LR, Kellams JJ, Willis DR, Hendrie HC. Implementing dementia care models in primary care settings: the aging brain care medical home (special supplement). Aging Ment Health. 2011;15(1):5–12. https://doi.org/10.1080/13607861003801052.
4. Collier R. Verdict still out on family health teams. CMAJ. 2011;183(10):1131–2. https://doi.org/10.1503/cmaj.109-3864.
5. Lee L, Kasperski MJ, Weston WW. Building capacity for dementia care. Training program to develop primary care memory clinics. Can Fam Physician. 2011;57(7):e249–52.
6. Bradford A, Kunik ME, Schulz P, Williams SP, Singh H. Missed and delayed diagnosis of dementia in primary care: prevalence and contributing factors. Alzheimer Dis Assoc Disord. 2009;23(4):306–14. https://doi.org/10.1097/WAD.0b013e3181a6bebc.
7. Passmore AP, Craig DA. The future of memory clinics. Psychiatr Bull. 2004;28:375–7.
8. Lee L, Hillier LM, Stolee P, Heckman G, Gagnon M, McAiney CA, Harvey D. Enhancing dementia care: a primary care-based memory clinic. JAGS. 2010; 58(11):2197–204.
9. Dewing J, Dijk S. What is the current state of care for older people with dementia in general hospitals? A literature review. Dementia (London). 2016;15(1):106–24. https://doi.org/10.1177/1471301213520172.
10. Rasmussen H, Hellzen O. The meaning of long-term caregiving for patients with frontal lobe dementia. Int J Qual Stud Health Well-being. 2013;8 https://doi.org/10.3402/qhw.v8i0.19860.
11. Moore AE, Nair K, Patterson C, White J, House S, Kadhim-Saleh A, Riva J. Physician and nurse perspectives of interprofessional and integrated primary care-based program for seniors. J Res Interprof Pract Educ. 2013; 3(1):103–21.
12. Van Manen M. Researching lived experience: human science for an action sensitive pedagogy. London: The Althouse Press; 1990.
13. Creswell JW. Qualitative inquiry & research design. Choosing among five approaches. 2nd ed. Thousand Oaks: Sage Publications, Inc; 2007.
14. Colaizzi PF. Psychological research as the phenomenologist views it. In: Valle RS, King M, editors. Existential-phenomenological alternatives for psychology. New York: Oxford University Press; 1978. p. 48–71.
15. Bradley EH, Curry LA, Devers KJ. Qualitative data analysis for health services research: developing taxonomy, themes, and theory. Health Serv Res. 2007; 42(4):1758–72. https://doi.org/10.1111/j.1474-6773.2006.00684.x.
16. Bridges J, Wilkinson C. Achieving dignity for older people with dementia in hospital. Nurs Stand. 2011;25(29):42–7.
17. Nolan L. Caring connections with older persons with dementia in an acute hospital setting–a hermeneutic interpretation of the staff nurse's experience. Int J Older People Nursing. 2006;1(4):208–15. https://doi.org/10.1111/j.1748-3743.2006.00033.x.
18. Alzheimer Society of Canada. (2011). Guidelines for care: person-centred care of people with dementia living in care homes. Retrieved from: http://www.alzheimer.ca/sites/default/files/files/national/culture-change/culture_change_framework_e.pdf. Accessed 7 May 2018.
19. Pimlott NJ, Persaud M, Drummond N, Cohen CA, Silvius JL, Seigel K, et al. Family physicians and dementia in Canada part 2. Understanding the challenges of dementia care. Can Fam Physician. 2009;55(5):508–9.

20. Warnock C. Breaking bad news: issues relating to nursing practice. Nurs Stand. 2014;28(45):51–8.
21. Wilkinson H, Whittington R, Perry L, Eames C. Examining the relationship between burnout and empathy in healthcare professionals: a systematic review. Burnout Research. 2017;6:18–29.
22. Byszewski AM, Molnar FJ, Aminzadeh F. The impact of disclosure of unfitness to drive in persons with newly diagnosed dementia: patient and caregiver perspectives. Clin Gerontol. 2010;33:152–63. https://doi.org/10.1080/07317110903552198.
23. Goldman J, Meuser J, Rogers J, Lawrie L, Reeves S. Interprofessional collaboration in family health teams an Ontario-based study. Can Fam Physician. 2010;56(10):e368–74.
24. Johansson G, Eklund K, Gosman-Hedstrom G. Multidisciplinary team, working with elderly persons living in the community: a systematic literature review. Scand J Occup Ther. 2010;17(2):101–16. https://doi.org/10.1080/11038120902978096.
25. Broda A, Bieber A, Meyer G, Hopper L, Joyce R, Irving K, et al. Perspectives of policy and political decision makers on access to formal dementia care: expert interviews in eight European countries. BMC Health Serv Res. 2017;17:518.
26. Mandville-Anstey SA, Ward P, Grainger P, Foley V. Nursing students' knowledge and attitudes toward caring for older adults. Perspectives. 2014;37(2):6–14.
27. Meiboom AA, de Vries H, Hertogh CMPM, Scheele F. Why medical students do not choose a career in geriatrics: a systematic review. BMC Med Educ. 2015;15:101. https://doi.org/10.1186/s12909-015-0384-4.
28. Koch T, Iliffe S. Rapid appraisal of barriers to the diagnosis and management of patients with dementia in primary care: a systematic review. BMC Fam Pract. 2010;11:52. https://doi.org/10.1186/1471-2296-11-52.

16

Relationship between self-efficacy, self-care behaviour and glycaemic control among patients with type 2 diabetes mellitus in the Malaysian primary care setting

Zahirah Tharek[1], Anis Safura Ramli[1,2*], David Leonard Whitford[3], Zaliha Ismail[4], Maryam Mohd Zulkifli[5], Siti Khuzaimah Ahmad Sharoni[6], Asrul Akmal Shafie[7] and Thevaraajan Jayaraman[8]

Abstract

Background: Self-efficacy has been shown to be positively correlated with self-care behaviour and glycaemic control among patients with type 2 diabetes mellitus. However, such evidence is lacking in the Malaysian primary care setting. The objectives of this study were to i) determine the levels of self-efficacy, self-care behaviour and glycaemic control among patients with type 2 diabetes mellitus in the Malaysian primary care setting ii) determine the relationship between self-efficacy, self-care behaviour and glycaemic control iii) determine the factors associated with glycaemic control.

Methods: This was a cross-sectional study involving patients with type 2 diabetes mellitus from two public primary care clinics in Malaysia. Self-efficacy and self-care behaviour levels were measured using previously translated and validated DMSES and SDSCA questionnaires in Malay versions, respectively. Glycaemic control was measured using HbA_{1c}.

Results: A total of 340 patients with type 2 diabetes mellitus were recruited. The total mean (±SD) of self-efficacy and self-care behaviour scores were 7.33 (±2.25) and 3.76 (±1.87), respectively. A positive relationship was found between self-efficacy and self-care behaviour (*r* 0.538, $P < 0.001$). Higher self-efficacy score was shown to be correlated with lower HbA_{1c} (*r* – 0.41, $P < 0.001$). Multiple linear regression analysis demonstrated that higher self-efficacy scores (*b* – 0.398; 95% CI: -0.024, – 0.014; $P < 0.001$), shorter duration of diabetes (*b* 0.177; 95% CI: 0.002, 0.007; $P < 0.001$) and smaller waist circumference (*b* 0.135; 95% CI: 0.006, 0.035; $P = 0.006$), were significantly associated with good glycaemic control.

Conclusion: This study demonstrated that higher self-efficacy was correlated with improved self-care behaviour and better glycaemic control. Findings of this study suggest the importance of including routine use of self-efficacy measures in the management of type 2 diabetes mellitus in primary care.

Keywords: Type 2 diabetes mellitus, Self-efficacy, Self-care behaviour, Primary care, Malaysia

Background

Type 2 Diabetes Mellitus (T2DM) has become a major burden not just to individuals but also to the health care systems both nationally and internationally. Globally, 387 million people have T2DM in 2014 and this is expected to rise to 592 million by 2035 [1]. The prevalence of T2DM in Malaysia has dramatically escalated over the past five decades. The Malaysian National Health Morbidity Survey (NHMS) 2011 showed an almost 20-fold increase in the prevalence of registered T2DM from 0.65% in 1960 to 15.2% in 2011 [2]. Analysis of the National Diabetes Registry (NDR) has shown that majority of patients with T2DM have co-existing cardiovascular (CV) risk factors such as hypertension which was found in 70.1% of patients followed by dyslipidaemia in 55.1% [3]. Local evidence also showed that majority (52.6%) of patients with T2DM received sub-optimal management of these CV risk factors,

* Correspondence: rossanis_yuzadi@yahoo.co.uk
[1]Discipline of Primary Care Medicine, Faculty of Medicine, Universiti Teknologi MARA (UiTM), Selayang Campus, Jalan Prima Selayang 7, 68100 Batu Caves, Selangor, Malaysia
[2]Institute of Pathology, Laboratory and Forensic Medicine (I-PPerForM), Universiti Teknologi MARA (UiTM), Sungai Buloh Campus, Jalan Hospital, 47000 Sungai Buloh, Selangor, Malaysia
Full list of author information is available at the end of the article

resulting in poor control [4]. T2DM poses a significant healthcare burden accounting for 16% of the Malaysian healthcare budget (2.4 billion Malaysian Ringgits), with the majority of resources being used to treat diabetes complications, which often arise from poor glycaemic control as well as poor control of the associated CV risk factors [5].

In Malaysia, majority of patients with T2DM are being managed in the primary care setting [6, 7]. In spite of the availability of national policies and programmes, including national clinical practice guidelines detailing treatment recommendations to improve diabetes care, the number of patients with good glycaemic control remains low [2–4].

The NDR project showed that the mean HbA_{1c} among patients with T2DM was 8.1% and only 23.8% achieved the glycaemic target of < 6.5% [3]. This highlights that it is important to look at patient factors as a mean to improve glycaemic control and the control of other associated CV risk factors to reduce complications alongside other aspects of the health care system.

Patient self-efficacy has been shown to be positively correlated with improving diabetes control via diabetes self-care [8–11]. Self-efficacy has been defined as one's ability to perform goal-directed behaviours in the presence of an obstacle or barrier [12]. Putting this concept into the context of T2DM, the goal-directed behaviours refers to self-care behaviours including adhering to self-monitoring of blood glucose (SMBG), dietary control, physical activity, foot care and medication intake as recommended. The self-efficacy concept translates into the level of self-confidence that the patients have in performing these recommended self-care behaviours. The integration of self-efficacy theory into the Health Belief Model (HBM) proposes that self-efficacy improves self-care behaviour which ultimately leads to better glycaemic control [13, 14].

Evidence is accumulating to show that glycaemic control could be improved with better self-efficacy and self-care behaviour among patients with T2DM [8–11]. In Malaysia, the only study supporting this was conducted in a university hospital setting [15]. However, characteristics of T2DM patients and healthcare delivery system in primary care may differ from secondary care in terms of patient's education level, health literacy and availability of trained healthcare personnel to deliver self-care support. In view of the lack of evidence in our primary care setting, there was a need to determine the role of self-efficacy and its relationship with self-care behaviour and glycaemic control among patients with T2DM in primary care. Therefore, the objectives of this study were to i) determine the levels of self-efficacy, self-care behaviour and glycaemic control among patients with T2DM in the Malaysian primary care setting ii) determine the relationship between self-efficacy, self-care behaviour and glycaemic control, and iii) determine the factors associated with glycaemic control.

Methods

Study design and setting

This was a cross-sectional study carried out at two public primary care clinics in the state of Selangor, Malaysia from August 2014 to September 2015. These clinics were selected because they were public primary care clinics located in urban areas with heavy patient load and good multiracial diversity. In addition, both clinics have a Non-Communicable Disease (NCD) clinic dedicated for T2DM providing a good pool for patient recruitment.

Study population

The study population was patients with T2DM who were receiving care at the two public primary care clinics. The inclusion criteria included T2DM patients aged ≥18 years old who have been diagnosed with T2DM for at least 1 year duration, received follow-up care at the primary care clinic at least twice within the last 1 year (to establish that the patient was a regular patient at the clinic) and were able to speak and understand Malay language. The exclusion criteria included those with Type 1 Diabetes Mellitus, pregnant, mental disorders associated with a loss of a sense of reality (schizophrenia, bipolar disorder, Alzheimer's disease, psychosis or dementia), any hearing or visual impairment that may impede patients from understanding instruction and completing the self-administered questionnaires, any literacy problems that may impede ability to give informed consent and/or any major complications that could interfere with self-care behaviours (such as being blind, suffered from debilitating strokes or coronary disease).

Sampling method

Patients with T2DM who attended the NCD clinics at the two primary care clinics were approached consecutively by the investigators and were given a patient information leaflet describing the study and its objectives. Those who were interested to participate were screened using the eligibility checklist according to the inclusion and exclusion criteria. Written informed consent was obtained from patients who fulfilled the inclusion and exclusion criteria. Participants were informed that they were free to withdraw from the study at any time.

Study tools

The tools for this study consisted of two sets of questionnaires which have been previously translated and validated: the Diabetes Management Self-Efficacy Scale (DMSES) Malay version [15] and the Summary of Diabetes Self-Care Activities Scale (SDSCA) Malay version [16].

The DMSES Malay version [15] was chosen to measure the self-efficacy levels in this study population because of its reliability (Cronbach's α of 0.951) and comprehensiveness in covering the domains in diabetes management.

The self-administered questionnaire consisted of 20 items with 11-point (0 to 10) Likert scale that measures 5 domains of participants' perceived self-efficacy in diabetes self-care activities i.e. dietary control, blood glucose monitoring, physical activity, foot-care and medication intake [15]. Overall, the scores range from 0 to 200 with higher scores indicating greater levels of self-efficacy [15].

The SDSCA Malay version [16] was chosen because of its reliability (Cronbach's α of 0.740), brevity and ease of scoring. It is a self-administered questionnaire comprising of 10 items with five subscale domains which measure the frequency of various self-care activities perform by a patient over the previous 7 days [16]. The five scale domains include general diet, specific diet, physical activity, blood glucose testing and foot-care. Response choices range from 0 to 7 giving a total score ranging from 0 to 70 [16]. Higher total scores indicate better performance of self-care behaviour [16].

The HbA_{1c} level taken within the 3 months prior to the extraction of the clinical data was used as a measure of glycaemic control of the study population. There was no HbA_{1c} missing data because patients without HbA_{1c} within the last 3 months were excluded from the study. Good glycaemic control is represented by $HbA_{1c} < 6.5\%$ in accordance with the Malaysian T2DM clinical practice guideline [17].

Data collection and study procedures

Data was collected by the investigators and staff nurses at the NCD clinic. All investigators and the staff nurses involved in this study were trained with regards to the study procedures prior to the conduct of the study to minimize variability in the method of data collection.

Demographic and anthropometric data collection

A standardised case report (CRF) form was used to collect socio-demographic information on the study subjects i.e. age, gender, ethnic group, educational attainment, occupation, duration of T2DM and smoking status, including the number of cigarettes smoked per day for current smokers. Those who never smoked or had quit smoking for more than 6 months were considered as non-smokers.

Anthropometric measurements included height, weight, body mass index (BMI), waist circumference (WC) and blood pressure (BP). Height and weight were measured using the Seca 769 Digital Medical Scale stadiometer. Weight was measured in light clothing, without shoes on the scale with a precision of 0.1 kg. Height was measured to 0.1 cm using the stretch stature method of the stadiometer and then converted to metres. BMI was calculated using the standard formula (weight in kg)/ (height in metres)^2. WC was measured to the nearest 0.1 cm using non-stretchable measuring tape with the subjects standing in a relaxed position and arms at the side. The measurement was taken at the midpoint between the lower rib margin (12th rib) and the iliac crest.

BP was measured twice, 2 min apart on the right arm in sitting position, using automatic digital blood pressure monitor (Omron HEM-757). Participants were made to rest for at least 5 min before the measurements were taken. Each participant was seated upright with his/her right arm supported at the heart level. The mean of the first and second systolic and diastolic measurements was reported as the BP value for individual participant.

Questionnaires administration

Participants were given a set of DMSES-Malay and SDSCA-Malay versions. Clear written and verbal instructions were given on how to fill up the questionnaires. They were requested to circle or tick which options suited them the most. Participants were encouraged to seek clarification from the investigators at any time should any queries arise. They were also reminded to answer the questionnaires themselves rather than getting help from their accompanying family members.

Participants were given a pen to complete the questionnaires at a corner of the clinic equipped with tables and chairs. The investigators ensured that participants did not interact with each other whilst answering the questionnaires. On average, participants took approximately 10 to 20 min to complete the questionnaires. Once they had finished, they handed the questionnaires to the investigators, who then checked the responses for completeness. Figure 1 illustrates the conduct of the study.

HbA_{1c} measurement

HbA_{1c} was measured using the Bio-Rad D-10 HPLC instrument available at the study sites. HbA_{1c} level that was taken within 3 months of the data collection date was retrieved from the patients' clinical notes.

Sample size calculation

Sample size was calculated using the single proportion formula with 5% precision and 95% confidence interval, where the proportion (P) was estimated based on the findings of a similar study in South East Asian population which showed that 32.7% had high self-efficacy score and 32.9% had good self-care behaviour score among T2DM subjects with good glycaemic control [18]. Therefore, using $Z = 1.96$, Δ (precision) = +/− 0.05, P = proportion of high self-efficacy (32.7%) or self-care behaviour (32.9%), would give a required sample size of 338 or 339, respectively. Considering additional 20% of refusal and non-eligibility rate, this study aimed to approach approximately 424 patients.

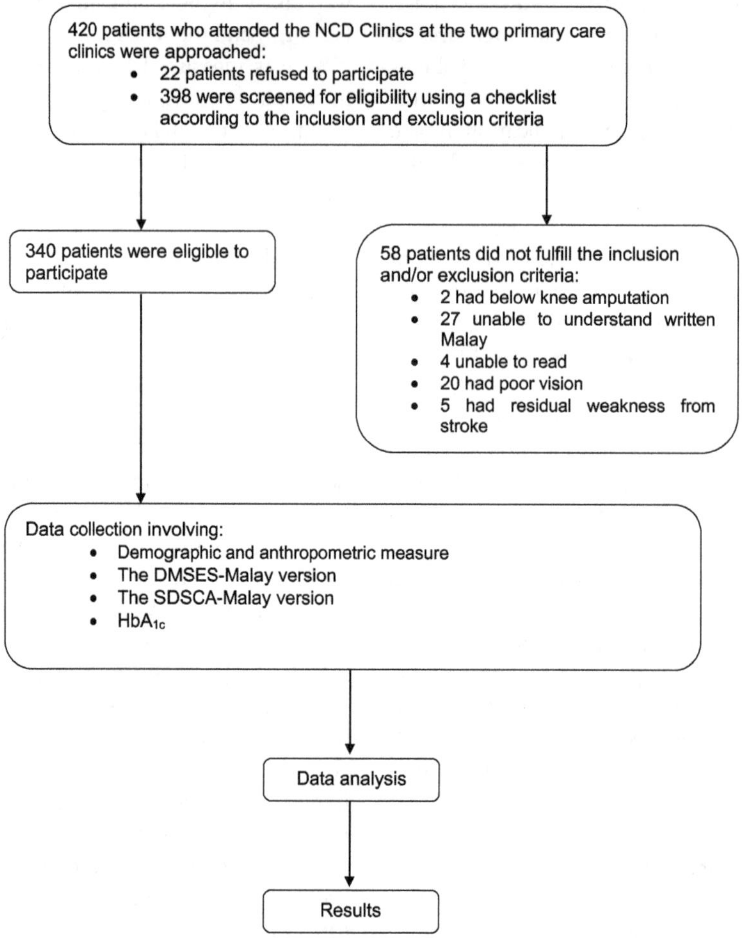

Fig. 1 Flow chart of the conduct of the study

Statistical analyses

Data was analysed using the Statistical Package for the Social Sciences (SPSS) version 21.0 (IBM). All continuous variables were described as mean (±SD) and number (n) and percentage (%) for dichotomous or nominal data. The score for item 4 of the SDSCA-Malay version was reversed as the question was negatively phrased. The levels of self-efficacy, self-care behaviour and glycaemic control were analysed using mean (±SD) as the data were normally distributed. The relationships between self-efficacy, self-care behaviour and glycaemic control were analysed using the Pearson's correlation test since the data were normally distributed. The coefficient of correlation (r) ranges from + 1.0 to − 1.0, where $r > 0$ indicates positive relationship, $r < 0$ indicates negative relationship while $r = 0$ indicates no relationship [19]. A value $r \geq 0.8$ or − 0.8 indicates strong relationship, r = 0.5–0.8 or − 0.5 to − 0.8 indicates moderate relationship and $r \leq 0.5$ or − 0.5 indicates weak relationship [19]. The factors associated with glycaemic control amongst the study population were analyzed by simple linear regression followed by multiple linear regressions since the data consisted of continuous variables. The independent variables that were entered into the simple linear regression were age, gender, BMI, duration of diabetes, BP, WC, SDSCA scores and DMSES scores. Variables with a P value of less than 0.25 by single linear regression were then included in the multiple linear regressions and these were duration of diabetes, WC, SDSCA scores and DMSES scores. A P value of less than 0.05 was considered statistically significant in the multiple linear regressions.

Results

A total of 420 patients with T2DM were approached and invited to enter the study. Out of this, 22 patients (5.2%) refused to participate and another 58 patients (13.8%) were not eligible to enter the study as they did not fulfill the inclusion and/or the exclusion criteria. Therefore, the recruitment rate for this study was 81% giving a total number of 340 eligible patients with T2DM who completed the questionnaires.

Characteristics of the study population

Table 1 shows the sociodemographic and clinical characteristics of the participants. The majority of the participants (58.8%) were female with an average age of 58.34 years old (±11.86, range 30–89). The participants were ethnically diverse, comprising of 61.5% Malays, 19.4% Chinese, 18.2% Indians and 0.9% of other ethnicity. Almost half of the participants (47.9%) were educated up to the secondary school level. The mean HbA1c was 7.99 (±1.71). Only 13.5% had good glycaemic control (HbA_{1c} < 6.5).

Levels of self-efficacy and self-care behaviour

Tables 2 and 3 shows the total mean scores of self-efficacy and self-care behaviour of the participants. The total mean scores (±SD) for self-efficacy and self-care behaviour were 7.33 (±2.25) and 3.76 (±1.87) respectively.

Table 2 illustrates the mean scores (±SD) for each DMSES subscale domains and items. The highest subscale domain score of 8.78 (±1.76) was for 'medications and follow-up' and the lowest subscale score of 6.60 (±2.97) was for 'blood glucose monitoring'.

Table 3 shows the mean subscale scores for five SDSCA subscale domains among the patients with T2DM. The highest mean subscale domain score of 5.73 (±1.53) was for 'general diet' and the lowest mean subscale domain score of 1.19 (±1.87) was for 'blood glucose testing'.

Relationships between self-efficacy with self-care behaviour and glycaemic control

Table 4 shows the correlation between self-efficacy, self-care behaviour scores and glycaemic control. There was a moderate positive correlation between self-efficacy and self-care behaviour (r 0.538, P < 0.001). A weak negative relationship was found between self-efficacy and HbA_{1c} (r – 0.41, P < 0.001). The scatter plots depicting these relationships are provided in Additional files 1 and 2.

Factors associated with glycaemic control

Table 5 shows the multiple linear regression model summaries of factors associated with good glycaemic control. Model 3 was the best fit model as it accounted for 21.7% of the variation compared to Model 1 (16.8%) and Model 2 (19.9%). DMSES score was negatively correlated with HbA_{1c} while the duration of T2DM and WC were positively correlated.

Table 6 presents the final multiple linear regression analysis in determining the factors associated with good glycaemic control. There were three variables with P < 0.05 which accounted for 21% (coefficient of determination, R^2 = 0.210) of the variation in HbA_{1c} between individuals. These were DMSES scores, duration of T2DM and WC. The analysis demonstrated that higher self-efficacy scores (b – 0.398; 95% CI: -0.024, – 0.014; P < 0.001), shorter duration of diabetes (b 0.177; 95% CI: 0.002, 0.007; P < 0.001)

Table 1 Sociodemographic and clinical characteristics of the patients with T2DM (n = 340)

Variables	n (%)	Mean (±SD)
Age (years)		58.34 (±11.86)
30–39	19 (5.6)	
40–49	63 (18.5)	
50–59	94 (27.6)	
≥ 60	164 (48.2)	
Gender		
Male	140 (41.2)	
Female	200 (58.8)	–
Ethnicity		
Malay	209 (61.5)	
Chinese	66 (19.4)	–
Indian	62 (18.2)	
Others	3 (0.9)	
Education level		
None	15 (4.4)	
Primary school (age 7 to 12)	119 (35)	–
Secondary school (age 13 to 17)	163 (47.9)	
Tertiary (college/ university)	43 (12.6)	
Occupation		
Employed	138 (40.6)	
Unemployed/Pensioner	202 (49.5)	–
Smoking status		
Smokers	40 (11.8)	–
Non-smokers	300 (88.2)	
BMI (kg/m^2)		28.53 (±5.29)
Normal (< 23)	48 (14.1)	
Abnormal (≥ 23)	291 (85.6)	
Waist circumference (cm)		
Male		91.52 (±9.89)
Normal (< 90)	64 (45.7)	
Abnormal (≥ 90)	76 (54.3)	
Female		88.30 (±11.95)
Normal (< 80)	39 (19.5)	
Abnormal (≥ 80)	161 (80.5)	
Blood pressure (mmHg)		
Controlled (< 140/80)	135 (39.7)	–
Uncontrolled (≥140/80)	205 (60.3)	
Glycaemic control (%)		
Controlled (HbA_{1c} < 6.5)	46 (13.5)	7.99 (±1.71)
Uncontrolled (HbA_{1c} ≥ 6.5)	294 (86.5)	

Table 2 The mean DMSES subscale scores among patients with T2DM (n = 340)

Subscale domains	Subscale items		Mean (±SD)
	Items (scale 0 = cannot do, 10 = certainly can do)		
Blood glucose monitoring	1	I am able to check my blood sugar if necessary	5.43 (±3.97)
	2	I am able to correct blood sugar when the sugar level is too high (e.g. eat different foods)	7.19 (±2.49)
	3	I am able to correct my blood sugar when the blood sugar level is too low (e.g. eat different foods)	7.19 (±2.45)
	Total mean subscale domain score		6.60 (±2.97)
Eating plan	4	I am able to choose the correct foods	7.47 (±2.09)
	5	I am able to choose different foods and stick to a healthy eating pattern	7.39 (±2.20)
	6	I am able to keep my weight under control	7.11 (±2.24)
	9	I am able to adjust my eating plan when ill	7.33 (±2.29)
	10	I am able to follow a healthy eating pattern most of the time	7.28 (±2.20)
	13	I am able to follow a healthy eating pattern when I am away from home	6.82 (±2.38)
	14	I am able to adjust my eating plan when I am away from home	7.09 (±2.20)
	15	I am able to follow a healthy eating pattern during the festive periods	6.14 (±2.57)
	16	I am able to follow a healthy eating pattern during wedding ceremonies or at a party	6.24 (±2.5)
	17	I am able to adjust my eating plan when I am feeling stressed or anxious	7.12 (±2.30)
	Total mean subscale domain score		7.00 (±1.97)
Physical activity	8	I am able to do enough exercise	7.12 (±2.3)
	11	I am able to do more exercise if the doctor advises me to	6.79 (±2.42)
	12	When I do more exercise, I am able to adjust my eating plan	6.66 (±2.44)
	Total mean subscale domain score		6.85 (±2.19)
Foot care	7	I am able to examine my feet for cuts	7.40 (±2.36)
Medications and follow-up	19	I am able to take my medication as prescribed	8.77 (±1.68)
	20	I am able to maintain my medication when I am ill	8.68 (±1.85)
	18	I am able to visit my doctor four times a year to monitor my diabetes according to treatment plan to monitor my diabetes	8.88 (±1.74)
	Total mean subscale domain score		8.78 (±1.76)
Total mean DMSES score			7.33 (±2.25)

and smaller waist circumference (b 0.135; 95% CI: 0.006, 0.035; P = 0.006) were significantly associated with good glycaemic control.

Therefore, the final prediction equation of the model for glycaemic control among patients with T2DM was:

Glycaemic control = 8.522–0.398*(DMSES score) + 0.177*(duration of T2DM) + 0.135*(waist circumference]

The regression analysis have shown that an increase of DMSES score by one would reduce the HbA1c by 0.398%, an increase in duration of T2DM by 1 year would increase the HbA1c by 0.177% and an increase in WC by 1 cm would increase the HbA1c by 0.135%.

Discussion

This was the first study evaluating the relationship between self-efficacy, self-care behaviour and glycaemic control among patients with type 2 diabetes mellitus in the Malaysian primary care setting.

Levels of self-efficacy, self-care behaviour, and glycaemic control

This study demonstrated a moderately high mean self-efficacy score (7.33) and participants were found to be most self-efficacious in tasks relating to medication intake and least self-efficacious in blood glucose testing. These findings were comparable with the study conducted in a hospital setting in Malaysia which showed a mean self-efficacy score of 7.57, where the highest score was for medication intake [15]. On the contrary, their study population was least efficacious in their eating plan [15]. Similar findings were found in a Jordanian study which showed a mean self-efficacy score of 7.26 with the highest score for efficacy to carry out medication intake [20]. Their participants were least confident in performing physical activity [20]. A likely explanation for the highest self-efficacy for medication intake is that this is a straightforward task which does not require much effort to perform. The low self-efficacy score in performing blood

Table 3 The mean SDSCA subscale scores among the patients with T2DM ($n = 340$)

Subscale domains	Subscale items		Mean (±SD)
	Self-management behaviours over the previous 7 days		
General diet	1	Follow a healthy eating plan in the last week	5.71 (±1.62)
	2	Follow a healthy eating plan (on average per week, over the past month)	5.75 (±1.53)
	Total mean subscale domain score		5.73 (±1.53)
Specific diet	3	Eats five or more servings of fruits and vegetables	5.41 (±1.83)
	4	Eats high-fat foods (reverse scoring item)	4.18 (±1.60)
	Total mean subscale domain score		4.80 (±1.18)
Physical activity	5	Participates in at least 30 min of exercise	4.60 (±2.32)
	6	Participates in specific exercise session	2.09 (±2.33)
	Total mean subscale domain score		3.35 (±1.85)
Blood glucose testing	7	Tests for blood sugar	1.18 (±1.89)
	8	Tests your blood sugar acording to the number of times recommended by your health care providers	1.19 (±1.915)
	Total mean subscale domain score		1.19 (±1.87)
Foot care	9	Check your feet	4.00 (±3.07)
	10	Inspect the inside of your shoes	3.48 (±3.18)
	Total mean subscale domain score		3.74 (±2.94)
Total mean SDSCA score			3.76 (±1.87)

glucose testing in our study population highlighted the need to educate patients on self-monitoring of blood glucose (SMBG) to increase their self-efficacy to perform this task.

A moderate level of self-care behaviour (3.76) was found among the participants in our study. Participants reported practicing general dietary restriction the most and blood glucose testing the least. It is also interesting to note that blood glucose testing was also the task which the participants in this study were found to be least self-efficacious to perform. These findings were comparable to the Jordanian study which found similar level of self-care behaviour with a mean of 3.74, and blood glucose testing was also found to be the least frequently reported self-care behaviour in their study population [20]. The low self-care behaviour for blood glucose testing in our study population may be explained by the unavailability of affordable glucometer or glucose strips, even among those who are on insulin. These equipments are not available on prescriptions in public primary care clinics in Malaysia. Findings of this study further highlights the need to increase the availability of affordable blood glucose testing equipments especially for those on insulin, as well as to enhance self-behaviour skills to perform this task.

Table 4 Simple linear correlation between DMSES score with SDSCA score and HbA_{1c}

	DMSES score Pearson's correlation (r)	P value[a]
SDSCA score	0.538	<0.001
HbA_{1c}	−0.410	<0.001

[a] Correlation is significant at P value < 0.01

Our study highlights that only 13.5% of the participants achieved the glycaemic target of < 6.5% with mean HbA_{1c} of 7.99%, indicating difficult challenges physicians face in achieving glycaemic control among patients with T2DM in primary care. This finding is similar to the local study conducted in a teaching hospital which showed that only 15.5% of their study population achieved HbA1c of < 6.5% [15]. However, our finding is lower than the NDR report in 2012 which showed that 23.8% of patients with T2DM achieved good glycaemic control [3]. These findings highlight that our T2DM population largely has poor glycaemic control which leads to high complication rates. Rigorous efforts should focus on finding cost-effective methods to improve glycaemic control among patients with T2DM. Identification of factors associated with poor glycaemic control would help clinicians and policy makers to strategise for effective interventions.

Relationships between self-efficacy with self-care behaviour and glycaemic control

A positive correlation between self-efficacy and self-care behaviour was demonstrated in patients with T2DM in this study, and this finding is similar to the study conducted in a hospital setting in Malaysia [15]. This is further supported by several other studies showing that high self-efficacy level was associated with better self-care behaviour [21, 22]. A review on the role of self-efficacy in

Table 5 Multiple linear regression model summaries of factors associated with good glycaemic control

Variables in the model				R^2
	WC Coefficients (95% CI)	Duration DM Coefficients (95% CI)	DMSES Coefficients (95% CI)	
Model 1			−0.410 (−0.024, − 0.015)	0.168
Model 2		0.174 (0.002–0.007)	−0.411 (− 0.024, − 0.015)	0.199
Model 3	0.135 (0.006–0.35)	0.177 (0.002–0.007)	− 0.398 (− 0.024, − 0.014)	0.217

diabetes care showed that self-efficacy provides a suitable framework for understanding and predicting commitment towards self-care behaviours and effectiveness of self-management in diabetes treatment [23].

A negative relationship was found between self-efficacy and HbA_{1c} in this study. This indicates that higher self-efficacy scores were significantly correlated with better glycaemic control. Similar findings were demonstrated in a study amongst Turkish patients with T2DM which showed that self-efficacy had a modest negative correlation with glycaemic control [24]. Another study proved that an increase in diabetes self-efficacy over time was related to an improvement in glycaemic control [25]. A cross-sectional study in Myanmar has shown that patients with a high self-efficacy level were 5.29 times more likely to have better glycaemic control than those with a fair or low self-efficacy level [18].

Factors associated with good glycaemic control

This study shows that better self-efficacy, shorter duration of T2DM and smaller WC were significantly associated with good glycaemic control. Similar findings were identified by a study in Jordan where an increased duration of diabetes, not following eating plan as recommended by dietitians, negative attitude towards diabetes, and increased barriers to adherence scale scores were associated with poor diabetic control [25]. From this result, it can be expected that patients with low self-efficacy and longer duration of diabetes would have poor glycaemic control. Therefore intervention should be targeted in these groups of patients.

Strengths and limitations of the study

The main strength of this study is the novelty of its findings in demonstrating significant relationships between self-efficacy, self-care behaviour and glycaemic control among patients with T2DM in the Malaysian primary care setting. Additional strength is the utilisation of valid and reliable tools which have been translated and validated for the Malaysian population. Limitations of this study include the non-probability sampling method which could be vulnerable to sampling bias. However, efforts were made to invite all patients with T2DM in the waiting area to participate in this study during the data collection period. This study also selected T2DM patients who received follow-up care at the clinic at least twice within the last 1 year to establish that the patients were regular patients at the clinic. This was to ensure that subsequent intervention can be targeted towards this group of patients. Self-efficacy, self-care behaviour and glycaemic control may be better in this group of patients compared to the defaulters. Findings of this study may not be generalisable to other primary care clinics in Malaysia as it was conducted in two primary care clinics in urban areas. Other limitations include the self-report method used to measure self-care behaviour, rather than more direct measures such as direct observations of the self-care behaviours. However, although self-report provides an estimate of health behaviours, it represents the most practical method of health behaviour measurement [26]. Finally, this study did not explore other potential factors which may affect glycaemic control such as education level, smoking status, presence of co-morbidities, types of medications, dietary intake and physical activity. Therefore, the multiple linear regression results should be interpreted with caution.

Implications for clinical practice and future research

This study shows that better self-efficacy is a major determinant of good glycaemic control. Findings of this study suggest the importance to include routine use of self-efficacy measures in the management of T2DM in primary care aiming to improve glycaemic control. Assessment of self-efficacy in patients with T2DM should be an important first step in the development of individually tailored interventions. These interventions should also focus on

Table 6 Factors associated with good glycaemic control by multiple linear regressions

Variables	Standardized coefficients Beta (*b*) (95% CI)	t statistics	*P* value[a]
DMSES score	- 0.398 (− 0.024, − 0.014)	−8.201	< 0.001
Duration of T2DM	0.177 (0.002, 0.007)	3.664	< 0.001
Waist Circumference	0.135 (0.006, 0.035)	2.791	0.006

[a] Multiple linear regression coefficient of determination, $R^2 = 0.210$. The model was adjusted simultaneously for all variables included in the model. The model reasonably fits well. Model assumptions were met. There was no interaction and multicollinearity problem

enhancing self-efficacy to improve self-management of diabetes. Efforts should be made by primary care providers to enhance their patients' self-efficacy in order to improve their self-care behaviour, and ultimately, glycaemic control. Primary care providers should be trained to provide self-management support to their patients with T2DM in order to increase self-efficacy and self-care practice. However, further research using systematic random sampling of patients with T2DM in a larger number of public primary care clinics in Malaysia is needed to confirm the findings of this study.

Self-efficacy and self-care behaviour of patients with T2DM would also vary over time and investigating such variations is beyond the scope of this study. Future research should include prospective cohort studies to investigate the longitudinal causal effects of self-efficacy on changes in diabetes self-care behaviour and glycaemic control. In addition, further research should also explore facilitators and barriers influencing self-efficacy and self-care behaviour. Such evidence is required to guide policy change and resource allocations in the Malaysian public primary care setting.

Conclusions

In conclusion, this study has demonstrated that higher self-efficacy was correlated with better self-care behaviour and glycaemic control. Higher self-efficacy score, shorter duration of T2DM and smaller WC were identified as significant predictors of good glycaemic control. Despite its limitations, this study is the only study which explored such relationships among T2DM patients in the Malaysian primary care setting. Findings of this study highlight the importance to measure self-efficacy in order to develop individual self-management intervention programmes for patients with T2DM in primary care, with the aim of improving glycaemic control and reducing major complications.

Abbreviations

BMI: Body mass index; BP: Blood pressure; CRF: Case report form; CV: Cardiovascular; DMSES: Diabetes Management Self-Efficacy Scale; HbA_{1c}: Glycated Haemoglobin; HBM: Health Belief Model; NCD: Non-Communicable Disease; NDR: National Diabetes Registry; NHMS: National Health Morbidity Survey; SDSCA: Summary of Diabetes Self-Care Activities Scale; SMBG: Self-monitoring of blood glucose; T2DM: Type 2 Diabetes Mellitus; WC: Waist circumference

Acknowledgements

The authors wish to thank YBhg. Datuk Dr. Noor Hisham Abdullah, Director General of Health, Malaysia, for the permission to publish this manuscript. The authors also wish to thank the Family Medicine Specialists of Klinik Kesihatan Taman Ehsan (KKTE); Dr. Rosnah Mat Isa and Klinik Kesihatan Sungai Buloh (KKSB); Dr. Jemah Sajari as well as the nurses and support staff of the Non-communicable Diseases Unit of KKTE and KKSB who provided facilities and assistance during the data collection.

Funding

This study was funded by the Ministry of Higher Education (MOHE) Malaysia: Research Acculturation Grant Scheme (RAGS) no. 600-RMI/RAGS 5/3 (60/2014). The funding body did not play any role in the design of the study, or in data collection, analysis or interpretation, or in writing the manuscript.

Authors' contributions

ZT, ASR, DLW and ZI conceptualized and designed the study. ZT, ASR, MMZ and TJ acquired the funding. ASR, DLW and ZI supervised and coordinated the study. ZT and MMZ acquired the data. ZT, DLW and ZI analysed and interpreted the data. ZT, ASR, DLW and ZI drafted the manuscript. AAS, SKAS, MMZ and TJ revised it critically for important intellectual content. All authors have read and given approval of the final manuscript. Each author has participated sufficiently in the work to take public responsibility for appropriate portions of the content as described above. All authors agreed to be accountable for all aspects of the work to ensure that questions related to the accuracy or integrity of any part of the work would be appropriately investigated and resolved.

Consent for publication

Participants' consent for publication is not applicable as person's individual data was neither provided nor presented in the manuscript.

Competing interests

All authors declare that they have no competing interests.

Author details

[1]Discipline of Primary Care Medicine, Faculty of Medicine, Universiti Teknologi MARA (UiTM), Selayang Campus, Jalan Prima Selayang 7, 68100 Batu Caves, Selangor, Malaysia. [2]Institute of Pathology, Laboratory and Forensic Medicine (I-PPerForM), Universiti Teknologi MARA (UiTM), Sungai Buloh Campus, Jalan Hospital, 47000 Sungai Buloh, Selangor, Malaysia. [3]Department of General Practice, Royal College of Surgeons in Ireland (RCSI), Mercer Building, Noel Purcell Walk, Dublin, Republic of Ireland. [4]Discipline of Population Health and Preventive Medicine, Faculty of Medicine, Universiti Teknologi MARA (UiTM), Sungai Buloh Campus, Jalan Hospital, 47000 Sungai Buloh, Selangor, Malaysia. [5]Department of Family Medicine, School of Medical Sciences, Universiti Sains Malaysia (USM), 16150 Kubang Kerian, Kelantan, Malaysia. [6]Department of Nursing, Faculty of Health Sciences, Universiti Teknologi MARA (UiTM), Puncak Alam Campus, 42300 Bandar Puncak Alam, Selangor, Malaysia. [7]Discipline of Social and Administrative Pharmacy, School of Pharmaceutical Sciences, Universiti Sains Malaysia (USM), 11800 Penang, Malaysia. [8]Discipline of Medicine, Faculty of Medicine, Universiti Teknologi MARA, Sungai Buloh Campus, Jalan Hospital, 47000 Sungai Buloh, Selangor, Malaysia.

References

1. International Diabetes Federation. IDF Diabetes Atlas. 7th ed. Brussels: International Diabetes Federation; 2015. [file:///C:/Users/Hp%20Pavilion/Downloads/IDF_Atlas%202015_UK.pdf].
2. Institute for Public Health, Ministry of Health, Malaysia. National Health and morbidity survey 2011 (NHMS 2011) vol II: non-communicable disease. Kuala Lumpur: Institute for Public Health; 2011. [file:///C:/Users/Hp%20Pavilion/Downloads/NHMS_2011_FACT_SHEET%20(1).pdf].
3. National Diabetes Registry Report. Non-communicable disease section, disease control division. Minist Health Malaysia. 2009-2012;1:1–48.
4. Mastura I, Chew BH, Lee PY, Cheong AT, Sazlina SG, Jamaiyah H, Syed Alwi SAR, Sri Wahyu T, Zaiton A. Control and treatment profiles of 70,889 adult type 2 diabetes mellitus patients in Malaysia - a cross sectional survey in 2009. Int J Collab Res Internal Med Public Health. 2011;3:98–113.
5. Zhang P, Zhang X, Brown J, Vistisen D, Sicree R, Shaw J, Nichols G. Global healthcare expenditure on diabetes for 2010 and 2030. Diabetes Res Clin Pract. 2010;87(3):293–301. https://doi.org/10.1016/j.diabres.2010.01.026.
6. Mimi O, Tong SF, Nordin S, Teng CL, Khoo EM, Abdul-Rahman A, Zailinawati AH, Lee VKM, Chen WS, Shihabudin WM, Noridah MS, Fauziah ZE. A comparison of morbidity patterns in public and private primary care clinics in Malaysia. Malaysian Fam Physician. 2011;6(1):19–25.
7. Ramli AS, Taher SW. Managing chronic diseases in the Malaysian primary health care – a need for change. Malaysian Fam Physician. 2008;3(1):7–13.
8. Gao J, Wang J, Zheng P, Haardorfer R, Kegler MC, Zhu Y, Fu H. Effects of self-care, self-efficacy, social support on glycaemic control in adults with type 2 diabetes. BMC Fam Pract. 2013;66(14):1–6.

9. Sarkar U, Fisher L, Schillinger D. Is self-efficacy associated with diabetes self-management across race/ ethnicity and health literacy? Diabetes Care. 2006;29:823–9.
10. Beckerle CM, Lavin MA. Association of self-efficacy and self-care with glycaemic control in diabetes. Diabetes Spectr. 2013;26(3):172–7.
11. Walker RJ, Smalls BL, Hernandaz-Tejada MA, Campbell JA, Egede LE. Effect of diabetes self-efficacy on glycaemic control, medication adherence, self-care behaviour and quality of life in a predominantly low-income, minority population. Ethn Dis. 2014;24(3):349–55.
12. Bandura A. Self efficacy. New York: The exercise of control; 1994.
13. Janz NK, Becker MH. The health belief model: a decade later. Health Educ Q. 1984;11(1):1–47.
14. Rosenstock IM, Strecher VJ, Becker MH. Social learning theory and health belief model. Health Educ Q. 1988;15(2):175–83.
15. Ahmad Sharoni SK, Wu SFV. Self-efficacy and self-care behaviour of Malaysian patients with type 2 diabetes: a cross sectional survey. Nurs Health Sci. 2012;14:38–45.
16. Jalaludin MY, Fuziah MZ, Hong JYH, Mohamad Adam B, Jamaiyah H. Reliability and validity of the revised summary of diabetes self-care activities (SDSCA) for Malaysian children and adolescents. Malaysian Fam Physician. 2012;7(2&3):10–20.
17. Health Technology Assessment Section. Medical development division Ministry of Health, Malaysia. Clinical practice guideline on the Management of Type 2 diabetes mellitus. 5th ed. Putrajaya: Ministry of Health, Malaysia; 2015. http://www.moh.gov.my/penerbitan/CPG/CPG%20T2DM%202015.pdf.
18. Nyunt SW, Howteerakul N, Suwannapong N, Rajatanun T. Self-efficacy, self-care behaviours and glycaemic control among type 2 diabetes patients attending two private clinics in Yangon, Myanmar. Southeast Asian J Trop Med Public Health. 2010;4(41):943–51.
19. Machin D, Campbell MJ, Walters SJ. Medical statistics: a textbook for the health sciences. 4th ed. West Sussex: Wiley Ltd; 2007. p. 151–6. chapter 9, correlation, linear and logistic regression.
20. Al-Khawaldeh OA, Al-Hassan MA, Froelicher ES. Self-efficacy, self-management and glycaemic control in adults with type 2 diabetes mellitus. J Diabetes Complicat. 2012;26:10–6.
21. Wendling S, Beadle V. The relationship between self-efficacy and diabetic foot self-care. J ClinTranslat Endocrinol. 2015;2(1):37–41.
22. Depalma MT, Trahan LH, Eliza JM, Wagner AE. The relationship between diabetes self-efficacy and diabetes self-care in American Indians and Alaska natives. Am Indian Alsk Native Ment Health Res. 2015;22(2):1–22.
23. Mohebi S, Azadbakht L, Feizi A, Sharifirad G, Kargar M. Review the key role of self-efficacy in diabetes care. J Educ Health Promot. 2013;2:1–7.
24. Gulhan C, Erdogan S. Influence of psychosocial factors on self-care behaviours and glycaemic control in Turkish patients with type 2 diabetes mellitus. J Transcult Nurs. 2014;1(25):51–9.
25. Khattab M, Khader YS, Al-Khawaldeh A, Ailouni K. Factors associated with poor glycaemic control among patients with type 2 diabetes. J Diabetes Complicat. 2010;4(2):84–9.
26. Glasgow RE, Ory MG, Klesges LM, Cifuentes M, Fernald DH, Green LA. Practical and relevant self-report measures of patient health behaviours for primary care research. Ann Fam Med. 2005;3(1):73–81.

17

Patient empowerment and general self-efficacy in patients with coronary heart disease

Anita Kärner Köhler[1*], Pia Tingström[2], Tiny Jaarsma[1] and Staffan Nilsson[2,3]

Abstract

Background: In managing a life with coronary heart disease and the possibility of planning and following a rehabilitation plan, patients' empowerment and self-efficacy are considered important. However, currently there is limited data on levels of empowerment among patients with coronary heart disease, and demographic and clinical characteristics associated with patient empowerment are not known.

The purpose of this study was to assess the level of patient empowerment and general self-efficacy in patients six to 12 months after the cardiac event. We also aimed to explore the relationship between patient empowerment, general self-efficacy and other related factors such as quality of life and demographic variables.

Methods: A sample of 157 cardiac patients (78% male; age 68 ± 8.5 years) was recruited from a Swedish hospital. Patient empowerment was assessed using the SWE-CES-10. Additional data was collected on general self-efficacy and well-being (EQ5D and Ladder of Life). Demographic and clinical variables were collected from medical records and interviews.

Results: The mean levels of patient empowerment and general self-efficacy on a 0–4 scale were 3.69 (±0.54) and 3.13 (±0.52) respectively, and the relationship between patient empowerment and general self-efficacy was weak ($r = 0.38$). In a simple linear regression, patient empowerment and general self-efficacy were significantly correlated with marital status, current self-rated health and future well-being. Multiple linear regressions on patient empowerment (Model 1) and general self-efficacy (Model 2) showed an independent significant association between patient empowerment and current self-rated health. General self-efficacy was not independently associated with any of the variables.

Conclusions: Patients with a diagnosis of coronary heart disease reported high levels of empowerment and general self-efficacy at six to 12 months after the event. Clinical and demographic variables were not independently associated with empowerment or low general self-efficacy. Patient empowerment and general self-efficacy were not mutually interchangeable, and therefore both need to be measured when planning for secondary prevention in primary health care.

Keywords: Patient empowerment, General self-efficacy, Coronary heart disease, Self-rated health, Well-being, Primary health care

* Correspondence: anita.karner@liu.se
[1]Department of Social and Welfare Studies (ISV/OMV), Linköping University, Norrköping, Sweden
Full list of author information is available at the end of the article

Background

Coronary heart disease is the major cause of premature death among men and women in Europe [1]. Yearly, around 30,000 Swedes suffer a myocardial infarction [2] and among patients who survive, about 20% suffer a secondary cardiovascular event in the first year. Around 50% of major coronary events occur among those with a previous diagnosis of myocardial infarction [3]. Regular exercise, smoking cessation and the use of cardiovascular preventive drugs are effective preventive actions that reduce mortality and re-infarction rates [4]. Yet, risk factors remain significant in patients, even after initiation of secondary prevention. A study of patients with coronary heart disease showed that 48.6% continued to smoke 1.35 years in median time after the cardiovascular event, almost two out of three patients were physically inactive, 38% were obese, more than 40% had hypertension and 80.5% had hypercholesterolemia [5].

Cardiac rehabilitation and secondary prevention, which are confirmed to be effective and safe in the management of clinically stable patients with coronary heart disease, are two other kinds of support accessible during the recovery process. Therefore, it is problematic that only 20–50% of the eligible patients [6] attend cardiac rehabilitation programmes that could facilitate smoking cessation and taking up physical exercise, which are really effective preventive actions [7] that reduce mortality after myocardial infarction [8, 9].

For patients recovering from a myocardial infarction, restenosis after percutaneous coronary intervention, or coronary artery bypass surgery, achieving control of their own health has been viewed as a struggle, including negotiating the management of daily problems [10]. Bodily experiences make cardiac patients uncertain and frightened of recurrence and death. Patients' questions about how long the effects of the cardiac surgery will last also demonstrate their uncertainty. It seems that after revascularisation, patients are not always aware that they are chronically ill, and this may have consequences for the management and practice of self-care [11]. Additionally, patients experience, for example, constraining somatic and social incentives, affecting their capacity to perform physical activity and to follow programmes of drug treatment [12]. If patients felt safe and in control based on their understanding of their heart disease during cardiac rehabilitation and were inclined to manage self-care with support, their recovery could proceed more smoothly. Patients' recovery after coronary heart disease seems complex and challenging, and we need to know more about key factors that facilitate this recovery.

Patient empowerment (PE) is viewed as a key factor for improving health outcomes, enhancing communication between patients and health professionals, bringing about better adherence to treatment regimes, and ensuring the efficient use of primary health resources. This is outlined as a specific intention by the World Health Organization's (WHO) Regional Office for Europe in Health 2020 [13]. According to this policy framework, which provides main strategies and priorities to support European action for health and well-being, people are increasingly seen as co-producers of their own health, and need to be empowered to take control of the determinants of their own health [13]. The WHO defines PE as a process where patients understand their role, are given the knowledge and skills by the health care provider to perform a task in an environment where there is an awareness of community and cultural differences, and where patients are encouraged to participate [14]. A recent concept analysis of PE stated that:

> *"Individual patient empowerment is a process that enables patients to exert more influence over their individual health by increasing their capacities to gain more control over issues they themselves define as important* [15] (p. 1927)."

Moreover, Castro et al. [15] found that PE is situated on several levels (micro-, meso- and macro-) and could be approached by the patient, the health care provider or the health care system.

Self-efficacy (SE), a concept derived from social cognitive theory, concerns people's beliefs in their capacity to exercise control over events that affect their lives [16]. SE beliefs influence how people think, feel, motivate themselves and act [17]. It has been viewed as relevant in relation to the fact that people and populations who believe they will succeed are more likely to attempt a new behaviour. To achieve SE, a person might perform a task that was previously successful within their capabilities (mastery experience), watch someone with whom they can identify performing a task successfully (social modelling), receive positive feedback/verbal persuasion relating to the task from someone or interpret physiological or affective states, with some or all of these factors being present before SE is accomplished [18]. SE is a well-studied concept within cardiac rehabilitation. Relationships between perceived SE [19] and personal goals during cardiac rehabilitation have been positively associated with physical exercise six and 12 months after discharge [20], with food choices after a tailored one-year intervention at an outpatient clinic [21], with smoking habits two to four weeks after discharge [22], and with health-related quality of life two years post-MI [23]. General SE (GSE) has received attention in research, and it is defined as the belief in one's competence to cope with a broad range of stressful and challenging demands. GSE appears to be a universal construct yielding meaningful relations with other psychological constructs and having a positive impact on health behaviours [24]. Patients with high GSE recovered better one week after cardiac surgery and experienced a higher quality of life six months later compared with their low-GSE counterparts [25]. Thus, it is important to consider GSE when predicting behavioural intentions and health behaviour change after an event of coronary heart disease.

We argue that GSE and PE are important to consider at an individual level, for managing life with coronary heart disease, as well as at an organisational level, for arranging secondary cardiac rehabilitation in primary health care. However, PE is not well-studied in cardiac rehabilitation.

We therefore assessed the level of GSE and PE in patients who had been diagnosed with coronary heart disease six to 12 months ago. Based on previous literature and theoretical foundation we also explored the relation between other related factors such as gender, age marital status, education, well-being, self-rated health, cardiovascular risk factors and diseases, in relation to PE and GSE.

Methods

Setting

In this cross-sectional study, we recruited patients with coronary heart disease in south-east Sweden between September 2011 and November 2014. A detailed description of the study procedures is given in a design article [26], but a summary is provided below.

Recruitment

The patients were invited to the COR-PRIM study, an ongoing five-year prospective single- centre randomised controlled study (NCT01462799), performed in a primary health care setting in south-eastern Sweden. The current analysis uses the baseline data of the patients. The recruitment was conducted by the Vrinnevi Hospital heart unit in Norrköping, Sweden, from the electronic medical record, based on the following criteria: Inclusion criteria were: (i) patients with coronary heart disease verified by myocardial infarction and/or percutaneous coronary intervention and/or coronary artery bypass surgery six to 12 months before the planned start of the interventions, (ii) patients who were stable regarding their cardiac condition and taking optimised cardiac medication that had not substantially changed during the previous month, (iii) patients who had completed heart school in hospital, and were listed at one of six specific primary health care centres. Exclusion criteria were: planned coronary artery bypass surgery or other conditions demanding continuing cardiologic care; for example: ongoing contact with heart failure clinic due to drug titration, life expectancy ≤ one year, documented psychiatric disease causing difficulties in cooperating with other people, obvious abuse of alcohol or narcotics. Patients were also excluded if they were unable to read or communicate in the Swedish language.

The patients were informed about the study during a visit to a nurse. The nurse asked the patients if the researcher in charge of the project could contact them by letter and telephone call in order to further inform them and discuss possible recruitment with them. Of 446 patients invited, 157 consented to participate (response rate 35%), completed and sent back questionnaires at baseline before randomisation and before any intervention was started (Fig. 1).

Patient questionnaires

Patient empowerment was assessed by the SWE-CES-10 questionnaire, which was developed to survey PE in patients with coronary heart disease. This questionnaire was originally based on the SWE-DES-23, which is a valid and reliable tool for assessing PE in diabetes mellitus (DM) and rheumatic disease (RA) [27–29]. The SWE-DES-23 was shortened to become the SWE-DES-SF-10 and was found to be reliable in relation to the original version. The author of the scale allowed us to replace the word 'diabetes' with 'heart disease' in all 10 items and agreed that further psychometric testing was not needed before using the scale in patients with cardiac disease. The SWE-CES-10 has four subscales assessing different components of patient empowerment: 1) Goal achievement and overcoming barriers to goal achievement, 2) Self-awareness, 3) Managing stress, 4) Assessing dissatisfaction and readiness to change. The items are scored on a five-point Likert scale ranging from 'strongly disagree' (1) to 'strongly agree' (5). A higher value indicates a stronger empowerment [30].

Self-efficacy was assessed by the General Self-Efficacy Scale (GSES, Additional file 1) [31], on which items are scored on a four-point Likert scale ranging from 'not at all true' (1) to 'exactly true' (4). A higher score indicates a higher GSE, which predicts the ability to cope with daily problems and the ability to adapt after experiencing various stressful life events [32]. High reliability, stability and construct validity of the GSES scale are confirmed in earlier studies [33, 34].

Well-being was assessed by the Cantril Ladder, a single-item indicator of well-being. This scale is presented as a ladder with steps numbered from zero at the bottom to 10 at the top, where 10 represents the best possible life for the participant, and zero the worst. The participants are asked on which step of the ladder they feel they stood one year ago, on which step they stand at present, and on which step they will stand one year in the future. The Ladder of Life has been used in large population studies, and tested for reliability, concurrent and predictive validity [35]. It has also been used in

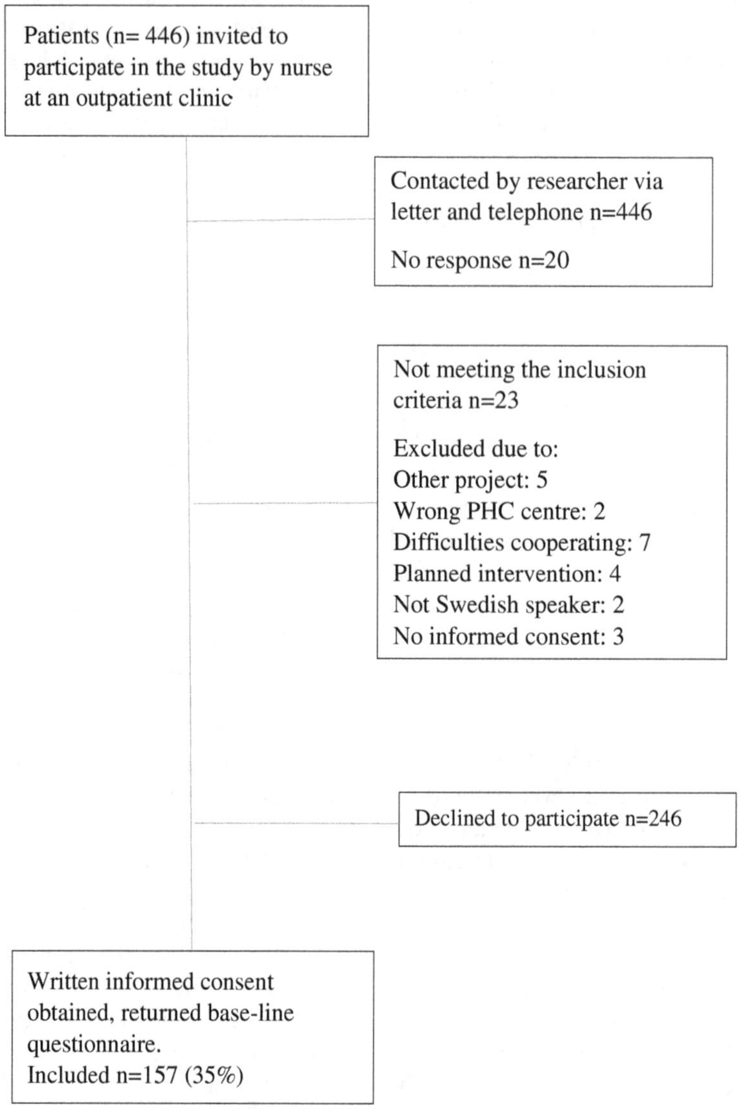

Fig. 1 Sampling frame

elderly patients recovering from an acute coronary event [36] and in a randomised study of patients with coronary heart disease [37].

Self-rated health was measured by the Visual Analogue Scale within the EQ5D (Additional file 2). It produces scores of 0–100, with higher scores indicating a better overall quality of life [38].The EQ5D is considered to be a reliable and valid instrument for use in patients with stable coronary heart disease [39].

Demographic and clinical data

Patients' baseline data on: type of cardiovascular event, days of treatment of hypertension and hyperlipidaemia, smoking, presence of comorbidities (DM, hypertension, chronic obstructive pulmonary disease, stroke, heart failure) were collected from the Swedeheart® register and the medical records about two weeks after discharge from the hospital. Age, sex, education, residential area, job position and marital status were collected from patient questionnaires (Table 1). The patients were also asked to self-report, in free text their diseases. Cardiovascular diseases and DM were excluded. Self-reported comorbidity was categorised by the researchers as: comorbidities of all kinds or comorbidity affecting mobility. This was done in order to catch the total experience of burden of disease.

Statistical analyses

Descriptive statistics were used to characterise the study population. Means, medians and standard deviations are presented for patients' baseline data involving clinical and demographical measures. Chi-square tests were used

Table 1 Baseline characteristics of patients suffering from a coronary heart disease event 6–12 months ago. Comparison of self-reported high or low patient empowerment (SWE-CES-10[1]) and general self-efficacy (GSES[a])

	Total $n = 157$ n (%), mean (SD)	SWE-CES-10 ≤ 3.6 $n = 77$ n (%), mean (SD)	SWE-CES-10 > 3.6 $n = 72$ n (%), mean (SD)	*p*-value	GSES ≤ 2.95 $n = 48$ n (%), mean (SD)	GSES > 2.95 $n = 98$ n (%), mean (SD)	*p*-value
Gender, M/F	122/35	58/19	58/14	0.442	36/12	76/22	0.732
Age, years	68.7 (8.5)	68.4 (8.6)	68.7 (8.4)	0.828	68.7	68.8	0.919
Residential area							
City	74 (47.1)	39 (50.6)	30 (41.7)		24 (50.0)	43 (43.9)	
Rural or small town	83 (52.9)	38 (49.4)	42 (48.3)	0.272	24 (50.0)	55 (56.1)	0.486
Education							
Compulsory education[b]	84 (53.5)	40 (51.9)	39 (54.2)		25 (52.1)	54 (55.1)	
Upper secondary school	31 (19.7)	14 (18.2)	16 (22.2)		10 (20.8)	20 (20.4)	
University	38 (24.2)	21 (27.3)	17 (23.6)	0.493	13 (27.1)	23 (23.5)	0.869
Job position							
Employed	26 (16.9)	10 (13.0)	16 (22.2)		9 (18.8)	15 (15.3)	
Self-employed	15 (9.7)	10 (13.0)	5 (6.9)		4 (8.3)	10 (10.2)	
Disabled pensioner	9 (5.8)	6 (7.8)	3 (4.2)		5 (10.4)	4 (4.1)	
Retired pensioner	104 (67.5)	50 (64.9)	48 (66.7)	0.295	30 (62.5)	68 (69.4)	0.531
Marital status							
Cohabitating	115 (73.2)	53 (68.8)	59 (81.9)		33 (68.8)	75 (76.5)	
Living alone	40 (25.5)	24 (31.2)	13 (18.1)	0.064	15 (31.3)	23 (23.5)	0.314
Time from cardiac event to start of study group, days	284 (74)	274 (75)	291 (70)	0.147	277 (67)	289 (78)	0.362
Smoking, current	19 (12.1)	10 (13.0)	8 (11.1)	0.726	7 (14.6)	10 (10.2)	0.438
Cardiac event one year before study inclusion[c]							
Myocardial infarction	86 (54.8)	43 (55.8)	41 (56.9)		25 (52.1)	56 (57.1)	
Other	71 (45.2)	34 (44.2)	31 (43.1)	0.892	23 (47.9)	42 (42.9)	0.563
Cardiac event one year before study inclusion							
PCI only	110 (70.1)	55 (71.4)	50 (69.4)		34 (70.8)	68 (69.4)	
CABG, CABG+PCI or MI without revascularisation	47(29.9)	22 (28.6)	22 (30.6)	0.791	14 (29.2)	30 (30.6)	0.858
Number of previous myocardial infarctions							
1	15 (10.1)	9 (11.7)	6 (8.3)		4 (8.3)	8 (8.2)	
2	3 (2.0)	1 (1.3)	2 (2.8)		2 (4.2)	1 (1.0)	
3	2 (1.3)	1 (1.3)	1 (1.4)	0.841	0 (0)	2 (2.0)	0.468
Angina pectoris, diagnosed	47 (29.9)	26 (33.8)	19 (26.4)	0.327	17 (35.4)	28 (28.6)	0.400
CCS[d]							
I	98 (62.4)	53 (75.7)	41 (64.1)		26(61.9)	66 (73.3)	
II	27 (17.2)	9 (12.9)	16 (25.0)		9 (21.4)	17 (18.9)	
III	11 (7.0)	6 (8.6)	5 (7.8)		5 (11.9)	5 (5.6)	
IV	4 (2.5)	2 (2.9)	2 (3.1)	0.345	2 (4.8)	2 (2.2)	0.430
Diabetes Mellitus	25 (15.9)	9 (11.7)	14 (19.4)	0.190	11 (22.9)	13 (13.3)	0.139
Hypertension	75 (47.8)	37 (48.1)	36 (50.0)	0.812	26 (54.2)	47 (48.0)	0.481
Medication for hypertension before study start, days	1376 (649–2094)[e]	1542 (673–2107)[e]	1270 (645–1883)[e]	0.383	1459 (649–2149)[e]	1187 (649–1912)[e]	0.641
COPD[f]	15 (9.6)	9 (11.7)	6 (8.3)	0.496	5 (10.3)	9 (9.2)	0.812

Table 1 Baseline characteristics of patients suffering from a coronary heart disease event 6–12 months ago. Comparison of self-reported high or low patient empowerment (SWE-CES-10[1]) and general self-efficacy (GSES[a]) *(Continued)*

	Total $n = 157$ n (%), mean (SD)	SWE-CES-10 ≤ 3.6 $n = 77$ n (%), mean (SD)	SWE-CES-10 > 3.6 $n = 72$ n (%), mean (SD)	p-value	GSES ≤ 2.95 $n = 48$ n (%), mean (SD)	GSES > 2.95 $n = 98$ n (%), mean (SD)	p-value
Hyperlipidaemia	56 (35.7)	31 (40.3)	24 (33.3)	0.381	23 (47.9)	29 (29.6)	0.030
Days with treatment for hyperlipidaemia before study start	1038 (420–1884)[e]	695 (338–2156)[e]	1150(507–1799)[e]	0.513	1061 (341–1740)[e]	1067 (456–2038)[e]	0.324
Comorbidity, all kinds	60 (38.2)	26 (33.8)	31 (43.1)	0.244	16 (33.3)	40 (40.8)	0.382
Comorbidity, affecting mobility	17 (10.8)	10 (13.0)	7 (9.7)	0.531	6 (12.5)	9 (9.2)	0.535

[a]Dichotomized
[b]Less than 10 years in school
[c]Current, basis for study inclusion
[d]Canadian Cardiovascular Society scale for grading angina pectoris
[e]Median (IQR)
[f]Chronic obstructive pulmonary disease

to compare dichotomised variables. The SWE-CES-10 (Patient Empowerment Scale) was dichotomised based on the median value in the present sample (md = 3.6). For GSES (Additional file 1), the mean value for population data [40] was used as a cut-off value (m = 2.95) when dichotomised. Simple linear and multiple regression models were used where the two main outcome variables, GSES and PE, were considered dependent. In order not to overlook effects, the SWE-CES-10 and GSES variables were used as continuous variables in multiple linear regression analysis (Model 1 and 2). Simple linear regressions tested the association of PE and GSES with sex, age, marital status, education, well-being (Cantril's Ladder) and self-rated health (EQ5D). The significant variables from the simple linear regressions, together with sex and age, were used in Models 1 and 2. A *p*-value < 0.05 was considered significant.

Results

Of the individuals included, three quarters were men, and the mean age for the whole group was 68.7 (±8.5) (range 47–87) years (Table 1). There were equal proportions living in rural or small town areas or in the city. Half of the group (54.8%) had suffered a myocardial infarction, and 70.1% of all participants had been treated with percutaneous coronary intervention. Twenty participants had had a previous myocardial infarction. In total, 29.9% of the participants had been diagnosed with angina pectoris, with 2.5% having severe angina (CCS IV). The mean value for the participants' ($n = 149$) self-rated total PE was 3.69 (±0.54) (theoretical range 1 low and 5 high). Mean values for subscales were: Goal achievement 3.76 (±0.65), Self-awareness 3.90 (±0.99), Managing stress 3.47 (±0.86), Readiness to change 3.57 (±0.76). The mean value for GSES was 3.13 (±0.52) ($n = 146$). Distributions are shown in Figs. 2 and 3.

The correlation between the SWE-CES and GSES was, $r = 0.381$ ($p < 0.000$). When SWE-CES and GSES were dichotomised, there were no significant differences between participants rating high or low on these variables, with the exception of hyperlipidaemia and GSE (Table 1).

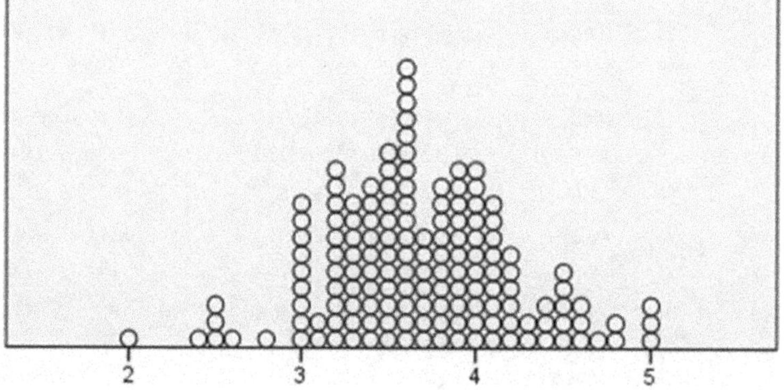

Fig. 2 Distribution of empowerment SWE-CES. Scale 1–5 ($n = 150$)

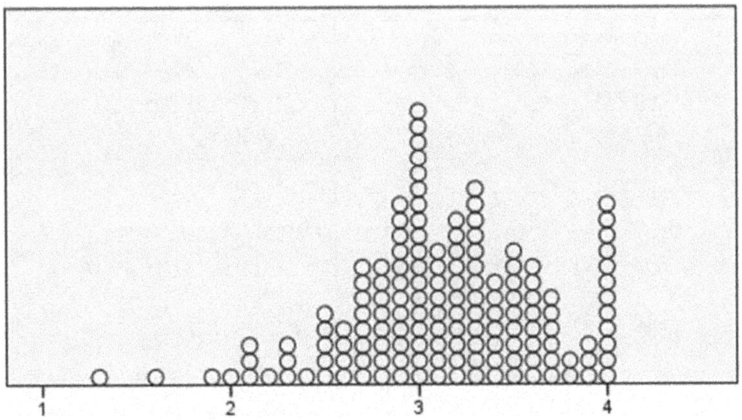

Fig. 3 Distribution of self-efficacy. Scale 1–4 ($n = 144$)

Patient empowerment, general self-efficacy and related variables

Gender, age, marital status, education, self-rated health and well-being were considered to be possibly related to PE. All of these variables were first tested with simple linear regression. The variables that were significantly related to PE, together with gender and age, were used in the multiple linear regression model. Consequently, the variable 'education' was excluded from Model 1. The same procedures as applied in PE were used when analysing GSES. There were significant correlations between PE and marital status, self-rated health (EQ5D) and well-being (Ladder of Life) in a simple linear regression. In the multiple linear regression, Model 1, the association between PE and self-rated health (EQ5D) remained significant (Table 2). For GSE, there were significant univariate correlations for all variables except age and education. We excluded education in the multiple linear model. In the multiple linear regression, Model 2, none of the variables were significantly associated with GSE (Table 3).

Discussion

This is the first study assessing PE and GSE and related variables in a cardiac population. The levels of GSE and PE were high, and GSE in this group was similar when compared to a general population [40, 41] as well as for patients with other chronic illnesses [34]. This might indicate that levels of PE or GSE are not related to chronic conditions.

The main message of this study is that we were not able to find demographic and clinical variables that could be used as predictors of low PE or GSE. We cannot predict how patients with coronary heart disease rate PE or GSE based on variables such as age, sex, marital status, or type of cardiovascular event. We found a significant association between self-rated health and PE. The higher the patients rated their health, the higher the PE. However, self-rated health was not related to GSE. Our findings do not support the hypothesis of Bravo et al. (2015), who suggested that patients scoring high for PE would have better reported outcomes, e.g. be better adapted to their condition; have better quality of life; report higher levels of well-being and

Table 2 Simple and multiple correlation for patient empowerment (SWE-CES-10[a]). R^2 0.125, adjusted R^2 0.091

	Simple linear regression				Multiple linear regression			
Independent variables	Unstandardized Beta coefficient	95% CI		p-value	Unstandardized Beta coefficient	95% CI		p-value
Gender, M[b]/F	−0.174	−0.382	0.034	0.100	−0.92	−0.302	0.119	0.392
Age, years	0.004	−0.007	0.014	0.474	0.008	−0.002	0.018	0.114
Education	−0.016	−0.115	0.082	0.743	NA	NA	NA	NA
Cohabitating[b]/ Living alone	0.201	−0.400	−0.003	0.047	−0.088	−0.295	0.120	0.405
Current self-rated health (scale 0–100)[c]	0.010	0.005	0.014	< 0.001	0.007	0.002	0.013	0.014
Well-being (scale 0–10)[d]	0.060	0.014	0.106	0.011	0.021	−0.035	0.076	0.463

[a]Continuous variable, [b]Reference, [c] EQ5D, [d] Ladder of life, *NA* Not applicable

Table 3 Simple and multiple correlation for dependent variable general self-efficacy (GSES[a]). R^2 0.111, adjusted R^2 0.076

	Simple linear regression				Multiple linear regression			
Independent variables	Unstandardised Beta coefficient	95% CI		*p*-value	Unstandardised Beta coefficient	95% CI		*p*-value
Gender, M[a]/F	−0.202	−0.0399	−0.005	0.045	− 0.145	−0.350	0.061	0.166
Age, years	0.000	−0.010	0.010	0.960	0.005	−0.006	0.015	0.371
Education	0.024	−0.074	0.123	0.628	NA	NA	NA	NA
Cohabitating[b]/ Living alone	−0.246	−0.434	−0.057	0.011	− 0.111	−0.317	0.095	0.288
Current self-rated health (scale 0–100)[c]	0.008	0.004	0.013	< 0.001	0.004	−0.002	0.010	0.178
Well-being (scale 0–10)[d]	0.065	0.021	0.109	0.004	0.040	−0.015	0.095	0.149

[a]Continuous variable, [b]Reference, [c] EQ5D, [d] Ladder of life, *NA* Not applicable

satisfaction with life and achieve some independence in relation to their health care [42].

The mean level of PE in total did not differ from other studies on chronic diseases, such as rheumatoid arthritis (RA) [43] and DM [28]. On some of the subscales of PE, the cardiac population scored higher compared to RA on self-awareness (3.90) vs (3.5) and lower compared to RA/DM on readiness to change (3.57) vs. (3.7); higher compared to DM on goal- achievement (3.76) vs (3.64) [28, 43]. An interpretation of this finding could be that the cardiac population know enough for making self-care choices, and when and where to get support if needed. They are goal- oriented and can over-come barriers to reach the goals. However, part of the self-care causes dissatisfaction and to some extent they are cautiously awaiting self-care change. This might be due to lack of motivation despite them being knowledgeable.

According to the literature review [18], few studies have investigated the connection between SE and PE. We found a weak correlation between PE and GSE, indicating that these cannot replace each other. GSE was not related to educational level, civil status or well-being, either. It is vital for people to acquire SE in order to be able to handle adversity and the struggles they encounter in life [17]. We therefore argue that it is important to identify patients with low GSE and PE, as this might place them at risk of failing to reach goals in their cardiac rehabilitation plan. By measuring PE and GSE, we can identify the patients that are in need of support during cardiac rehabilitation. As addressed by WHO, PE is a key factor for improving health outcomes, enhancing communication between patients and health professionals, and adherence to treatment regimens [13].

There is a paradigm shift taking place, as clinical encounters have traditionally focussed on persuading patients to comply with taking medication as prescribed [44], and PE is aiming instead at a collaboration between health care professionals and patients, assisting the latter in becoming self-aware of the considerations, needs and barriers to changing their lifestyle, managing their illness, and using resources to solve problems in their daily lives [45]. There is convincing evidence that empowerment-based self-management interventions can improve PE and also health outcomes. For example, PE was significantly stronger among people with RA diseases after problem-based learning programmes compared to a control group six months post-intervention [43]. A meta-analysis of empowerment-based interventions showed improvements in HbA1C, SE and empowerment levels in patients with chronic metabolic diseases [46]. Such interventions can be designed to facilitate patients' self-management, and PE is also considered as a valuable measurable patient-reported outcome for depression, DM and asthma [47, 48] and, among survivors from cancer, using information technology to improve PE [49]. However, further randomised trials are needed to evaluate the effects of interventions aimed at improving GSE and PE to change/manage self-care. Longitudinal trials could help us to define at what scores additional support is warranted [26].

Strengths and limitations

The present study has some limitations. Firstly, we used cross-sectional data that was collected during an intervention study. However, despite this shortcoming, this is to our knowledge the first study that has investigated PE in patients with coronary heart disease.

Secondly, we were unable to include more than half of the invited patients in the study. Some gave reasons such as feeling too old, living abroad for half of the year, difficulties in travelling to the group meetings, or social circumstances, but we did not structurally collect data on the non-participants, as in accordance with ethical legislation, reasons for non-participation could not be collected. We cannot therefore say whether the participants differ significantly from the non-participants. In total, 35% of eligible patients were enrolled and that may be considered as a small number, and as highly selected, as they from the start were positive and wanted to take part in the COR-PRIM-study [26], which is quite a demanding programme, with group discussions in primary care over a period of one year and a long follow-up time of five years. Internal drop-outs were low, and in comparison with Jelinek et al. [6] who enrolled 20–50% of eligible patients to cardiac rehabilitation, the number of participants in our study is not low.

Conclusion

PE and GSE are not mutually interchangeable, and therefore both need to be measured when planning for secondary prevention in primary health care. The results showed that we cannot predict a high-risk group based on demographic variables, e.g. patients' sex, age, marital status or education. Therefore, in order to support PE and GSE, all patients need to be offered follow-up, and we are inclined to say that it should be personalised, with a focus on the patients' beliefs, needs and goals.

Abbreviations

COR-PRIM: Coronary heart disease-primary care; CR: Cardiac rehabilitation; EQ5D: European Quality of Life–Five Dimensions; GSE (S): General Self-Efficacy (Scale); PE: Patient Empowerment; SE: Self-efficacy; SWE-CES: Swedish Cardiac Empowerment Scale

Acknowledgements

The authors would like to thank all patients for their helpful collaboration. We also thank Sanna Lindgren, Elisabeth Svensson, Anita Pehrsson, Anneli Rudenäs, Melina Appel, Victoria Grönlund and Tina Ednarsson for their valuable assistance, which made it possible to conduct this study.

Funding

This study is funded by the Swedish Heart and Lung Association, project number E091/10, E122/11, E083/12, E103/13 and The County Council/ Region Östergötland, Sweden, project number LIO-92281, LIO-125151, LIO-27535, LIO-354951, LIO- 433801. The funders were not involved in the study design, in the collection, analysis, and interpretation of the data, in the writing of the report, or in the decision to submit the article for publication.

Authors' contributions

AKK participated in the design and coordination of the study, collected all data, contributed to data analysis and drafted the manuscript. PT participated in the design of the study, in data analysis, and made substantial contributions to drafting the manuscript. TJ led on the design, helped to interpret during data analysis, and made substantial contributions to drafting the manuscript. SN participated in the design of the study, in data analysis and made contributions to drafting the manuscript. All authors read and approved the final manuscript.

Competing interests

The authors declare that they have no competing interests.

Author details

[1]Department of Social and Welfare Studies (ISV/OMV), Linköping University, Norrköping, Sweden. [2]Department of Medical and Health Sciences (IMH), Linköping University, Linköping, Sweden. [3]Primary Health Care, Region Östergötland, Linköping, Sweden.

References

1. Hartley A, Marshall D, Salciccioli J, Sikkel M, Maruthappu M, Shalhoub J. Trends in mortality from ischemic heart disease and cerebrovascular disease in Europe: 1980-2009. Circulation. 2016;133(20):1916–26.
2. Socialstyrelsen: Statistik om hjärtinfarkter 2016. In: Hälso- och sjukvård; 2017. Retrieved 2018-05-17 from http://www.socialstyrelsen.se/publikationer2017/2017-10-23.
3. Jernberg T, Hasvold P, Henriksson M, Hjelm H, Thuresson M, Janzon M. Cardiovascular risk in post-myocardial infarction patients: nationwide real world data demonstrate the importance of a long-term perspective. Eur Heart J. 2015;36(19):1163–70.
4. Perk J, De Backer G, Gohlke H, Graham I, Reiner Z, Vershuren WMM, Albus C, Benlian P, Boysen G, Cifkova R, et al. European guidelines on cardiovascular disease prevention in clinicl practice (version 2012). Eur Heart J. 2012;33:1635–701.
5. Kotseva K, Wood D, De Bacquer D, De Backer G, Rydén L, Jennings C, Gyberg V, Amouyel P, Bruthans J, Castro Conde A, et al. EUROASPIRE IV: a European Society of Cardiology survey on the lifestyle, risk factor and therapeutic management of coronary patients from 24 European countries. Eur J Prev Cardiol. 2015;23(6):636–48.
6. Jelinek M, Thomson D, Ski C, Bunker S, Vale M. 40 years of cardiac rehabilitation and secondary prevention in post-cardiac ischaemic patients. Are we still in the wilderness? Int J Cardiol. 2015;179:153–9.
7. Anderson LJ, Taylor RS. Cardiac rehabilitation for people with heart disease: an overview of Cochrane systematic reviews. Int. J Cardiol. 2014;17:348–61.
8. Critchley J, Capewell S. Smoking cessation for the secondary prevention of coronary heart disease. Cochrane Database Syst Rev. 2003;4:CD003041.
9. Wilson K, Gibson N, Willan A, Cook D. Effect of smoking cessation on mortality after myocardial infarction: meta-analysis of cohort studies. Arch Intern Med. 2000;160(7):939–44.
10. Kristofferzon M-L, Löfmark R, Carlsson M. Striving for balance in daily life: experiences of Swedish women and men shortly after a myocardial infarction. J Clin Nurs. 2007;16:391–401.
11. Odell A, Grip L, Hallberg R-M. Restenosis after percutaneous coronary intervention (PCI): experiences from the patients' perspective. Eur J Cardiovasc Nurs. 2006;5:150–7.
12. Kärner A, Tingstrom P, Abrandt Dahlgren M, Bergdahl B. Incentives for lifestyle changes in patients with coronary heart disesae. J Adv Nurs. 2005; 51(3):261–75.
13. WHO/Europe: Health 2020: the European policy for health and well-being - About Health 2020: Retrieved 2018-05-17 from http://www.euro.who.int/en/health-topics/health-policy/health-2020-the-european-policy-for-health-and-well-being/about-health-2020.
14. WHO: Patient empowerment and health care. In.; 2009: Retrieved 2017-12-07 from http://www.ncbi.nlm.nih.gov/books/NBK144022/
15. Castro EM, Van Regenmortel T, Vanhaecht K, Sermeus W, Van Hecke A. Patient empowerment, patient participation and patient-centeredness in hospital care: a concept analysis based on a literature review. Patient Educ Couns. 2016;99:1923–39.
16. Bandura A. Self-efficacy in changing societies. Cambridge: Cambridge University Press; 1995.
17. Zulkosky K. Self-efficacy: a concept analysis. Nurs Forum. 2009;44(2):93–102.
18. Rawlett K. Journey from self-efficacy to empowerment. Health Care. 2014;2(1):1–9.
19. Schwarzer R, Fuchs R. Changing risk behaviors and adopting health behaviors: the role of self-efficacy beliefs. In: Bandura A, editor. Self-efficacy in changing societies. Cambride: Cambridge University press; 1995. p. 258–88.
20. Slovinec D'Angelo M, Pelletier L, Reid R, Huta V. The roles of self-efficacy and motivation in the prediction of short- and long term adherence to exercise among patients with coronary heart disease. Health Psychol. 2014; 33(11):1344–53.
21. Sol B, van der Graaf Y, van Petersen R, Visseren F. The effects of self-efficacy on cardiovascular lifestyle. Eur J Cardiovasc Nurs. 2011;10:180–6.
22. Bakker E, Nijkamp M, Sloot C, Berndt N, Bolman C. Intention to abstain from smoking among cardiac rehabilitation patients - The role of attitudes, self-efficacy and craving. J Cardiovasc Nurs. 2015;30(2):172–9.
23. Brink E, Alsén P, Herliz J, Kjellgren K, Cliffordson C. General self-efficacy and health-related quality of life after myocardial infarction. Psychol, Healt & Med. 2012;17(3):346–55.
24. Bandura A. Exercise of personal and collective efficacy in changing societies. In: Bandura A, editor. Self-efficacy in changing societies. Cambridge: Cambridge university press; 1995.

25. Schröder KEE, Schwarzer R, Konertz W. Coping as a mediator in recovery from cardiac surgery. Psychol Health. 1998;13(1):83–97.
26. Kärner A, Nilsson S, J T, Andersson A, Wiréhn A-B, Wodlin P, Hjelmfors L, Tingstrom P. The effect of problem-based learning in patient education after an event of CORONARY heart disease - a randomised study in PRIMARY health care: design and methodology of the COR-PRIM study. BMC Fam Pract. 2012;13(110):1–9.
27. Arvidsson S, Bergman S, Arvidsson B, Fridlund B, Tingström P. Psychometric properties of the Swedish rheumatic disease empowerment scale, SWE-RES-23. Musculoskeletal Care. 2012;10:101–9.
28. Leksell J, Funnel M, Sandberg G, Smide B, Wiklund G, Wikblad K. Psychometric properties of the Swedish diabetes empowerment scale. Scand J Caring Sci. 2007;21:247–52.
29. Barr PJ, Scholl I, Bravo P, Faber MJ, Elwyn G, McAllister M: Assessment of patient empowerment - a systematic review of measures. PLoS One. 2015;10(5): e0126553. https://doi.org/10.1371/journal.pone.0126553.
30. Anderson R, Fitzgerald J, Gruppen L, Funnel MM, Oh M: the diabetes empowerment scale- short-form (DES_SF). Diabetes Care 2013, 26(5):1641–1642.
31. Koskinen- Hagman M, Schwarzer R, Jerusalem M: Swedish version of the general self-efficacy scale. In., vol. 2017: http://userpage.fu-berlin.de/health/swedish.htm; 1999.
32. Schwarzer R, Jerusalem M. Generalized self-efficacy scale. In: Weinman J, Wright S, Johnston M, editors. Measures in health psychology: A user's portfolio Causal and control beliefs. Windsor UK: NFER-NELSON; 1995. p. 35–7.
33. Leganger A, Kraft P, RØysamb E: perceived self-efficacy in health behaviour research: conceptualisation, measurement and correlates. Psychol Health 2000, 15(1):51–69.
34. Luszczynska A, Scholz U, Schwarzer R. The general Sel-efficacy scale: multicultural validation studies. Aust J Psychol. 2005;139(5):439–57.
35. Andrews F, Withey S. Social indicators of well-being: American's perceptions of life quality. New York: Plenum; 1976.
36. Ståhle A, Mattsson E, Rydén L, Unden AL, Nordlander R. Improved physical fitness and quality of life following training of elderly patients after acute coronary events. A 1 year follow-up randomized controlled study. Eur Heart J. 1999;20(20):1475–84.
37. Tingström P, Kamwendo K, Bergdahl B. Effects of a problem-based learning rehabilitation programme on quality of life in patients with coronary artery disease. Eur J Cardiovasc Nurs. 2005;4:324–30.
38. The EuroQol G: EuroQol* - a new facility for the measurement of health-related quality of life. Health Policy 1990, 16:199–208.
39. De Smedt D, Clays E, Doyle F, Kotseva K, Prugger C, Pająk A, Jennings C, Wood D, De Bacquer D. Validity and reliability of three commonly used quality of life measures in a large European population of coronary heart disease patients. Int J Cardiol. 2013;167(5):2294–9.
40. Scholz U, Gutierrez Dona B, Sud S, Schwarzer R. Is general self-efficacy a universal construct? Psychometric findings from 25 countries. Eur J Psychol Ass. 2002;18(3):242–51.
41. Swarzer, R. Renner, B. Health-specific self-efficacy scales. 2014. https://www.researchgate.net/publication/251801350_Health-Specific_Self. Efficacy_Scales. Accessed 2017-11-10.
42. Bravo P, Edwards A, Barr PJ, Scholl I, Elwyn G, McAllister M. Conceptualising patient empowerment: a mixed methods study. BMC Health Serv Res. 2015; 15(1):1–14.
43. Arvidsson S, Bergman S, Arvidsson B, Fridlund B, Tingström P. Effects of a self-care promotion problem-based learning programme in people with rheumatic diseases: a randomized controlled study. J Adv Nurs. 2012;67(7): 1500–14.
44. Funnell MM. Patient empowerment: what does it really mean? Patient Educ Couns. 2016;99(12):1921–2.
45. Anderson RM, Funnel MM. Patient empowerment: reflections on the challenge of fostering the adoption of a new paradigm. Patient Educ Couns. 2005;57:153–7.
46. Kuo CC, Lin CC, Tsai FM. Effectiveness of empowerment-based self-management interventions on patients with chronic metaboloc diseases: a systematic review and meta-analysis. Evid Based Nurs. 2014;2014(11):5.
47. McAllister M, Dunn G, Payne K, Davies K, Todd C. Patient empowerment: the need to consider it as a measurable patient- reported outcome for chronic conditions. BMC Health Serv Res. 2012;12:157.
48. Tsai A, Morton S, Mangione C, Keeler E. A meta-analysis of interventions to improve care for chronic illnesses. Am J Manag Care. 2005;11:478–88.
49. Groen W, Kuijpers W, Oldenburg H, Wouters M, Aaronson N, Harten W. Empowerment of cancer survivors through information technology: an intergrative review. J Med Internet Res. 2015;17(11):e270.

Substitution of care for chronic heart failure from the hospital to the general practice: patients' perspectives

J. A. Wildeboer[1], A. R. T. van de Ven[2] and D. de Boer[3*]

Abstract

Background: Shifting care from the secondary to the primary system may present an opportunity to ensure that the increasing number of patients with chronic heart failure (CHF) receive high-quality care while containing costs. However, shifting from secondary to primary care might seem radical to patients. A qualitative insight into patients' issues, preferences, expectations and needs may help arrange a smooth transition from secondary to primary care for CHF patients. The aim of this exploratory study is therefore to gain insights into the way CHF patients in secondary care perceive the possibility of substitution of CHF care from secondary to primary care.

Methods: In total, fifteen semi-structured interviews were conducted with CHF patients. Topics discussed during the interviews were the advantages and disadvantages, attitudes of patients, preferences regarding the substitution and trust in the GP and cardiologist. A thematic analysis was performed.

Results: The minority of the patients welcomed the idea of substitution. Against that, the majority of the patients had various concerns. This attitude was mainly influenced by two main themes, confidence and security and accessibility. Most patients had more confidence in secondary than in primary care because of the greater level of knowledge and more possibilities for examination in secondary care and because of good relationships and positive previous experiences in secondary care. Patients also indicated that the general practice is geographically more easily accessible than the hospital.

Conclusion: Patients had various concerns regarding the substitution of care for chronic heart failure. Addressing these concerns by informing them appropriately may contribute to a smooth and patient-friendly substitution from secondary to primary care. The fears and needs of patients could also be taken into account by policymakers when optimising the way substitution is organised, or when substitution is introduced.

Keywords: Substitution, Patients' attitudes, Chronic heart failure

Background

Heart failure is a chronic condition with a high prevalence and a high morbidity and mortality [1, 2]. Worldwide, the prevalence of chronic heart failure (CHF) is 23 million [3]. The prevalence of CHF has increased over recent decades and is expected to increase further in the coming years [1, 4, 5]. The costs of CHF are considerable [6, 7]. In western society, CHF comprises 1–2% of all healthcare costs. The majority of these costs are for frequent, long-lasting and repeated hospitalisations [7].

Changes in healthcare and treatment for CHF are needed in order to ensure that the increasing number of patients with CHF receive high-quality care and to reduce the associated costs [8, 9]. Substitution, which optimises the care process by shifting care is a change that could be implemented to handle this problem [8, 9]. Substitution is defined as "the replacement of all or part of an existing healthcare facility by all or part of another facility, in which the original function will be fulfilled for a similar patient population" (p.9) [9].

Currently, CHF patients are under treatment in secondary care. Stable CHF patients visit their heart failure nurse and cardiologist both twice a year for a routine

* Correspondence: d.deboer@nivel.nl
[3]NIVEL, Otterstraat 118-124, 3518 CR Utrecht, Netherlands
Full list of author information is available at the end of the article

check. The Dutch government is interested in strategies to decrease the healthcare costs and to provide high quality of care [10], and substitution is one of these strategies. Substituting CHF care to primary care may be a more sustainable and a cost-efficient approach of treating stable CHF patients. Treating patients in primary care is less expensive than treating patients in secondary care due to the specialist and more expensive care that is provided in secondary care [9]. However, a solid primary care is necessary in order to treat patients in primary care. In the Netherlands, the primary care is well developed and organised and substitution of CHF care for stable patients would be possible.

The substitution approach is still evolving in the Netherlands and has recently been applied on a small scale in a number of regions and hospitals in the treatment of CHF [11, 12]. In the case of a shift from secondary to primary care, the general practitioner (GP) becomes the central care provider instead of the medical specialist. This might seem to be a radical shift to patients who are currently being treated in secondary care. To date only quantitative studies have been done to investigate patients' preferences for substitution. Those studies showed that patients prefer medical specialists for complex treatments and GPs for less complex treatments [9, 13]. A qualitative insight into patients' issues, preferences, expectations and needs relating to substitution of care will increase our understanding of how patients perceive this. In addition, such understanding can help to optimise the way in which substitution is organised from the patients' perspective, which can help improve the quality of care. The aim of this exploratory study is therefore to gain insights into the way CHF patients in secondary care perceive the possibility of substitution of CHF care from secondary to primary care.

Research question

How do chronic heart failure patients in secondary care perceive the possibility of substitution of their CHF care from secondary to primary care?

Method

Study design

Semi-structured interviews were conducted in this qualitative study to investigate how patients perceive substitution of CHF care. A topic list that was covered in the interviews included the advantages and disadvantages of substitution, attitudes of patients towards substitution, the relationships with the cardiologist and GP, trust in the cardiologist and GP, and patients' preferences in the matter (Additional file 1). Furthermore, probing questions were prepared. The topic list for the interviews was based on a theoretical model by Sixma et al. (1998) and six elements that determine quality of care according to the WHO [14, 15]. This conceptual model states that patients' perspectives can be identified by assessing the needs and expectations of patients. By identifying the needs and expectations of the six elements that define quality of care (effectivity, efficiency, accessibility, acceptability equity and safety), patients' perspectives towards the substitution from secondary to primary care were identified.

Participants and data collection

A group of patients were recruited from the population of CHF patients at the St. Anna hospital in Geldrop in the Netherlands. Patients received an invitation letter followed by a phone call within a week. Convenience sampling was used to select participants. A total of 18 patients were approached and 15 patients agreed to participate. Participants were recruited until data saturation was achieved [16]. This group of participants was selected from a list of patients who had an appointment with the heart failure nurse at several days in 2016. Nine interviews were scheduled following a doctor's appointment in the hospital and six interviews were conducted by phone due to logistic reasons and patients' preferences. An independent researcher, who did not have a relation with the participants, conducted the interviews and to ensure confidentially only the researcher and the participant were present in the room. At the beginning of the interview, the idea of transferring CHF care to primary care was explained to patients. Essentially, this transfer of care would mean that patients visit the GP for their CHF care and only see the specialist in the hospital through a referral from the GP. All participants gave approval for the interview to be recorded and signed an informed consent form. Additionally, patients filled in a seven-question questionnaire about demographic information. After the interview, a summary of the interview was sent to all participants for verification. The majority of the participants approved the summary and in a single case several adjustments were made. All interviews lasted around 30 min.

Data analysis

The data analysis for this study was based on thematic analysis [17]. The recordings of the interviews were transcribed verbatim, using Express Scribe Transcription Software. These transcripts were coded by using MAXQDA 12. The conceptual model was used as a starting point of the analysis of the transcripts. The transcripts were coded by using the concepts of the conceptual framework. Thereafter, open coding was used to identify the important aspects within each concept [17, 18]. The first three interviews were coded separately by the main researcher and a colleague. Discrepancies between the researchers were discussed, which resulted in a number of small changes in the coding system. The themes, deriving from the open coding, were named and relationships between the themes were identified in consultation with the main researcher and a supervising researcher [18].

Results

Research population

The participants were 15 CHF patients from St. Anna Hospital. Nine patients (60%) were male and six patients (40%) were female. The average age was 74, ranging from 65 to 81. All patients were born in the Netherlands. Patients described their state of health on average as moderate. Four patients (27%) did not have any other conditions in addition to CHF and eleven patients (73%) had one or more comorbidities such as diabetes, other heart and vascular diseases, renal insufficiency and pulmonary hypertension. These characteristics of the research population are representative of the entire population of CHF patients in the Netherlands [19–21]. The majority of the patients were classified according the New York Heart Association (NYHA) classification in class II and a minority in class III. Class II refers to slight limitation of physical activity and comfortable at rest. Class III refers to marked limitation of physical activity and comfortable at rest [22]. No different results were found in the face-to-face or telephonic interviews.

General attitude towards repositioning

The majority of the patients had a negative attitude towards substitution of care. These patients had a better relationship with their cardiologist and/or specialist heart failure nurse than with their GP, which let them feel more at ease in the hospital. Furthermore, these patients had more confidence in the cardiologist because of the specialisation in heart conditions, and patients felt that their heart condition was a severe condition for which they preferred a specialised physician.

In contrast, a number of patients was positive about the substitution from secondary to primary care for the treatment of CHF. They saw the substitution as a natural form of progress and reasoned that the hospital is still always there if necessary. These patients also saw the geographical proximity of the GP as an advantage. Furthermore, these patients indicated that a general practice had a friendlier ambience than a hospital, which made them to feel more at ease. Despite the fact that some patients were positive, they also had some requirements for substitution of care. First, a yearly check-up with the cardiologist in addition to the check-ups in primary care. Furthermore, patients thought they should get the same amount of time in primary care as in secondary care for a consultation. Currently, a half-hour check-up consultation in secondary care was perceived as pleasant by patients. Usually patients have a ten-minute consultation in primary care, which is felt to be too short for a check-up consultation about heart failure. Lastly, the possibility of examination at the general practice was mentioned. It appeared that the possibility of having an ECG or ultrasound in primary care would provide a sense of security for patients:

> *"I'd prefer an ECG once a year, just for a bit of extra safety and confidence. My health status isn't that good, so an ECG would be reassuring to have once a year. Yes, that would be a point of concern for me if I have to go to the GP instead of the hospital."* (Interview 1)

Two themes that influenced the attitude towards the substitution of heart failure care arose from the data. Security and confidence turned out to be the main theme, appearing to consist of several subthemes. The second theme that arose was accessibility.

Confidence and security

Confidence and security appeared to be the most important concepts for patients in influencing the way they looked at substitution of heart failure care. Most patients had more confidence in their cardiologist than their GP in the specific case of heart failure. In addition, patients are currently treated for CHF in secondary care, which made them familiar with that situation. Accordingly, patients do not know what to expect from the new situation, whereas they have faith in the current situation. These broad observations became manifest in various ways in the following subthemes.

Knowledge

The knowledge and expertise of a cardiologist made patients feel safe. Patients had the idea that a lack of knowledge could mean that a GP or practice nurse cannot help them as effectively and may still refer them to the cardiologist. Visiting the GP or practice nurse as well as the cardiologist would be an additional burden on patients:

> *"I prefer the hospital because in the hospital I trust the people they are more specialised in heart conditions than a GP. They [GP] haven't studied for a specific part of the body, and that doesn't give me confidence... For cases like this, I have more confidence in a specialised physician than in a GP."* (Interview 14)

Burden of disease

Most patients see heart failure as a condition that is too severe for a GP or practice nurse. Patients therefore preferred a specialised caregiver who treats CHF. This was particularly the case for patients in unstable situations, although it was not limited to unstable patients. Patients in stable situations also indicated this as a point of concern:

> *"I have a serious condition and I think that it is too severe to see a GP or practice nurse for. I think just going to the cardiologist is better because heart failure is a serious illness."* (Interview 2)

Relationship with care provider

The relationship with the care provider had a major influence on the extent to which patients trust them. Because the good, long-term relationships that most patients had with their cardiologists, these patients trusted their cardiologists more than their GPs and practice nurses. Patients thought that the relationship with their cardiologist cannot be built up with someone else. One of the patients described it as follows:

> *"The cardiologist and the specialist heart failure nurse are on a pedestal for me and no one should touch that. I'd never want to lose those two. I trust them completely. They mean so much to me, I believe them instantly."* (Interview 7)

On the other hand, a number of patients had a better relationship with their GP than with their cardiologist. The ambience of a general practice was friendlier and more accessible than a hospital. Patients had been seeing their GP for many years and also knew their GP from the community where they lived. Patients who perceived a better relationship with their GP than with their cardiologist were generally more open to the idea of repositioning their heart failure care.

Past experiences with care provider

Past experiences with a care provider also influenced the degree of confidence patients had in a care provider. Except for one patient, all patients had very positive experiences with the heart failure clinic. The nurse at the heart failure clinic had enough time to answer questions and if necessary the opportunity to consult a cardiologist directly, who was available at the hospital. Furthermore, the majority of these patients indicated that they were approached with a touch of humour, which patients perceive as pleasant. The one patient who had not had good experiences with the heart failure clinic was dissatisfied with the accessibility of the heart failure clinic by phone.

A few patients had less pleasant experiences with their GP regarding their heart condition. These patients reported that they were not redirected appropriately to the hospital or were misdiagnosed. These past experiences reduced patients' confidence in their GPs with respect to their heart conditions:

> *"Yes, yes, I really didn't have much confidence in him [GP] because of things I've experienced before and that incident it was only confirmed it more. They don't inspire confidence."* (Interview 15)

In contrast, one patient mentioned that his GP responded well in an acute situation when an acquaintance had heart problems. This increased the confidence of this patient in his GP with respect to heart conditions.

Communication between care providers

Another aspect that affected trust is the communication between care providers. Patients felt that access within the hospital to various different care providers was easier, which gave them a sense of security. Patients felt safer if the cardiologist could get involved very quickly. This was experienced more in the hospital than at the general practice. However, some patients indicated that the connection between the GP and the hospital was also quick:

> *"I think the GP is capable enough of calling an ambulance if something goes wrong, and then you will be in the hospital very quickly... Those people [care providers] have contact very quickly and they consult each other directly if something's wrong."* (Interview 6)

In addition, patients said they should have the opportunity to be redirected from the GP back to the hospital, even if they were at the GP for treatment of CHF. This generated feelings of confidence. However, some patients were a bit concerned that referral to the hospital would mean appointments with several different physicians, which would be too much for them.

Possibilities for examination

The extra opportunities for examination in secondary care created feelings of confidence in the patients. Patients felt there were more possibilities for examinations in a hospital, where it is possible to get an ECG, ultrasound, MRI and other medical examinations.

> *"I think the cardiologist ultimately has more possibilities for examinations than a GP, I think. If the cardiologist thinks something's wrong, he can immediately decide to do an ECG or ultrasound, and at the GP that's more difficult."* (Interview 13)

Patients did not need examinations every time they visit the hospital, but they particularly preferred having the possibility as an option. This was seen as being available in a hospital but not in a general practice.

Accessibility

A frequently mentioned concept when talking about substitution of care is accessibility, in particular geographical accessibility. All patients who did not live in the same town as the hospital said that the general practice is geographically more easily accessible. A general practice was often in the same village where patients lived. This made it possible for patients to get to the GP on foot or by bike, if they were physically able:

> *"Ohhh yes, the trip to the GP instead of the journey to the hospital, that's an advantage, without a doubt. For the GP, I can just go by bike but for the hospital I have to go by car... For me the bike is just much easier."* (Interview 5)

Patients who lived in the same town as where the hospital is located indicated that distance and accessibility to the hospital were not an issue for them. However, this was not limited to patients who lived in the same town.

Discussion

Main findings

The aim of this study was to reveal the attitudes of CHF patients towards substitution of CHF care from secondary to primary care. The majority had various concerns about shifting CHF care, while a minority appeared to be more open to the idea of shifting their heart failure care to primary care. The considerations patients reported regarding the way they saw substitution could be attributed to confidence and security and accessibility. The confidence and security domain appeared to consist of several sub domains, including the level of knowledge of the care provider, the burden of disease, the relationship with the care provider, past experiences with care providers, communication between care providers and possibilities for examination. The main concepts, confidence and security and accessibility are in accordance with the conceptual model that was used in this study. However, the other elements were hardly raised by patients considering substitution of CHF care. Furthermore, the needs and perspectives of patients according to the model of Sixma et al., (1998) towards these two concepts were identified in this study.

The fact that confidence and security appeared to play a large role in patients' considerations regarding substitution of their care for CHF is consistent with previous literature. Firstly, confidence and security are important issues for patients in general [23, 24]. Secondly, for repositioning in particular, a study by Bodegom-Vos et al. (2013) demonstrated that patients' preferences for substitution of care are significantly affected by the type of medical intervention. Patients prefer medical specialists for more complex procedures, which would be the case for CHF. Lastly, the perceived severity of the condition – which would be high for CHF patients – may also partly explain why confidence and security are considered important in the context of repositioning [9, 13].

Within the main concept of security and confidence, several subdomains were identified in the present study that are consistent with previous research. For instance, a study by Tarrant et al. (2003) showed that when the relationship between physicians and patients is better, patients also feel more confident and safer with the physician [25]. This is in line with patients' experiences in this study. In addition, positive experiences in the past with a care provider helped patients trust a care provider [26]. As such, a good relationship with a GP and pleasant experiences were associated with patients being more open towards repositioning. Furthermore, patients appeared to associate the possibilities for examination with confidence, as they reported feeling more at ease if they knew that additional examinations could be performed if necessary. This is also demonstrated in the literature [27, 28]. Additionally, the association that patients reported between communication among care providers and trust is confirmed by the literature [29]. Patients trusted care providers more when there was clear communication between care providers.

Strengths and limitations

A strength of the study is that respondent validation was obtained in this study. This provided the opportunity to validate the researcher's interpretation of the data. This improved the validity of this study. Furthermore, this study is the first qualitative study, as far as we are aware, that extensively investigates patients' attitudes towards substitution of CHF care. To date, only quantitative studies have been conducted to investigate this [9, 13].

This study has also a limitation, all patients were treated by the same specialised heart failure nurse, which is a form of selection bias [30]. This could have influenced the results, as it was found that past experiences influenced how patients felt about repositioning. Additionally, both a strength and a limitation of the present study is that the severity of the CHF patients differed. The majority of the patients was classified according to the NYHA classification in class II, which are relative stable CHF patients, and a number of patients was classified in class III, which are more unstable patients. However, the substitution of CHF care that is being developed is currently focussed on patients in class II. This means that we collected the perspectives of a broader patient population than those for which the substitution is currently being developed. This is an advantage for the richness and diversity of the perspectives we collected, but is also a limitation as some concerns raised by patients in our study might be slightly pronounced due to the severity of their condition.

Potential implications

This study is to our knowledge the first qualitative study that investigated patients' attitudes to substitution for chronic conditions. Policymakers and medical professionals can take the fears and needs of patients into account when optimising the way in which substitution is organised, or when substitution is introduced. These policies should include patients' needs for confidence and safety, accessibility, time constraints in primary care and the relationship between patients and clinicians. Furthermore, security and confidence appeared to be a major influence on how patients' see substitution. Trust in primary care should therefore be taken into account when optimising the way in which substitution is organised. The aim of substitution is to ensure that an increasing number of patients receive high-quality of care and to reduce the associated costs. This study identified the challenges from a patients' perspective of substitution. In the upcoming years, these challenges should be taken into account and evaluated, since CHF patients have often fears and uncertainties about the development of their condition. Furthermore, these challenges should also be identified for other chronic conditions, which could possibly be suitable for substitution. This is important to consider in future policies on primary and secondary care to make the healthcare system as sustainable as possible. This study is a beginning towards a sustainable health system for CHF patients.

From literature, it is known that giving patients self-control will create feelings of security and confidence towards care givers [31, 32]. It is therefore likely that giving patients self-control in the way substitution is organised means that patients will have more trust in primary care and thereby be more positive towards repositioning. One option for giving control to patients is offering them a chance to visit the cardiologist once a year without a referral, if they think it is necessary. A pilot should show whether this works efficiently and whether it does indeed reduce patients' concerns about substitution.

After a discussion with various medical professionals in the field of CHF, it was concluded that most fears of patients are caused by a lack of knowledge. For instance, patients were afraid that there was a lack of knowledge and expertise in primary care. However, all GPs and practice nurses have to participate in an educational programme about the treatment of CHF before repositioning of CHF is commenced. Furthermore, patients were afraid that they would not have enough time at the GP for their check-up. However, patients also have 30 min for a consultation at their practice nurse for their CHF check-up. If patients knew this, the fear of a lack of knowledge might disappear. Patients' fears about substitution could therefore be (at least partially) resolved by providing information to patients. The information might help patients trust primary care more and thereby give them a more positive attitude towards substitution.

Conclusion

The present study showed that patients had various concerns about substitution of care for chronic heart failure. This means that it is important to combine changes in the organisation of care for chronic heart failure with strategies for reducing patients' concerns. Such strategies should be based on a proper assessment of the concerns that patients have and should ideally be jointly developed by patients or patients' representatives and healthcare professionals.

Abbreviations

CHF: Chronic Heart Failure; ECG: Electrocardiogram; GP: General Practitioner; NYHA: New York Heart Association; WHO: World Health Organisation

Acknowledgements

We would like to thank all patients for their willingness to participate in this study and sharing their personal stories. Without their openness, dedication and kindliness, this study could not have been completed. Furthermore, we would like to thank Nicole Jegerings for her assistance, enthusiasm and humour during recruitment of the participants.

Funding

No funding was received.

Authors' contributions

JW conducted the interviews with the patients and analysed and interpret the data regarding patients' perspectives towards the substitution of heart failure care. Furthermore, JW wrote the manuscript. DB supervised the project and commented on the manuscript at all stages. AV critically commented on the manuscript in different stages. All authors were involved in designing the project and discussed the results and implications. All authors read and approved the final manuscript.

Consent for publication

Not applicable: data are anonymous and cannot be traced back to individuals.

Competing interests

The authors declare that they have no competing interests.

Author details

[1]VU University Amsterdam, De Boelelaan 1105, 1081 HV Amsterdam, Netherlands. [2]St. Anna Hospital, Bogardeind 2, 5664 EH Geldrop, Netherlands. [3]NIVEL, Otterstraat 118-124, 3518 CR Utrecht, Netherlands.

References

1. Bui AL, Horwich TB, Fonarow GC. Epidemiology and risk profile of heart failure. Nature reviews. Cardiology. 2011;8(1):30–41.
2. Guha K, McDonagh T. Heart failure epidemiology: European perspective. Curr Cardiol Rev. 2013;9(2):123–7.
3. Lloyd-Jones D, Adams RJ, Brown TM, Carnethon M, Dai S, De Simone G, et al. Heart disease and stroke statistics–2010 update: a report from the American Heart Association. Circulation. 2010;121(7):e46–e215.

4. Ho KK, Pinsky JL, Kannel WB, Levy D, Pitt B. The epidemiology of heart failure: the Framingham Study. J Am Coll Cardiol. 1993;22(4s1):A6–A13.
5. Mosterd A, Hoes AW. Clinical epidemiology of heart failure. Heart. 2007; 93(9):1137–46.
6. Berry C, Murdoch DR, McMurray JJ. Economics of chronic heart failure. Eur J Heart Fail. 2001;3(3):283–91.
7. Braunschweig F, Cowie MR, Auricchio A. What are the costs of heart failure? Europace. 2011;13(suppl 2):ii13–i7.
8. Drewes H, Boom J, Graafmans W, Struijs J, Baan C. Effectiviteit van disease management. Een overzicht van de (internationale) literatuur. RIVM rapport. 2008;260131001:2-39.
9. CEv D, Korevaar J, JDd J, Koopmans B, Mv D, DHd B. Kennisvraag: ruimte voor substitutie? Verschuiving van de tweedelijns- naar eerstelijnszorg. NIVEL overzichtsstudies. 2013;
10. van Rooy Y, Kuipers E, Veldman D, Dekker J, Daniëls M, Rouvoet A, et al. Addendum 2018 onderhandelaarsakkoord medisch-specialistische zorg 2014 t/m 2017. The Hague: Ministry of Health, Welfare and Sport; 2017.
11. DJv V, Jaarsma T, Rutten FH, Jaarsma P, EK-vd P, Hulzebos HJ, et al. Zorg rondom hartfalen. Houten, the Netherlands: Bohn Stafleu van Loghum; 2015.
12. NVvC NVVC. Aangemelde regio's hartfalen: NVVC. Connect. 2015; Available from: http://www.nvvcconnect.nl/hartfalen/aangemelde-regio-s-hartfalen
13. van Bodegom-Vos L, De Jong JD, Spreeuwenberg P, Curfs EC, Groenewegen PP. Are patients' preferences for shifting services from medical specialists to general practitioners related to the type of medical intervention? Qual Prim Care. 2013; 21(2):81–95.
14. World Health Organisation. Quality of care: a process for making strategic choices in health systems. Geneva: World Health Organisation. 2006.
15. Sixma HJ, Kerssens JJ, Campen CV, Peters L. Quality of care from the patients' perspective: from theoretical concept to a new measuring instrument. Health Expect. 1998;1(2):82–95.
16. Guest G, Bunce A, Johnson L. How many interviews are enough? An experiment with data saturation and variability. Field methods. 2006; 18(1):59–82.
17. Braun V, Clarke V. Using thematic analysis in psychology. Qual Res Psychol. 2006;3(2):77–101.
18. Attride-Stirling J. Thematic networks: an analytic tool for qualitative research. Qual Res. 2001;1(3):385–405.
19. Rutten PE. Hoe vaak komt hartfalen voor en hoeveel mensen sterven eraan? Volksgezondheid Toekomst Verkenning, Nationaal Kompas Volksgezondheid. 2014;Bilthoven: RIVM. (Retrieved from https://www.volksgezondheidenzorg.info/onderwerp/hartfalen. Nationaal Kompas Volksgezondheid\Gezondheidstoestand\Ziekten en aandoeningen\Hartvaatstelsel\Hartfalen,). Accessed 20 Dec 2017.
20. Engelfriet P, Hoogenveen R, Poos M, Blokstra A, van Baal P, Verschuren W. Hartfalen: epidemiologie, risicofactoren en toekomst. RIVM rapport. 2012; 260401006:3-122.
21. Hoeymans N, Verheij RA, Schellevis FC, Baan CA. Multimorbiditeit en comorbiditeit in de Nederlandse bevolking-gegevens van huisartsenpraktijk. Ned Tijdschr Geneeskd. 2011;155:A3193.
22. Dolgin M, Fox AC, Gorlin R, Levin RI. Criteria Committee, Nomenclature and criteria for diagnosis of diseases of the heart and great vessels. New York Heart Association. 1994;Lippincott Williams and Wilkins.
23. Pearson SD, Raeke LH. Patients' trust in physicians: many theories, few measures, and little data. J Gen Intern Med. 2000;15(7):509–13.
24. Kao AC, Green DC, Davis NA, Koplan JP, Cleary PD. Patients' trust in their physicians. J Gen Intern Med. 1998;13(10):681–6.
25. Tarrant C, Stokes T, Baker R. Factors associated with patients' trust in their general practitioner: a cross-sectional survey. Br J Gen Pract. 2003;53(495): 798–800.
26. Goold SD. Trust, distrust and trustworthiness: lessons from the field. J Gen Intern Med. 2002;17(1):79–81.
27. Thom DH. Physician behaviors that predict patient trust. J Fam Pract. 2001; 50(4):323–8.
28. Thom DH, Campbell B. Patient-physician trust: an exploratory study. J Fam Pract. 1997;44(2):169–77.
29. Thom DH, Hall MA, Pawlson LG. Measuring patients' trust in physicians when assessing quality of care. Health Aff. 2004;23(4):124–32.
30. Collier D, Mahoney J. Insights and pitfalls: selection bias in qualitative research. World Politics. 1996;49(01):56–91.
31. Bonds DE, Camacho F, Bell RA, Duren-Winfield VT, Anderson RT, Goff DC. The association of patient trust and self-care among patients with diabetes mellitus. BMC Fam Pract. 2004;5(1):1–7.
32. Evans AM, Dillon KD, Goldin G, Krueger JI. Trust and self-control. Judgm Decis Mak. 2011;6(7):697.

Equitable resourcing of primary health care in remote communities in Australia's Northern Territory

John Wakerman[1,4], Lisa Sparrow[1,4*], Susan L Thomas[1,4], John S Humphreys[2,4] and Mike Jones[3,4]

Abstract

Background: Improved Primary Health Care (PHC) utilisation is central to reducing the unacceptable morbidity and mortality rates characterising populations living in remote communities. Despite poorer health, significant inequity characterises the funding of PHC services in Australia's most remote areas. This pilot study sought to ascertain what funding is required to ensure equitable access to sustainable, high quality primary health care irrespective of geographical remoteness of communities.

Methods: High performing remote Primary Health Care (PHC) services were selected using improvement measures from the Australian Primary Care Collaboratives Program and validated by health experts. Eleven PHC services provided data relating to the types of services provided, level of service utilisation, human resources, operating and capital expenses. A further four services that provide visiting PHC to remote communities provided information on the level and cost of these services. Demographic data for service catchment areas (including estimated resident population, age, Indigenous status, English spoken at home and workforce participation) were obtained from the Australian Bureau of Statistics 2011 census. Formal statistical inference (*p*-values) were derived in the linear regression via the nonparametric bootstrap.

Results: A direct linear relationship was observed between the total cost of resident PHC services and population, while cost per capita decreased with increasing population. Services in smaller communities had a higher number of nursing staff per 1000 residents and provided more consultations per capita than those in larger communities. The number of days of visiting services received by a community each year also increased with population. A linear regression with bootstrapped statistical inference predicted a significant regression equation where the cost of resident services per annum is equal to $1,251,893.92 + ($1698.83 x population) and the cost of resident and visiting services is equal to $1,378,870.85 + ($2600.00 x population).

Conclusions: The research findings provide empirical evidence based on real costs to guide funding for remote PHC services that takes into account the safety and equity requirements for a minimum viable service. This method can be used as a transparent, coordinated approach to ensure the equitable delivery of sustainable, high quality PHC in remote communities. This will in turn contribute to improved health outcomes.

Keywords: Primary health care, Remote, Equity, Access, Cost, Benchmark, Funding

* Correspondence: lisa.sparrow@flinders.edu.au
[1]Flinders Northern Territory, Casuarina, Australia
[4]Centre for Research Excellence in Rural and Remote Primary Health Care, Flinders University, Bedford Park, South Australia 5042, Australia
Full list of author information is available at the end of the article

Background

Although Australia is ranked consistently in the top ten Organisation for Economic Co-operation and Development (OECD) countries for life expectancy, it has the third highest regional disparity. For example, the Northern Territory's (NT) population of 244,900 people are spread over an area of 1.3 million square kilometres (more than twice that of France) and have a life expectancy 6.1 years less than those residing in the more densely populated Australian Capital Territory [1]. This disparity is largely due to the higher morbidity and mortality of populations living in remote communities, partly reflecting the high proportion of Aboriginal and/or Torres Strait Islander (hereafter as Indigenous) people resident there.

Reducing these unacceptable morbidity and mortality rates requires access to appropriate health services. The Primary Health Care (PHC) sector is crucial in preventing, detecting and managing illness and injury [2]. Improved PHC utilisation results in decreased morbidity and mortality, lower rates of hospitalisation and fewer costs [3]. Despite the high need for PHC in remote communities, funding for PHC does not match that of non-remote communities. For example, expenditure on General Practitioner (GP) services in very remote areas of Australia is just 57% of that in major cities [4]. At the same time, residents from remote areas of the NT are 50% more likely to be hospitalised than those from non-remote areas [5].

Medicare, the cornerstone of Australian PHC, is a fee-for-service funding model that reimburses general practitioners for services. In some cases, this funding is supplemented by performance incentive payments designed to encourage improved patient outcomes. Supported by relatively small contributions from state and federally funded community health, Indigenous health and mental health programs, *Medicare* underpins the majority of PHC in Australia. In remote areas, most services are provided not by GPs but by Remote Area Nurses (RAN) or Aboriginal Health Practitioners (AHP), resulting in less than a third of health clinic costs being claimable under Medicare [6]. The remuneration value placed on Medicare Benefits Schedule (MBS) items is derived from expenditures involved in running a typical Australian medical practice and does not reflect the safety and equity considerations associated with geographical remoteness. [4].

Current funding arrangements are inadequate, complex, administratively cumbersome and involve a large number of short term grants to many small organisations [7]. These funding arrangements are a product of history, lack transparency, and fail to account for variable populations, geographical classifications, differential health needs, and varied costs in different locations [8–10]. Zhao et al. (2006) demonstrated that the average cost of a face-to-face consultation with a medical officer in a remote context was approximately three times that of the corresponding MBS benefit fee [11]. Significant inequity characterises the funding of PHC services, particularly in the most remote areas of the country. To some degree, this disparity in expenditure is offset by Commonwealth funded grants to Aboriginal Controlled Community Health Organisations, which provide services to a large number of remote and very remote communities.

Responding to this inequity requires a transparent and systematic approach to funding that addresses population size, health need, geographical remoteness, and provides consumers with some understanding of the services they can reasonably expect to receive [8, 12]. Recommendations taking account of these factors have been made over many years, most notably by the National Health and Hospitals Reform Commission in 2009 [13, 14] and the OECD review of health care quality in Australia in 2015 [15]). Unfortunately these have gone largely unrealised.

Ensuring equitable health outcomes through more equitable access to PHC clearly requires equitable resourcing of these services so that they can respond appropriately to the needs of their catchment populations. This issue is complex, long-standing [16] and not unique to Australia. In developing countries there are few health services in rural and remote areas, and people experience a disproportionate burden of disease as a result [17]. The European Region is also faced with the challenge of providing quality health services at higher costs to the sparsely populated areas of Scandinavia. [18]. Our purpose here is not so much to review the extent of rural health inequities that characterise both developed and underdeveloped countries [19], but rather to consider how best to determine what level of PHC resourcing is required to benchmark core PHC services in communities of different sizes and composition in remote areas.

In an attempt to achieve this goal, important research has been undertaken to provide empirical evidence upon which policy-makers can develop more equitable funding models and workforce programs. Studies have defined which PHC services residents of rural and remote communities should be able to access [20], and have identified the population thresholds at which those services should be available from a resident (as opposed to visiting) service provider [21]. This study seeks to advance this research by investigating the resource levels required to deliver accessible, high quality PHC services in remote areas of the NT. In particular, this pilot study aimed to ascertain what funding is required to ensure equitable access to sustainable, high quality PHC irrespective of geographical isolation of the resident population in remote communities

Methods

Data from the Australian Primary Care Collaboratives Program (APCC) were used to identify high performing remote PHC services. Five improvement measures describing the management of type two diabetes and coronary heart disease (two of the most salient indicators of PHC) were used to measure service performance. Improvement measures for diabetes included the proportion of registered patients with an HbA1c ≤ 7.0 mmol/l, with measured total cholesterol <4.0 mmol/l or LDL ≤ 2.0 and with last recorded blood pressure ≤ 130/80. Measures for coronary heart disease included the proportion of patients prescribed an anti-platelet agent and a statin. Practices were assigned an average trend rating by the APCC, which indicated whether a practice had improved, declined or stayed the same over a 12 month period. Based on their rating, health services were selected for communities that fell within three different-sized population groups (100–500, 501–1000 and 1001 to 3000). From a total of 743 practices that had collected data over an 18 month period, 31 remote or very remote services were eligible for inclusion. Of these, 16 were selected on the basis of meeting high quality performance criteria validated by expert opinion.

Services were then invited to participate in the study with 11 agreeing. After acceptance, a survey tool was forwarded to participants for completion. Data collected for the 2013–14 financial year included the types of PHC services provided, as defined by Thomas et al. (2015) [20], whether the services were provided by resident or visiting personnel [21], level of service utilisation, operating and capital expenditure and information describing the context of service delivery (see Table 1). Costs attributed to Public Health and capital and corporate projects were excluded from the data. All costs were adjusted for inflation to 2013–14 amounts [22]. A follow-up site visit and interview were conducted with each service to validate the survey data and ensure an accurate understanding of the health service environment.

Data identifying the number, duration, type and costs of visiting PHC services to remote communities were obtained from four visiting service providers, three territory wide services and one regional service. Data were combined across two broad categories; technical services (requiring significant technical infrastructure and maintenance) and non-technical services. An average cost per day for the two categories of visiting services was calculated and applied to the annual number of visit-days reported to obtain an estimated cost of visiting services.

Population data relevant to the catchment of each participating health service were obtained from the Australian Bureau of Statistics 2011 Census [23] including estimated resident population, age, Indigenous status, English spoken at home and workforce participation (Table 1).

Due to non-normality in many of the study variables, statistical analysis of associations has been via simple linear and quadratic regression with formal statistical inference

Table 1 Summary of Remote Health Centre Characteristics

Expenditure	
• workforce or staff	• drugs, medical consumables and equipment
• professional development	• accounting / legal/ insurance expenses
• recruitment	• other
• communications	• corporate cost allocation
• vehicle operation	• capital and depreciation
• buildings	
ABS 2011 Population Demographics	
	• workforce Participation
• catchment population	• Socio-Economic Indexes for Areas (SEIFA)
• age	• travel time to nearest regional centre
• Indigenous status	• distance to nearest regional centre
• English spoken at home	• Australian Standard Geographical Classification – Remoteness Area (ASGC-RA)
Service Delivery	
• consultations per annum	• resident service provided
• patients currently registered	• visiting service provided
• patients seen in past 6 months	• regularity and duration of visiting services

(p-values) in the linear regression derived via the nonparametric bootstrap. Predictive ability of the resulting model was evaluated through the model R^2 by testing against actual and proposed remote health funding levels reported in the *"Evaluation of the Child Health Check Initiative and the Expanding Health Service Delivery Initiative: Final report"* [24].

Ethics approval was obtained from the Central Australian Human Research Ethics Committee (HREC-12-57). Data analysis was undertaken using IBM SPSS Statistics for Windows [25].

Results

Participant profile

The study included 11 remote NT health centres operated by four health service providers some of which provided outreach services to smaller communities or outstations. Catchment populations for these centres varied from 155 to 2124 and catchment areas extended to 64,000 km^2. Some centres experienced considerable changes in population due to tourism in the 'dry season' or due to restricted mobility in the 'wet season'.

Most residents in the service catchment populations were Indigenous, did not speak English at home and had low workforce participation. This demography changed slightly in those communities influenced by tourism and/

or mining. Based on the Australian Standard Geographical Classification Remote Areas (ASGC-RA), all communities, including island settings, were classified as RA4 (remote) or RA 5 (very remote). The distance from communities to a public hospital varied considerably from 2 km to 560 km.

All centres provided a similar range of services, consistent with the scope of practice of RANs, AHPs and remote GPs. Four centres did not offer 24 h emergency care. In all cases where podiatry, physiotherapy, speech pathology, psychology, audiology and occupational therapy were available, they were provided by a visiting health professional. Visiting services data covered 2063 visits by 23 different health professions to 80 different remote communities over 4705 days.

All services reported costs particular to their remote locality. Some related specifically to their geographical location, while others were similar across several remote sites. Examples include: overtime costs of $220,000 per year associated with a 24 h service, accommodation for staff at $40,000 per year, satellite internet connection to support patient information systems of over $50,000 (in a small service with a population under 300), air travel costs for staff of $150,000 per annum and freight costs of $20,000 per annum.

Resident services

Total costs of resident PHC services ranged from $955,603 to $4,830,823 per annum. There was a direct linear relationship with population size. A linear regression with bootstrapped statistical inference was calculated to predict the cost of resident services based on population size (Table 2, Fig. 1). A significant regression equation relationship was found. The cost of resident services is equal to $1,251,893.92 + ($1698.83 x population) per annum.

The cost of resident PHC services ranged from $2239 to $7346 per capita per annum, with larger services having significantly lower per capita costs (Table 2, Fig. 2). Figure 2 indicates non linearity where the reduction in cost per capita, with increasing population, levels off after a population of approximately 800 residents. A departure from a linear relationship is not clear in a quadratic regression with bootstrapped statistical inference (B = −6.318, p = 0.78), however would potentially become clearer with a larger sample.

The cost of resident PHC services per consultation showed considerably smaller range (between $157 and $372), and exhibited no significant association with population size (Table 2, Fig. 3).

Participating services provided between seven and 36 consults per capita per annum (Fig. 4). Smaller communities provided a significantly higher number of consultations per capita (Table 2).

The number of RANs per 1000 population showed an inverse relationship with population. While this relationship was not significant with a bootstrapped statistical inference (Table 2), statistical effect is indicated by the standardised coefficient (β = 0.657, p = 0.028) and a larger sample would be expected to show this relationship with greater certainty. Clinics in smaller communities had more resident nurses/clinical staff per 1000 population than larger communities. With the exception of one outlier, the number of nurses per 1000 population in participating services ranged from 2.8 to 12.7.

Visiting services

Visiting services included allied health, dental services, aged care assessment and case management services, alcohol and other drugs, and mental health and counselling services. The average total cost of delivering visiting PHC services was $4023.02 per day. The average cost per day was greater for services requiring significant infrastructure and maintenance (technical services) such as dental and audiology services ($6811.06) than for other allied health services ($2221.23). The mean duration of a visit was 2.28 days. The number of days of visiting services received per year increased significantly with population (Table 2, Fig. 5).

Visiting services provided the equivalent of between 0.5 and 1.6 full time staff per 1000 population, with the exception of one small community receiving the equivalent of five full time staff per 1000 population. The additional visiting services received by this community

Table 2 Summary of simple linear regression derived via the nonparametric bootstrap

Parameter	Intercept	Slope (SE)	p-value	Adjusted R^2
Total annual cost of resident services	1,251,893.92	1698.83 (58)	0.004	0.72
Cost per capita	6268.303	−2.315 (−0.321)	0.015	0.47
Cost per consultation	211.58	−0.022 (0.008)	0.698	−0.075
Consultations per capita	29.59	−0.011 (0.002)	0.032	0.570
RANs per 1000 population	13.40	−0.006 (−0.001)	0.149	0.369
Visiting days per annum	61.78	0.253 (0.005)	0.021	0.728
Total annual cost of resident and visiting services	1,378,870.85	2600.00 (112)	0.001	0.882

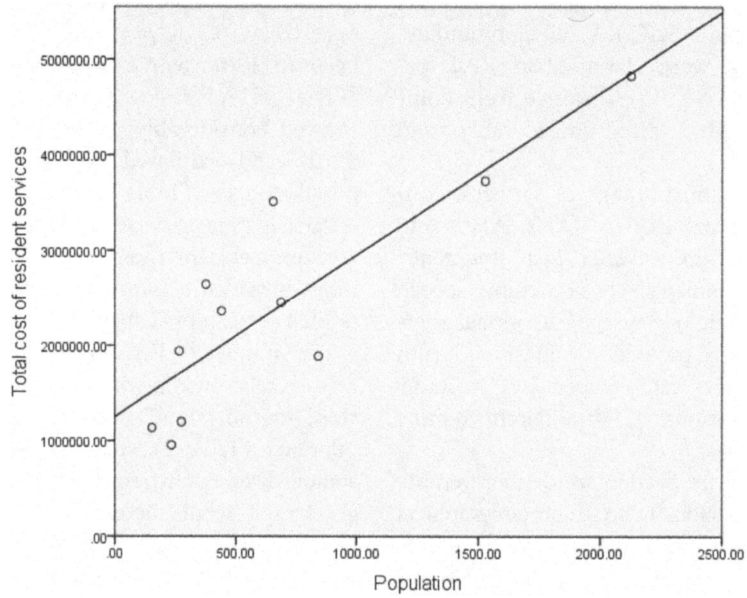

Fig. 1 Cost of Resident Services by Population: linear regression using total cost of resident services for 11 primary health care services is used to predict cost of resident primary health care using population size. A significant relationship between cost and population is shown where the cost of resident services rises by $1698.83 per head of population per annum

appear to have a compensatory effect to the relatively lower expenditure on resident services (see Fig. 6).

A linear regression with bootstrapped statistical inference was calculated to predict cost of resident and visiting services based on population size (Table 2, Fig. 7). A significant regression equation was found with the cost of resident and visiting services being equal to $1,378,870.85 + ($2600.00 x population) per annum.

Cost estimates were compared with estimates provided by a number of other studies [26], and the actual expenditure reported by the Productivity Commission [27] (Table 3).

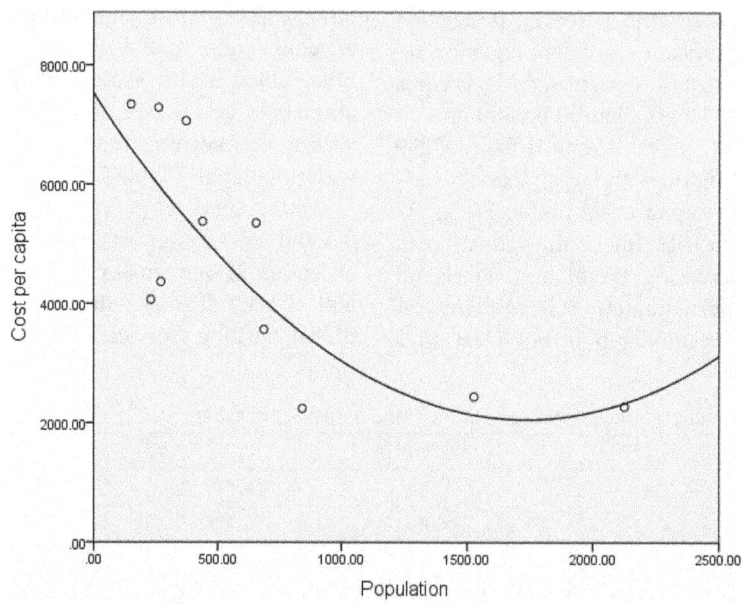

Fig. 2 Per Capita Cost of Resident Primary Health Care Services in 11 Remote Communitites: per capita costs were determined using total cost of resident services and catchment population for each the 11 remote primary health care services. The data suggest the per capita costs decrease with increasing population in a non-linear relationship. This departure from linearity failed to reach statistical significance but may be supported by a larger sample

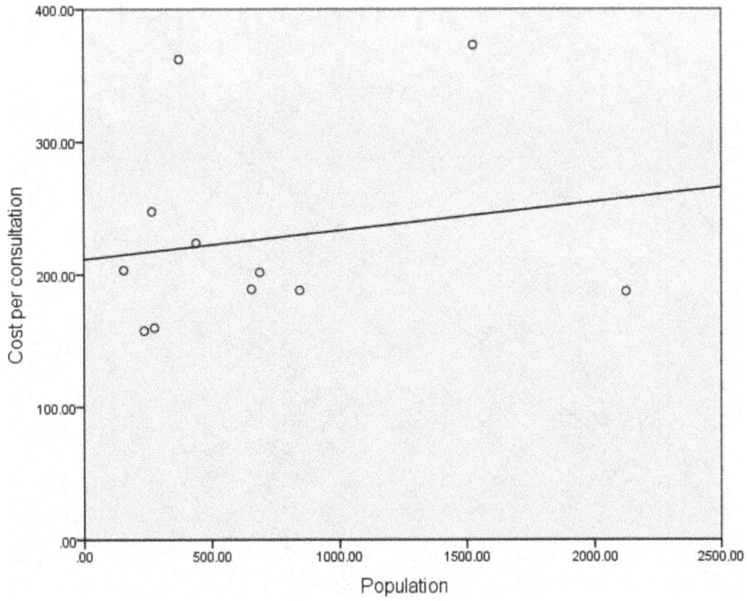

Fig. 3 Mean Cost of One Resident Primary Health consultation in 11 Remote Communities: mean cost per consultation was determined using total cost of resident services and the number of consults provided per annum for each the 11 remote primary health care services. Linear regression shows no clear relationship between cost per consultation and population

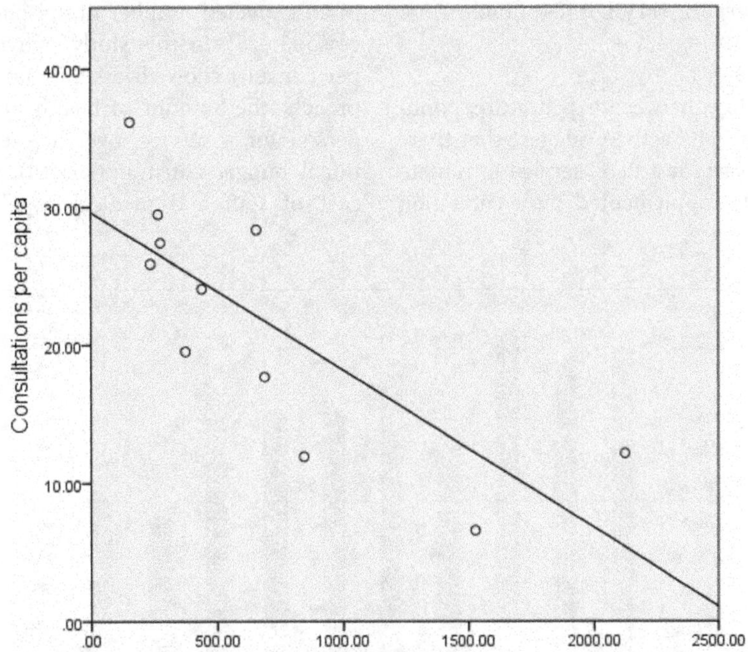

Fig. 4 Mean Number of Consultations Per Capita in 11 Remote Communities: The mean number of consultations per capita was determined using the number of consultations per year and the catchment population for each remote primary health care service. Linear regression demonstrates a significant relationship between the number of consultations per capita per year and the catchment population for 11 primary health care services

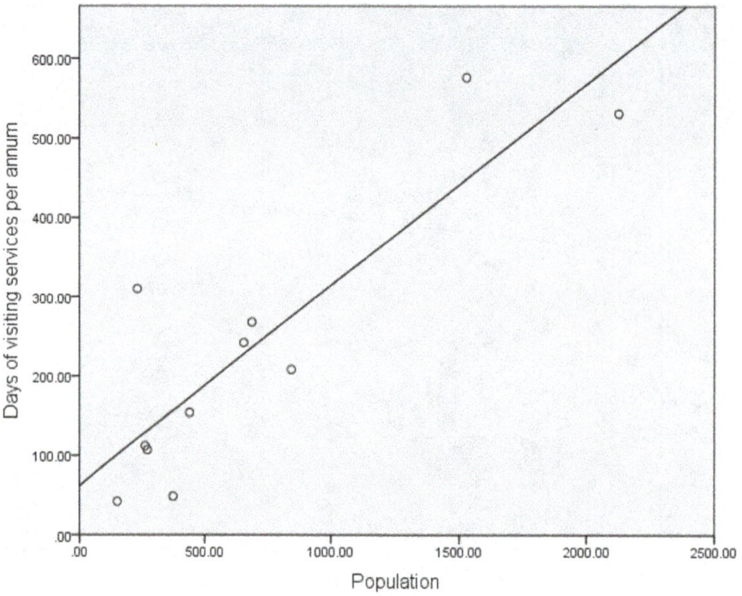

Fig. 5 Days of Visiting Services per Annum in 11 Remote Communities: The self reported number of days of visiting services provided to each of 11 remote primary health care services are presented in a simple linear regression showing a significant relationship with population where the number of visiting days per annum increases with the catchment population of the health service

Funding estimates, based on the predictive model developed in this study, were compared with data on health centre funding sourced from the *"Evaluation of the Child Health Check Initiative and the Expanding Health Service Delivery Initiative: Final report"* (EHSDI) [24] (Table 4).

Discussion

Analysis of the relationships between expenditure, population size and nature of PHC activity suggest that there is a minimum funding base for a PHC service in remote communities in the NT, supplemented by a capitation rate. The analysis suggests that economies of scale take effect in communities with a catchment population of approximately 800.

Activity based funding involves payment on the basis of an expected number of episodes of care at a rate per episode [28]. In this study, activity-based costings (cost per consult) showed less variation than a capitation approach (the amount of health funds to be assigned per person for a service, over a given time, subject to national budget constraints. [29]), particularly when only cost of staff and medical supplies were included. As

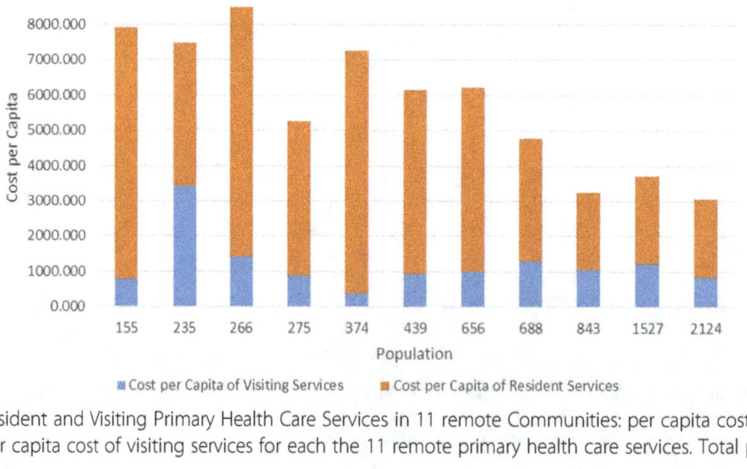

Fig. 6 Cost Per Capita of Resident and Visiting Primary Health Care Services in 11 remote Communities: per capita costs of resident services are shown cumulatively with per capita cost of visiting services for each the 11 remote primary health care services. Total per capita costs decrease with increasing population

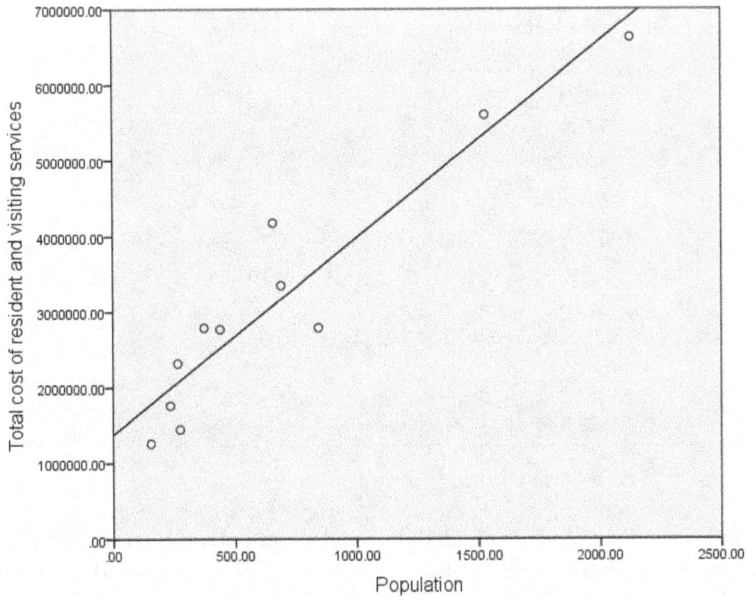

Fig. 7 Total Cost of Resident and Visiting Services per Annum by Population: linear regression in which total cost of resident services for 11 primary health care services is used to predict cost of resident and visiting primary health care using population size. A linear relationship between cost of resident and visiting services and population is shown, where cost increases by $2600 per head per annum

activity-based approaches foster a biomedical, episodic and piecemeal approach to patient care, focused solely on outputs rather than quality and outcomes, they are not appropriate as the sole funding criterion for remote contexts. Activity-based models may also threaten the viability of some PHC services due to their low volume of patients and the lack of flexibility required to meet local needs [15, 30].

Capitation cost is correlated with population size, offering some predictability. A significant correlation between the number of consults per capita and population might indicate that the higher cost of health services in smaller communities is associated with higher levels of service and fewer economies of scale, as well as reflecting variation in the pattern of need and epidemiology across remote communities. The finding that services with smaller catchment populations are providing significantly higher levels of service to their communities may be attributed to resourcing decisions for small health centres being determined more by safety and equity considerations than implied demand. That is, there is a minimum funding requirement to ensure safety of staff and

Table 3 Comparison with other estimates and actual expenditure

Study	Cost Per Consultation	Cost per Capita
Current study	227	4672
Ong et al. [26]	206	
Gador Whyte [33] Cost @ Min cost per CKD patient $4062 pa		4062
Zhao [11] Top Down Estimate per Consultation GP (inflation calculator applied to 2003/04 estimate)	220.55	
Zhao [11] Category 2 Single established disease, existing case (inflation calculator applied to 2003/04 $700)		918.97
AIHW [39] expenditure levels per episode of care for residents of remote and very remote areas	218	
Productivity Commission [27] - cost of community health services for Indigenous Australians during 2012/13 in the Northern Territory (inflation adjusted to 2013/14)		3647
Productivity Commission [27]- cost of community health services for Indigenous Australians real inflation adjusted average over 2008/09, 2010/11 and 2012/13 for the Northern Territory. (inflation adjusted to 2013/14)		6247
Evaluation of the Child Health Check Initiative and the Expanding Health Service Delivery Initiative [24] 2009–10 Average per capita EHSDI benchmark (across 10 remote sites) inflation adjusted to 2013/14		3822.67

Table 4 Comparison with EHSDI Actual and Benchmark Funding Levels

Population	Predicted income per Capita Proposed Model (2013/14)	EHSDI actual HSDA level funding (2009/10) - Inflation adjusted to 13/14	Difference	EHSDI HSDA level benchmark (inflation adjusted to 2013/2014)	Difference
2292	$2245.03	$2355.51	−4.92%	$3505.67	−56.15%
1527	$2518.67	$2706.52	−7.46%	$3283.81	−30.38%
2111	$2291.86	$3002.34	−31.00%	$3311.40	−44.49%
2124	$2288.23	$2730.80	−19.34%	$4017.83	−75.59%
688	$3518.44	$3559.76	−1.17%	$4358.91	−23.89%
1171	$2767.91	$2752.88	0.54%	$3578.52	−29.29%
926	$3050.77	$3440.54	−12.78%	$4431.76	−45.27%
348	$5296.23	$3077.39	41.89%	$3953.81	25.35%
235	$7026.04	$2928.38	58.32%	$3905.24	44.42%
Average	$3444.91	$2950.46	14.35%	$3816.33	−10.78%

residents in small isolated communities. Zhao et al. (2006) [11] report that the minimum feasible operation for a remote PHC centre included a half-time visiting medical officer, two RANs, one AHP and a minimum level of other supporting personnel. The cost of this is more than twice that of a typical practice on which the current MBS item costings are based.

This relationship between population (as a determinant of demand) and equity and safety considerations can be explained using the linear regression models in this study. Our modelling suggests a constant base level of funding per annum ($1,251,893.00 for resident services and $1,378,870.00 for resident and visiting services) that ensures quality and safety in addition to a per capita rate per annum which reflects community demand ($1698.83 for resident services and $2600.00 for resident and visiting services).

While the small number of large services in this study limit the conclusions that can be drawn from the observed levelling out of cost per capita in populations over 800, this observation was also noted by Zhao et al. (2010) [6] who identified that larger health centres, catering for populations greater than 700 start to see this efficiency gain.

Influenced by safety and equity considerations, efficiencies associated with scale decrease significantly for communities with populations under 200. Following the model derived in this study, the cost of resident PHC services increases by 79% as the population decreases from 200 ($7958 per capita) to 100 ($14,218 per capita). Estimates based on average staffing levels indicate that the minimum feasible service proposed by Zhao will meet the needs of populations up to 210–250. Cost effectiveness must be weighed against access and equity issues to determine the best models of care for such small populations. In many regions these communities are serviced by a minimum establishment of resident AHPs and/or an outreach service from larger neighbouring communities. In these cases the formula may be applied to the aggregate rather than individual community populations.

Comparison of results with other studies

The average cost per consult identified in this study was $227 and the average cost of resident services per capita per annum was $4672. Costs were comparable (within 18%) with inflation adjusted estimates by Ong, Gador Whyte (minimum cost per CKD patient), Zhao (top down estimated cost per consultation), AIHW (expenditure levels per episode of care for residents of remote and very remote areas), and Allen and Clarke. Zhao's estimated costs for per capita treatment of chronic disease were however significantly lower than the data in this study (Table 3).

Per capita cost of $4672 per annum was comparable with the Indigenous expenditure reports for the Northern Territory Community Health Services produced by the Productivity Commission [27, 31]. While the 2012/13 expenditure adjusted for inflation to 2013/14 was $3647 per capita (22% lower than the $4672 average identified in this study), the average inflation adjusted per capita expenditure across 2008/09, 2010/11 and 2012/13 was $6247 (34% higher than the average identified in this study), indicating a significant reduction in real terms of funding between 2008 and 2013.

Comparisons were made between estimated funding based on the predictive model developed in this study and data on health centre funding sourced from the "*Evaluation of the Child Health Check Initiative and the Expanding Health Service Delivery Initiative: Final report*" (EHSDI) [24]. Results indicated some consistency between the inflation-adjusted 2009/10 actual funding levels and those predicted by the 2013/14 model, although some services were identified as significantly under-resourced (Table 4).

The average funding under the model identified in this study varied by less than 15% from both the inflation adjusted actual 2009/10 and EHSDI benchmark funding level; although individual services vary significantly, particularly in relation to the EHSDI benchmark. EHSDI benchmarks were developed and applied to larger health service delivery areas. This benchmark was developed using national average MBS payment per capita and weightings for remoteness, English fluency and costs of service delivery in the NT. This approach does not address allocation of these resources between discreet services within the health service delivery area, nor economies of scale and so does not address the issues of minimum requirements for safety and equity identified in this study. As such there is greater disparity between EHSDI HSDA benchmarks as they are applied to individual services and those developed in this study, most noticeably in larger services where the effect of minimum requirements are dissipated by economies of scale.

The estimates derived from our model compare favourably with the majority of estimates found in other studies. These estimates were derived from a range of different methods, yet there is a broad consistency in the results.

Limitations

Although a bottom-up approach is a more precise and reliable approach to costing health services [32], it is time consuming and expensive [33]. Ultimately decisions about selecting a costing method involve a trade-off between accuracy and resources available. This pilot study utilised a 'top-down' approach, with a small number of participants but incorporated a high level of detail and context to improve comparability between service costs.

While the small sample size limited the reliability and generalisability of our results, they have enabled researchers to further understand the complex financial context characterising remote health service delivery. Thorough interrogation of data was required to ensure it met the requirements of the research question, provided adequate consistency across services to validate comparisons and to explain any anomalies.

Fiscal equalisation requires adjustments in order to account for the various impacts of population size, geographical remoteness, diseconomies of scale, population density, Indigeneity, socio-economic status, health status and other variables which impact on both demand for, and cost of, health services [34–36]. Noting the relative homogeneity of services (predominantly Indigenous, grant funded and the sole service in a discrete catchment area) and the lack of consistent and reliable local level data, this study was unable to adequately evaluate the impact of all of these variables on resource requirements.

Conclusions

Neither the Medicare system nor the current system of grants for funding remote PHC services provide an equitable approach to funding the health needs of Australians living in remote communities [6–9, 12, 37]. If we are to achieve equity in access to PHC for residents of remote areas, a transparent, planned and coordinated approach to funding is vital.

This study aimed to contribute to improved fiscal equalisation; an important response designed to address the problem of inequity in health care that spans all the dimensions of access [38]. The research findings contribute to an evidence base for funding remote PHC services that includes the safety and equity requirements for a minimum viable service. Although the sample size and unavailability of local level data provide some limitations, comparisons with other findings and approaches add some weight to the findings emanating from our model.

Any approach to resource the provision of PHC in remote communities will inevitably be constrained by the total resources available, not only how they are distributed. A consistent and rigorous approach to addressing clinical priorities, access and equity as they occur in small isolated communities located in remote environments will always be required. This study has demonstrated that a rigorous evidence-based and equitable approach to funding is possible and can underpin a transparent, reliable, planned and coordinated approach to the delivery of sustainable, high quality PHC in remote communities. More equitable access to PHC will contribute to reductions in the disproportionally high morbidity and mortality rates in these communities.

Abbreviations

AHP: Aboriginal Health Practitioner; AIHW: Australian Institute of Health and Welfare; APCC: Australian Primary Care Collaboratives; ASGC-RA: Australian Standard Geographical Classification – Remoteness Area; CKD: Chronic Kidney Disease; EHSDI: Expanding Health Service Delivery Initiative; FTE: Full Time Equivalent; GP: General Practitioner; HSDA: Health Service Delivery Area; MBS: Medical Benefits Scheme; OECD: Organisation for Economic Cooperation and Development; PHC: Primary Health Care; RA: Remoteness Area; RAN: Remote Area Nurse; SEIFA: Socio-Economic Indexes for Areas

Acknowledgments

The authors would like to acknowledge the important contribution of:
Participating organisations who offered open, honest and detailed insight into the financial and operational aspects of their service.
Dr. Jim Pearse, Director of Health Policy Analysis, Sydney, Australia. As a consultant, Dr. Pearse provided invaluable assistance in design of the data collection tool.
Mr. Pawel Scuza, statistical consultant, Flinders University who offered support with statistical analysis.

Funding

The research reported in this paper is a project of the Australian Primary Health Care Research Institute, which is supported by a grant from the Commonwealth of Australia as represented by the Department of Health. The information and opinions contained in it do not necessarily reflect the views or policy of the Australian Primary Health Care Research Institute or the Commonwealth of Australia (or the Department of Health).

Authors contributions

JW, JH and ST formulated the initial methodology including the selection of high performing services and development of data collection tools. JW, ST and LS undertook data collection and validation visits, LS and MJ undertook data analysis, LS drafted the manuscript. All authors reviewed, edited and approved the final manuscript.

Competing interests

The authors declare that they have no competing interests.

Consent for publication

Not applicable.

Author details

[1]Flinders Northern Territory, Casuarina, Australia. [2]School of Rural Health, Monash University, Melbourne, Australia. [3]Psychology Department, Macquarie University, Sydney, Australia. [4]Centre for Research Excellence in Rural and Remote Primary Health Care, Flinders University, Bedford Park, South Australia 5042, Australia.

References

1. OECD. OECD Regions at a Glance 2013. Paris: OECD Publishing; 2013. http://dx.doi.org/10.1787/reg_glance-2013-en.
2. Steering Committee for the Review of Government Service Provision. Report on Government services volume 2: health; community services; housing and homelessness. Canberra: Productivity Commission; 2013.
3. Zhao Y, Connors C, Lee AH, Liang W. Relationship between primary care visits and hospital admissions in remote indigenous patients with diabetes: a multivariate spline regression model. Diabetes Res Clin Pract. 2015;108(1):106–12.
4. Australian Institute of Health and Welfare. Australian health expenditure by remoteness - a comparison of remote, regional and city health expenditure, Health and welfare expenditure series. Canberra: AIHW; 2010.
5. Zhao Y, You J, Wright J, Guthridge SL, Lee AH. Health inequity in the Northern territory, Australia. Int J Equity Health. 2013;12:79. doi:10.1186/1475-9276-1112-1179.
6. Zhao Y, Malyon R. Cost drivers of remote clinics: remoteness and population size. Aust Health Rev. 2010;34(1):101–5. doi:10.1071/AH09685.
7. Moran M, Porter D, Curth-Bibb J. Funding indigenous organisations: improving governance performance through innovations in public finance management in remote Australia. Issues paper no 11. Canberra: AIHW and Melbourne: Australian Institute of Family Studies; 2014.
8. Alford K. Economic value of aboriginal community controlled health services. Canberra: National Aboriginal Community Controlled Health Organisation Press Club; 2014.
9. KPMG. Funding options to reform the distribution of OATSIH primary health care funding - consultation paper. Canberra: Department of Health and Ageing Government Advisory Services; 2012.
10. Wilson J. Remote area aboriginal health services managers: key practice challenges. Aust J Rural Health. 2001;9(3):138–40.
11. Zhao Y, Hanssens P, Byron P, Guthridge S. Cost estimates of primary health care activities for remote aboriginal communities in the Northern territory. Department of Health and Community Services: Darwin; 2006. http://digitallibrary.health.nt.gov.au/dspace/bitstream/10137/59/3/Primary_health_care_costs.pdf.
12. Wakerman J, Humphreys JS. Sustainable primary health care services in rural and remote areas: innovation and evidence. Aust J Rural Health. 2011;19(3):118–24.
13. National Health and Hospitals Reform Commission: A healthier future for all Australians-final report of the National Health and Hospitals Reform Commission. Canberra: Commonwealth of Australia; 2009.
14. National Health and Hospitals Reform Commission. A healthier future for all Australians interim report. Canberra: Commonwealth of Australia; 2009.
15. OECD. OECD reviews of health care quality: Australia 2015: raising standards. Paris: OECD Publishing; 2015.
16. Humphreys JS. Social provision and service delivery: problems of equity, health, and health care in rural Australia. Geoforum. 1988;19(3):323–38.
17. World Health Organisation. World Health Statistics 2016: monitoring health for the SDGs, sustainable development goals. Geneva: WHO publishing; 2016.
18. OECD. OECD territorial reviews: Northern sparsely populated areas. Paris: OECD Publishing; 2017.
19. Humphreys J, Solarsh G. Populations at special health risk: rural populations, The international encyclopedia of public health. Volume 5. 2nd ed. Oxford: Academic Press; 2017. p. 599–608.
20. Thomas SL, Wakerman J, Humphreys JS. What core primary health care services should be available to Australians living in rural and remote communities? BMC Fam Pract. 2014;15:143. doi:10.1186/1471-2296-1115-1143.
21. Thomas SL, Wakerman J, Humphreys JS. Ensuring equity of access to primary health care in rural and remote Australia. Int J Equity Health. 2015; 14(1):111. doi:10.1186/s12939-12015-10228-12931.
22. Reserve Bank of Australia. Inflation Calculator http://www.rba.gov.au/calculator/ Accessed 14 June 2016.
23. Australian Bureau of Statistics 2011. Community Profiles. http://www.abs.gov.au/websitedbs/censushome.nsf/home/communityprofiles?opendocument& navpos=230 Accessed 23 Oct. 2015.
24. Allen and Clarke. Evaluation of the Child health Check Initiative and the Expanding health service delivery Initiative: final report. Canberra: Department of Health and Ageing; 2011.
25. IBM Corp. IBM SPSS Statistics for windows. In., version 22 edn. IBM Corp: Armonk NY; 2013.
26. Ong KS, Carter R, Kelaher M, Anderson I. Differences in primary health care delivery to Australia's indigenous population: a template for use in economic evaluations. BMC Health Serv Res. 2012;12:307.
27. Australian Government Productivity Commission. 2014 Indigenous Expenditure Report Data Tables. http://www.pc.gov.au/research/ongoing/indigenous-expenditure-report/indigenous-expenditure-report-2014#data-tables: Accessed 23 Feb 2016.
28. PHCRIS: Primary Health Care Funding Models. PHCRIS Research Roundup. 33 edn: PHCRIS; 2013.
29. Rice N, Smith P. Approaches to capitation and risk adjustment in health care: an international survey. York: The University of York Centre for Health Economics; 1999.
30. Segal L. A vision for primary care - funding and other system factors for optimising the primary care contribution to the community's. Adelaide: University of South Australia; 2008.
31. SCRGSP (Steering Committee for the Review of Government Service Provision). 2014 indigenous expenditure report. Canberra: Productivity Commission; 2014. p. 2014.
32. Mogyorosy Z, Smith P. The main methodological issues in costing health care services: a literature review. York UK: University of York, Centre for Health Economics; 2005.
33. Gador-Whyte AP, Wakerman J, Campbell D, Lenthall S, Struber J, Hope A, et al. Cost of best-practice primary care management of chronic disease in a remote aboriginal community. Med J Aust. 2014;200(11):663–6.
34. McDermott R, Beaver C, Zhao Y. Outcomes-based resource allocation for indigenous health services: a model for Northern Australia. Health Policy. 1997;39(1):69–78.
35. Penno E, Gauld R, Audas R. How are population-based funding formulae for healthcare composed? A comparative analysis of seven models. BMC Health Serv Res. 2013;13:470. doi:10.1186/1472-6963-1113-1470.
36. Peacock S, Segal L. Equity and the funding of Australian health services prospects for weighted capitation. Centre for Health Program Evaluation: West Heidelberg; 1999.
37. Australian National Audit Office. Capacity development for indigenous service delivery: Department of Families, Housing, Community Services and Indigenous Affairs, Department of Education, employment, and workplace relations, Department of Health and Ageing. Commonwealth of Australia: Barton, A.C.T; 2012.
38. Russell DJ, Humphreys JS, Ward B, Chisholm M, Buykx P, McGrail M, et al. Helping policy-makers address rural health access problems. Aust J Rural Health. 2013;21(2):61–71.
39. Australian Institute of Health and Welfare. Australian health expenditure by remoteness: a comparison of remote, regional and city health expenditure, Health and welfare expenditure series no. 50. Cat. No. HWE 50. Canberra: Australian Institute of Health and Welfare; 2011.

Effectiveness of a motivational intervention on overweight/obese patients in the primary healthcare

Juan Jose Rodriguez-Cristobal[1], Carlos Alonso-Villaverde[2], Jose Ma Panisello[3], Pere Travé-Mercade[4], Francisca Rodriguez-Cortés[5], Josep Ramon Marsal[6] and Esther Peña[2,7*]

Abstract

Background: Overweight and obesity are common health problems which increase the risk of developing several serious health conditions. The main difficulty in the management of weight-loss lies in its maintenance, once it is achieved. The aim of this study was to investigate whether a motivational intervention, together with current clinical practice, was more efficient than a traditional intervention, in the treatment of overweight and obesity and whether this intervention reduces cardiovascular risk factors associated with overweight and obesity.

Methods: Multi-centre cluster randomized trial with a 24-month follow-up included 864 overweight/obese patients randomly assigned. Motivational intervention group (400 patients), delivered by a nurse trained by an expert psychologist, in 32 sessions, 1 to 12 fortnightly, and 13 to 32, monthly, on top of their standard programmed diet and exercise. The control group (446 patients), received the usual follow-up.

Results: Weight reduction was statistically significant in the second year with a mean reduction of 1.0 Kg in the control group and 2.5 Kg in the intervention group ($p = 0.\ 02$). While 18.1% of patients in the control group reduced their weight by more than 5%, this percentage rose to 26.9% in the intervention group, which is statistically significant ($p = 0.04$). Patients in the motivational intervention group had significantly greater improvements in triglycerides and APOB/APOA1ratio.

Conclusions: The results highlight the importance of the group motivational interview in the treatment of overweight /obese patients in primary care, and in the improvement of their associated cardiovascular risks factors.

Keywords: Overweight, Obesity, Motivational interview, Weight-loss, Cardiovascular risk factors

Background

The prevalence of obesity is increasing steadily in developing countries and has become a serious public health issue. According to the World Health Organization (WHO), at least 500 million people worldwide were obese in 2008. They also estimated that by 2015, approximately 2.3 billion adults would be overweight and more than 700 million would be obese [1].For instance, according to the SEEDO 2011 study, the prevalence of obesity (Body mass index (BMI) > 30) in Spain is 14.5% (13.3% in men and 15.7% amongst women) while the overall overweight and obesity (BMI>25) is 53% [2–4]. Overweight and obesity in adulthood decrease life expectancy significantly and increase individual, national, and global healthcare costs [5, 6]. Obesity was estimated to account for between 0.7 and 2.8% [7] of a country's total healthcare expenditures in several developed countries. When costs associated with being overweight (BMI > 25) were also included, the

* Correspondence: epena@csic-iccc.org
[2]Cardiovascular Research Center, CSIC-ICCC, Hospital de la Santa Creu i Sant Pau (UAB), IIB-Sant Pau, Barcelona, Spain
[7]Cardiovascular Research Center, Hospital de la Santa Creu i Sant Pau, C/ Sant Antoni Ma Claret, 167 08025 Barcelona, Spain
Full list of author information is available at the end of the article

upper limit of this range increased to 9.1% [8] of total healthcare expenditures. The true costs are undoubtedly much greater as not all obesity-related conditions are included in the calculations. There is currently clear scientific evidence that obesity is a strong predictor of the risk of metabolic disorders such as dyslipidemia, hypertension, and diabetes, as well as a cause for potential premature mortality [9, 10]. Overweight and obesity are largely preventable. Favorable environments and communities are essential in determining people's choices and in promoting healthier food choices and regular physical activity, and therefore preventing obesity [9, 11]. However, while significant weight loss can be achieved in a short-term, weight loss is notoriously difficult to sustain in the long term and it is for this reason that the research that would benefit these patients is of fundamental importance [4, 12]. It is crucial that patients integrate these life-habit changes into their lives. The Cochrane database study analyzed different studies aimed evaluate the effects of interactive computer-based interventions for weight loss or weight maintenance in overweight or obese people. The study concluded by saying that, compared to in-person interventions, interactive computer-based interventions result in smaller weight losses and lower levels of weight maintenance [13].

New guidelines released by the American College of Cardiology, American Heart Association Task Force on Practice Guidelines and The Obesity Society for the Management of overweight and obesity in adults that examined interventions to improve the maintenance of lost weight notify that, for all the trials that reported weight losses for two or more follow up evaluation periods, weight losses were consistently smaller in the long-term follow ups than at the 6- or 12-month assessments. These results indicate that further study is needed on facilitating maintenance of weight loss [14, 15].

Behavioural/ lifestyle interventions are effective at promoting initial weight loss [16–18]. However, successful in weight loss maintenance is often more difficult to achieve. Extended patient-therapist contact provides the opportunity to reinforce behavioral skills, support problem solving and providing continued accountability and motivation, and seems to be a key to diminish the weight regain [15].

The aim of this study (IMOAP: Group motivational intervention in overweight/obese patients in primary prevention of cardiovascular disease in the primary healthcare area) was primarily to assess whether a motivational group intervention (delivered by a nurse trained by an expert psychologist), was more effective than an isolated traditional intervention on weight loss and its maintenance, in overweight and obese patients. This was calculated as the percentage of patients reducing their weight by 5% and maintenance over time. And secondly, to determine whether this intervention was more effective in reducing cardiovascular risk factors associated with overweight and obesity.

Methods

Study design

This study design has been published elsewhere [19]. Briefly, this was a multi-centre cluster randomized trial of an intervention in overweight and obese patients, with a follow up of 24 months. Basic areas were randomly assigned to either control or intervention group as per a computer generated randomization schedule. The coordinators have contacted the Basic Health Areas (BHA), to explain the protocol and confirm their participation. Patients were recruited always as the five first who meet the inclusion criteria after centers were randomized. To avoid overburden the doctors, and nursing staff, patient recruitment and follow up were done in stages during the first six months of the study. The coordinators have contacted the BHA (24 clusters), to explain the protocol and confirm their participation. The distribution was: Intervention (12 clusters)/controls (12 clusters) with 20 patient of average size per cluster. The number of subjects necessary to divide into two independent groups has been calculated [19]. Basic Health Areas that dealt with the intervention groups received specific nursing-staff training from expert psychologists, consisting of a basic training strategy, and focusing on group motivation for life-style changes in overweight and obese patients. The training consisted of a number of workshops where role-play techniques were used to reinforce the concepts. The first patient was entered on September 2008. The final visit for the last randomized participant was planned for the last trimester 2010, with final study reports in the first trimester of 2013. Exclusion Criteria were: patients with severe clinical pathology (bedridden, dementia, advanced neoplasia, etc.), patients with secondary obesity (hypothyroidism, Cushing's disease, etc), patients with severe sensorial disorders capable of interfering with the motivational intervention, and patients with serious psychiatric disorders. They were included sequentially, from the beginning of the study. To avoid possible biases in the patients recruitment and follow up, and not overburden the nursing staff, the inclusion were developed in stages during the first six months of the study to the first two patients who met the inclusion requirements of the study and who present none of the exclusion criteria. This was carrying out superior quality control, using smaller sample size than would be possible if we randomized the patients.

Screening and randomization

Patients included were aged between 30 and 70 years with overweight (BMI>25) or obese (BMI>30) of both genders, registered in the medical history (MH) or recently diagnosed.

The Jordi Gol i Gurina Foundation Ethics Committee in Barcelona approved the study and it was carried out in compliance with the Helsinki Declaration. Each IMOAP participant provided informed written consent using procedures reviewed and approved by the Ethics Committee review board.

Control group

Four hundred and forty six participants followed the usual intervention, according to the protocols in each centre. Patients were visited every 3 months and doctors always included advice on life-style changes, physical exercise, hypo-caloric diet containing 1,200-1,500 kcal, and anthropometric measurements (weight, height and waist circumference). Follow-up blood tests by a healthcare professional were carried out at baseline, at 12-month and at 24-month follow-ups (triglycerides, APOA1, APOB-100, HDL cholesterol, and LDL cholesterol). In Additional file 1: Figure S1 is described the content of their visits.

Motivational intervention group

Four hundred participants received the identical treatment as in the control group plus a group motivational intervention every 15 days, once fortnightly during weeks 1 to 12, and then monthly from week 13 to 32. Each session would last for one hour, for a 24-month follow-up period, with a total of 32 interventions, as described above. In Additional file 2: Figure S2 is described the contents of their visit.

Outcomes and assessments

The primary outcome was the change in body weight at months 12 and 24 as compared with the control group. This was calculated as the percentage of patients reducing their weight by 5% and maintenance over time. Secondary outcomes included weight change in the intervention group as compared with control group and the percentage of participants whose initial weight was decreased by 5% or more at 12 and 24 months and by 10% or more at 12 and 24 months.

A wide range of interviews, physical examinations, and laboratory data were collected. The weight measurement (Kg) and waist measurement (cm) was always taken under the same conditions. Body Mass Index was calculated as: Weight in kilograms divided by height in meters squared (m^2) (Kg/m^2). The cardiovascular risk factors were also assessed: Hypertension was defined as either blood pressure readings of above 140/90 mm Hg on three occasions; Diabetes Mellitus: By case history or two prandial glycaemia readings > 126 mg/dl; -Smoking: n° packets/year.

Statistical analysis

A complete cases analysis was performed. For quantitative variables, mean and standard deviation were used, whereas for the qualitative ones, proportions were used. The data analysis included an evaluation of the initial comparability of the patients receiving the two types of treatment using bi-variant techniques; the Chi-Square for the proportions and, in the case of the mean, the Student's t-distribution or its nonparametric equivalent when necessary, by point estimation with a confidence interval of 95%. The effect of the treatment was estimated using a mixed lineal model. The clusters were defined by the primary centers whose gave care to the patients. A random-intercept model was adjusted. The intra-cluster correlation coefficient (ICC) also was calculated for the continuous bodyweight outcome.

Results

Baseline characteristics of the study participants

One thousand and two hundred patients were initially included. Eight hundred and forty six patients were randomized (77.19%women and 22.81% men). 52.72% formed the control group and 47.28% joined the intervention group. Mean age (±SD) was 55.49 ± 11.5 and 57.69 ± 22.1 years, with a mean body weight of 87.1 ±14.8 Kg, and 85.5 ± 13.9 Kg and a mean BMI of 34.1 ±4.8 and 34.1±4.8 (control and intervention group, respectively) (Table 1). There were no statistically significant differences in any demographic or lifestyle variables between the study groups at base-line. Approximately 60 and 47% of the participants in intervention and control group respectively had their weight measured at 24 months (Fig. 1).

Weight loss

Body weight changes were evaluated at 12 and 24 months and are presented in Table 2. In the first year, participants in the control group lost a mean 1.3 Kg, those in the motivational intervention group lost a mean 1.8 Kg. The weight reductions were greater in the intervention group but did not reach statistical significance. In the second year, patients in the control group presented a loss of 1 Kg while the reduction in the Motivational Interventional group was 2.5 Kg this difference was statistically significant (p=0.02).

A 5% reduction of the weight in the motivational group intervention in the first year was one of the objectives set. We found that a higher number of patients reached this goal in the Motivational Interventional group than in the control group (22.6 versus 16.6 %) (Fig. 2). This difference was not statistically significant (p=0.09). In the second year the reduction in the control group was 18.1 versus 26.9 % in the Motivational

Table 1 Baseline characteristics

	Usual Care (*n* = 446)	Motivational Intervention (*n* = 400)	All (*n* = 846)
	mean (SD)	*mean (SD)*	*mean (SD)*
Gender[a]			
Male	122 (27.4%)	71 (17.8%)	193 (22.8%)
Female	324 (72.6%)	329 (82.3%)	653 (77.2%)
Weight in Kg.			
At baseline	87.1 (14.8)	85.5 (13.9)	86.3 (14.4)
Height in cm.	159.8 (9.2)	158.4 (8.3)	159.1 (8.8)
BMI in Kg/m2	34.1 (4.8)	34.1 (4.8)	34.1 (4.8)
Waist circumference in cm.	107.7 (11.5)	107.6 (10.8)	107.7 (11.2)
SBP in mmHg	130.8 (14.8)	132.6 (15.2)	131.7 (15)
DBP in mmHg	78.7 (10.3)	79.3 (9.7)	79 (10)
Obesity[a]	374 (83.9%)	353 (88.3%)	727 (85.9%)
Diabetes[a]	76 (17%)	69 (17.3%)	145 (17.1%)
Hyperlipidemia[a]	269 (60.3%)	240 (60%)	509 (60.2%)
Smoking Habit[a]			
Never	298 (72.2%)	289 (77.3%)	587 (74.6%)
Current	54 (13.1%)	39 (10.4%)	93 (11.8%)
Ex-smoker	61 (14.8%)	46 (12.3%)	107 (13.6%)
Alcohol intake[a]	9 (2%)	3 (0.8%)	12 (1.4%)
Ischemic Heart Disease[a]	6 (3.2%)	1 (0.7%)	7 (2.2%)
Heart Failure[a]	6 (3.2%)	3 (2.2%)	9 (2.8%)
Transient Ischemic Attack[a]	1 (0.5%)	0 (0%)	1 (0.3%)
Neoplasm[a]	4 (2.1%)	3 (2.2%)	7 (2.2%)

[a]: n (%) and Chi-square Test, *SBP* Systolic Blood Pressure, *DBP* Diastolic Blood Pressure

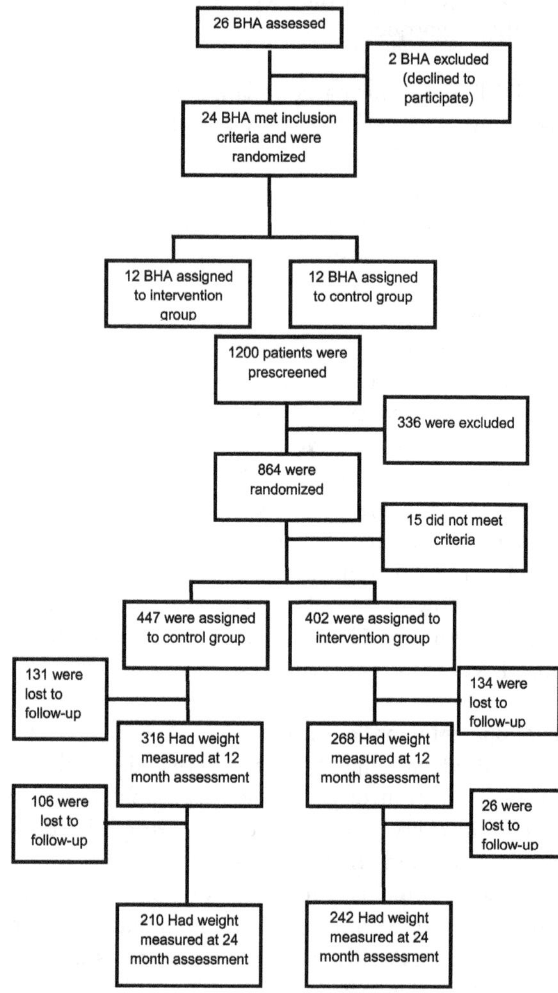

Fig. 1 CONSORT flow diagram. Flow diagram of the progress through the phases of a parallel randomized trial of two groups

Interventional group. This difference was statistically significant (p=0.04) (Fig. 2).

Weight loss of 10% was achieved by 4% in the control group and 6.7% of patients in the Motivational Interventional group (p = 0.1), which did not reach statistical significance after 1 year of intervention. Nor were losses significant in the second year (5 vs 8%; p=0.27) (Fig. 2).

The ICC was 0.08 for the bodyweight, so only the 8% of the variability was due by the center.

Changes in cardiovascular risk factors

Participants who received the group motivational intervention had significantly greater improvements in triglycerides (p<0.0001) and apoB-100 (p<0.05) at the end of the second year, and in apoA1 (p<0.001; p<0.05) and apoB/apoA1 ratio (p<0.01; p<0.001) at the end of the first and also if the second year (Table 3).

Discussion

The main finding of this study was that in a motivational intervention group significantly more patients achieved a reduction of 5% or more of the initial weight, which is a common criterion for clinically meaningful weight loss [20–22]. Interventions that focus on changing eating habits and increasing daily physical activity in order to promote a healthy lifestyle are the best options to address overweight and obesity. In addition, other components of cognitive-conductive therapy from the behavioral perspective have shown to be relevant to be included in interventions targeting at overweight and obesity in order to improve their effectiveness and promote the maintenance of the obtained results. Moreover regarding the effectiveness of these interventions to reduce weight, evidence has found satisfactory results, achieving reductions between 5 and 10% of the initial weight [23–25].

Table 2 Weight reduction between intervention groups

	Usual Care			Motivational Intervention			Fixed Model			Multi-level Model		
	N	Mean	SE	N	Mean	SE	OR	CI 95%	*p*	OR	CI 95%	*p*
Weight Baseline (kg)	428	87.1	0.7	393	85.5	0.7						
Weight. 1 Year (kg)	316	85.9	0.8	287	83.7	0.9						
Weight difference (kg)	302	1.3	0.1	283	1.8	0.4	0.45[a]	−0.47; 1.36	0.33	0.63[a]	−0.46; 1.73	0.26
Weight ≤ Baseline[b]		179	59.3%		175	61.8%	1.11	0.80; 1.55	0.53	1.18	0.78; 1.83	0.44
Weight Loss ≥ 5%[b]		50	16.6%		64	22.6%	1.47	0.98; 2.23	0.06	1.53	0.93; 2.56	0.09
Weight Loss ≥ 10%[b]		12	4.0%		19	6.7%	1.74	0.84; 3.75	0.14	1.86	0.83; 4.80	0.15
Weight. 2 Years (kg)	210	84.9	0.9	242	83.2	1						
Weight difference (kg)	199	1.0	0.4	238	2.5	0.5	1.53[a]	0.31; 2.74	0.01	1.82[a]	0.32; 3.35	0.02
Weight ≤ Baseline[b]		111	55.8%		156	65.5%	1.51	1.02; 2.22	0.04	1.62	0.98; 2.77	0.06
Weight Loss ≥ 5%[b]		36	18.1%		64	26.9%	1.67	1.06; 2.66	0.03	1.74	1.03; 3.07	0.04
Weight Loss ≥ 10%[b]		10	5.0%		19	8.0%	1.64	0.76; 3.75	0.22	1.67	0.67; 4.53	0.27

For each follow-up were calculated four variables:
a) Weight difference was calculated as the weight in each visit minus the baseline weight, expressed in kg
b) Weight ≤ Baseline Weight: If the weight in the visit was lower than the baseline weight
c) Weight loss ≥ 5%: If the relative percentage loss of weight (weight difference/baseline weight) was ≥ 5%
d) Weight loss ≥ 10%: If the relative percentage loss of weight (weight difference/baseline weight) was ≥ 10%
[a]differences of means
[b]n(%) and chi-square Test. *Kg* Kilograms, p: Mann-Whitney Test

This reduction was achieved in 22.6% of patients in the intervention group at the end of the first year but did not reach statistical significance. This loss was not only maintained in the second year but actually increased to 26.9% of patients and reached statically significance (p=0.04). Moreover, our findings suggest that the use of adequately motivational intervention for weight loss is also effective improving cardiovascular risks factors of obese/overweight patients. Furthermore, the significant increase in weight loss at year 2 in the intervention group could point out the efficacy of the group motivational approach among patients.

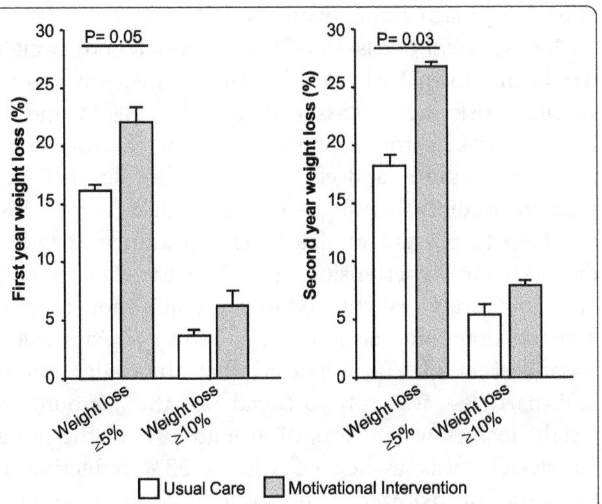

Fig. 2 Effect of interventions on weight change. 5–10% of weight loss successful by group-*p* value for the comparison between

Weight loss in the intervention group was greater than the weight loss observed in other primary care studies [15, 19, 26, 27] but smaller than the weight loss observed by Wadden et al. in the first year of the study [20]. Nevertheless, an important difference was that, unlike the Wadden study, the loss recorded in our study was maintained in the second year. This group motivational intervention, added to usual care, has been shown to be a valid technique and should form a part of routine treatment in primary care in the future.

A variety of individual and group strategies have been used to enhance adherence in weight loss management. In a study conducted in 20 primary healthcare centers in Great Britain, investigators have demonstrated that weigh loss in 883 patients at high risk of cardiovascular disease through modifying fat intake, physical activity and smoking, had greatest benefit in the intervention group [28].

Shawk et al [29] performed a meta-analyses that include 36 clinical studies to assess the effects of psychological interventions that combined with dietary and exercise strategies, they concluded that combination of all strategies was more useful. Of all these thirty six studies only one was conducted in Spain in diabetic obese patients [30].

Smith-West et al [31] in a randomized, controlled study where all participants received an 18-month, group-based behavioral obesity treatment showed that obesity treatment was most beneficial when was adjunct to behavioral motivational interviewing for women with type 2 diabetes. Motivational interviewing was designed

Table 3 Changes in cardiovascular risk factors

	Usual care			Motivational intervention		
	Baseline[1] mean ± SD [1vs4] p-value=	12 months[2] mean ± SD [2vs5]p-value=	24 months[3] mean ± SD [3vs6]p-value=	Baseline[4] mean ± SD	12 months[5] mean ± SD	24 months[6] mean ± SD
Cholesterol	208.5 ± 39.8 *0.17*	206.4 ± 34.9 *0.78*	206.7 ± 33.6 *0.41*	211.5 ± 36.6	207.5 ± 36.4	203.8 ± 36
Triglycerides	135.4 ± (81.6) *0.21*	134.7 ± 66.7 *0.08*	135.4 ± 65.6 *0.0001*	133.9 ± 93.9	127.6 ± 61.1	125.9 ± 65.1
HDL Cholesterol	54.6 ± 13.1 *0.66*	53.4 ± 13.5 *0.68*	54.2 ± 13.7 *0.41*	55.3 ± 13.4	53.8 ± 11.9	55.4 ± 14.3
LDL Cholesterol	131.6 ± 31.3 0.06	128.4 ± 33.8 *0.08*	126.4 ± 32.5 *0.06*	127.6 ± 32.6	125.9 ± 32.5	124.5 ± 35.9
APO A1	1.6 ± 0.3 *0.15*	1.6 ± 0.4 *0.0002*	1.5 ± 0.3 *0.04*	1.6 ± 0.3	1.7 ± 0.3	1.8 ± 0.3
APO B-100	1 ± 0.2 *0.10*	1 ± 0.2 *0.30*	0.9 ± 0.2 *0.05*	1 ± 0.2	0.9 ± 0.2	0.8 ± 0.2
APOB-100/ APO-A1	0.62 ± 0.2 *0.07*	0.62 ± 0.3 *0.002*	0.55 ± 0.3 0.0003	0.62 ± 0.3	0.52 ± 0.3	0.44 ± 0.3
SBP	130.8 ± 14.8 0.24	129.7 ± 15 *0.29*	131.7 ± 15.4 *0.57*	132.6 ± 15.2	130.9 ± 14.1	132.1 ± 14
DBP	78.7 ± 10.3 *0.44*	78.6 ± 9 0.12	77.0 ± 9.2 *0.17*	79.3 ± 9.7	78.2 ± 9.1	78.0 ± 8.8

SBP Systolic Blood Pressure, *DBP* Diastolic Blood Pressure. *P-value*: Mann-Whitney test
[1]UsualCare-Baseline
[2]Usual Care-12 months
[3]Usual Care-24 months
[4]Motivational intervention-Baseline
[5]Motivational Intervention-12 months
[6]Motivational Intervention-24 months

to help participants resolve ambivalent feelings that they may have about changing their behavior. Those in the traditional intervention group lost 3.1, 2.7, and 1.7 Kg at 6, 12, and 18 months, respectively. The addition of motivational interviewing increased weight loss significantly at each time point by 1.6 to 2.1 Kg.

The strengths of this study include the randomized design, and the provision of interventions by primary care therapist who treated overweight and obese patients in their ordinary local practices. This was a group intervention which permitted patient access to treatment, carried out by professionals in their own centers on patients whom they usually treat, without the need for external professionals. Patients received a hygiene-dietetic approach without pharmacological treatment. It is important to point out the high number of patients in the sample. Limitations included a considerable number of patients lost to follow-up. The higher drop-out rate (52.25 % completed the final visit at 2 years) observed in our study are in line with those reported in recent studies with a similar treatment duration. We did not specifically investigated the reason of drop-out and it is not possible perform a missing data analysis, but the majority of these losses were attributed to visit missing, patient deaths or changes in their address or in their general physician, which caused difficulties in their following-up. This is one of the major weak points in the follow-up of obese patients, similar to that found in other intervention trials, although far from the 86% of patients who completed the Wadden study [20]. It is notable that, in our study, adherence was better in the intervention group than in the control group with significantly fewer losses in the second year (33 vs 7%). This confirms the long-term efficacy of the group motivational approach among patients.

Modest weight loss—5 –10% of initial body weight has been shown to have a beneficial effect on cardiovascular risk factors associated with obesity and to improve risk factor clustering, such as improvements in blood pressure, and cholesterol [32]. Lifestyle intervention studies also suggest that modest weight loss can help to prevent or delay the appearance of type 2 diabetes and hypertension [33]. The beneficial effects of a moderate weight reduction apply not only in hypertension but also in the serum lipids levels. Vasankari et al [34] reported that the reduction of LDL-particles was proportional to the amount of weight lost. A weight loss of around 10% of the initial bodyweight was associated with a 33% reduction in the ratio of oxidized LDL to total LDL. A modest weight reduction has been shown to be beneficial in reducing the clustering of major cardiovascular risk factors. Individuals in the Framingham cohort, who lost at least 2.25 kg over 16 years, had a 40 –50% reduction in their total risk factor score. Recent retrospective analyses [35] from 401 patients conclude that patients losing only 5–10 % showed improvement on triglycerides, total cholesterol, and LDL cholesterol. This study supports the recommendation that 5–10 % weight loss may improve cardiovascular risk factors.

Conclusion

Our study shows that combining usual care with group-based motivational interventions by a trained nurse, in addition to the regular follow-up appointments with a doctor currently offered to obese patients, significantly increases the maintenance of weight loss. Furthermore, also provides evidence that we may need to improve clinical practice and focus our efforts on psychological aspects that contribute to weight loss in obese and overweight patients. Even if this requires organizational changes, an effort should be made given that the benefits we have achieved justify this type of intervention.

Abbreviations

BHA: Basic Health Areas; BMI: Body mass index; ICC: Intra-cluster correlation coefficient; IDIAP: Instituto de Investigación en Atención Primaria; IMOAP: Group motivational intervention in overweight/obese patients in primary prevention of cardiovascular disease in the primary healthcare area; WHO: World Health Organization

Acknowledgements

The authors are grateful to the Sociedad Española de Arteriosclerosis and to the Cardiovascular Research Center, CSIC-ICCC, Hospital de la Santa Creu i Sant Pau for their support to the project. The authors would like to thank F. Flor, and J. Almeda for his statistical advice. The authors would like to thank A. Muñoz for her collaboration in the project. The authors would like to acknowledge the patients and the researchers and the basic areas participants in the IMOAP group [19].

Funding

This work was supported in part by grants from Fondo de Investigaciones Sanitarias de la Seguridad Social FIS (PI 070087 to JJR).

Authors' contributions

JjR-C researched data, contributed to discussion, reviewed manuscript, read and approved the final version. CA-V contributed to discussion, reviewed manuscript, read and approved the final version. JmP contributed to discussion, reviewed manuscript, read and approved the final version. PT-M contributed to discussion, reviewed manuscript, read and approved the final version. FR-C contributed to discussion, reviewed manuscript, read and approved the final version. JrM contributed to discussion, reviewed manuscript, read and approved the final version. EP participated in conception and design, contributed to discussion, reviewed manuscript, read and approved the final version.

Competing interests

The authors declare that they have no competing interests.

Consent for publication

Not applicable.

Author details

[1]Centre Atenció Primària Florida Sud. Direcció Atenció Primària Costa de Ponent-ICS. L'Hospitalet, Institut Universitari d'Investigació en Atenció Primària Jordi Gol (IDIAP Jordi Gol), Barcelona, Spain. [2]Cardiovascular Research Center, CSIC-ICCC, Hospital de la Santa Creu i Sant Pau (UAB), IIB-Sant Pau, Barcelona, Spain. [3]FUFOSA (Fundación Fomento Salud), Barcelona, Spain. [4]Univestitat de Barcelona, Facultad de Farmacia, Barcelona, Spain. [5]Unitat de Salut Mental Collblanc, L'Hospitalet del Llobregat, Barcelona, Spain. [6]Cardiovascular Department, Epidemiology Unit, University Hospital Vall d'Hebron. Lleida Research Support Unit, Primary Care Research Institut (IDIAP) Jordi Gol, Autonomus University of Barcelona, Barcelona, Catalonia, Spain. [7]Cardiovascular Research Center, Hospital de la Santa Creu i Sant Pau, C/ Sant Antoni Ma Claret, 167 08025 Barcelona, Spain.

References

1. Obesity. Preventing and managing the global epidemic. Report of a WHO consultation. World Health Organ Tech Rep Ser. 2000;894:1–253. i-xii
2. Gargallo Fernandez M, Basulto Marset J, Breton Lesmes I, Quiles Izquierdo J, Formiguera Sala X, Salas-Salvado J, group F-Sc: Evidence-based nutritional recommendations for the prevention and treatment of overweight and obesity in adults (FESNAD-SEEDO consensus document). Methodology and executive summary (I/III). Nutr Hosp. 2012;27(3):789-799.
3. Gargallo Fernandez M, Quiles Izquierdo J, Basulto Marset J, Breton Lesmes I, Formiguera Sala X, Salas-Salvado J, group F-Sc: Evidence-based nutritional recommendations for the prevention and treatment of overweight and obesity in adults (FESNAD-SEEDO consensus document). The role of diet in obesity prevention (II/III). Nutr Hosp. 2012;27(3):800-832.
4. Aranceta J, Perez Rodrigo C, Serra Majem L, Ribas Barba L, Quiles Izquierdo J, Vioque J, et al. Prevalence of obesity in Spain: results of the SEEDO 2000 study. Med Clin. 2003;120(16):608–12.
5. Peeters A, Barendregt JJ, Willekens F, Mackenbach JP, Al Mamun A, Bonneux L, Nedcom tNE, Demography Compression of Morbidity Research G: Obesity in adulthood and its consequences for life expectancy: a life-table analysis. Ann Intern Med 2003, 138(1):24-32.
6. Peeters A, Bonneux L, Nusselder WJ, De Laet C, Barendregt JJ. Adult obesity and the burden of disability throughout life. Obes Res. 2004;12(7):1145–51.
7. Long DA, Reed R, Lehman G. The cost of lifestyle health risks: obesity. Journal of occupational and environmental medicine / American College of Occupational and Environmental Medicine. 2006;48(3):244–51.
8. Finkelstein EA, Fiebelkorn IC, Wang G. National medical spending attributable to overweight and obesity: how much, and who's paying? Health Aff. 2003;(Suppl Web Exclusives:W3):219–26.
9. Diet. Nutrition and the prevention of chronic diseases. World Health Organ Tech Rep Ser. 2003;916:1–149. i-viii, backcover
10. Swinburn B, Gill T, Kumanyika S. Obesity prevention: a proposed framework for translating evidence into action. Obesity reviews : an official journal of the International Association for the Study of Obesity. 2005;6(1):23–33.
11. Linmans JJ, Spigt MG, Deneer L, Lucas AE, de Bakker M, Gidding LG, et al. Effect of lifestyle intervention for people with diabetes or prediabetes in real-world primary care: propensity score analysis. BMC Fam Pract. 2011;12:95.
12. Casazza K, Fontaine KR, Astrup A, Birch LL, Brown AW, Bohan Brown MM, et al. Myths, presumptions, and facts about obesity. N Engl J Med. 2013;368(5):446–54.
13. Wieland LS, Falzon L, Sciamanna CN, Trudeau KJ, Brodney S, Schwartz JE, et al. Interactive computer-based interventions for weight loss or weight maintenance in overweight or obese people. The Cochrane database of systematic reviews. 2012;8:CD007675.
14. Jensen MD, Ryan DH, Apovian CM, Ard JD, Comuzzie AG, Donato KA, et al. 2013 AHA/ACC/TOS guideline for the management of overweight and obesity in adults: a report of the American College of Cardiology/American Heart Association task Force on practice guidelines and the Obesity Society. J Am Coll Cardiol. 2014;63(25 Pt B):2985–3023.
15. Look ARG, Wing RR. Long-term effects of a lifestyle intervention on weight and cardiovascular risk factors in individuals with type 2 diabetes mellitus: four-year results of the look AHEAD trial. Arch Intern Med. 2010;170(17):1566–75.
16. Brown A, Gouldstone A, Fox E, Field A, Todd W, Shakher J, et al. Description and preliminary results from a structured specialist behavioural weight management group intervention: specialist lifestyle management (SLiM) programme. BMJ Open. 2015;5(4):e007217.
17. Blackford K, Jancey J, Lee AH, James AP, Howat P, Hills AP, et al. A randomised controlled trial of a physical activity and nutrition program

targeting middle-aged adults at risk of metabolic syndrome in a disadvantaged rural community. BMC Public Health. 2015;15:284.
18. Fioravanti G, Rotella F, Cresci B, Pala L, De Vita G, Mannucci E, et al. Motivational enhancement therapy in obese patients: a promising application. Obesity research & clinical practice. 2015;9(5):536–8.
19. Rodriguez Cristobal JJ, Panisello Royo JM, Alonso-Villaverde Grote C, Perez Santos JM, Munoz Lloret A, Rodriguez Cortes F, et al. Group motivational intervention in overweight/obese patients in primary prevention of cardiovascular disease in the primary healthcare area. BMC Fam Pract. 2010;11:23.
20. Wadden TA, Volger S, Sarwer DB, Vetter ML, Tsai AG, Berkowitz RI, et al. A two-year randomized trial of obesity treatment in primary care practice. N Engl J Med. 2011;365(21):1969–79.
21. Martin PD, Dutton GR, Rhode PC, Horswell RL, Ryan DH, Brantley PJ. Weight loss maintenance following a primary care intervention for low-income minority women. Obesity. 2008;16(11):2462–7.
22. Ockene IS, Hebert JR, Ockene JK, Saperia GM, Stanek E, Nicolosi R, et al. Effect of physician-delivered nutrition counseling training and an office-support program on saturated fat intake, weight, and serum lipid measurements in a hyperlipidemic population: Worcester area trial for Counseling in Hyperlipidemia (WATCH). Arch Intern Med. 1999;159(7):725–31.
23. Christian JG, Tsai AG, Bessesen DH. Interpreting weight losses from lifestyle modification trials: using categorical data. Int J Obes. 2010;34(1):207–9.
24. Rossner S. Defining success in obesity management. Int J Obes Relat Metab Disord. 1997;21(Suppl 1):S2–4.
25. Jensen MD, Ryan DH, Apovian CM, Ard JD, Comuzzie AG, Donato KA, et al. AHA/ACC/TOS guideline for the management of overweight and obesity in adults: a report of the American College of Cardiology/American Heart Association task Force on practice guidelines and the Obesity Society. Circulation. 2014;129(25 Suppl 2):S102–38.
26. Gargallo Fernandez Manuel M, Breton Lesmes I, Basulto Marset J, Quiles Izquierdo J, Formiguera Sala X, Salas-Salvado J, group F-Sc: Evidence-based nutritional recommendations for the prevention and treatment of overweight and obesity in adults (FESNAD-SEEDO consensus document). The role of diet in obesity treatment (III/III). Nutricion hospitalaria 2012, 27(3):833-864.
27. Kumanyika S, Fassbender J, Phipps E, Tan-Torres S, Localio R, Morales KH, et al. Design, recruitment and start up of a primary care weight loss trial targeting African American and Hispanic adults. Contemporary clinical trials. 2011;32(2):215–24.
28. Steptoe A, Kerry S, Rink E, Hilton S. The impact of behavioral counseling on stage of change in fat intake, physical activity, and cigarette smoking in adults at increased risk of coronary heart disease. Am J Public Health. 2001; 91(2):265–9.
29. Shaw K, O'Rourke P, Del Mar C, Kenardy J. Psychological interventions for overweight or obesity. The Cochrane database of systematic reviews. 2005; 2:CD003818.
30. Carral F, Aguilar M, Olveira G, Mangas A, Domenech I, Torres I. Increased hospital expenditures in diabetic patients hospitalized for cardiovascular diseases. J Diabetes Complicat. 2003;17(6):331–6.
31. West DS, DiLillo V, Bursac Z, Gore SA, Greene PG. Motivational interviewing improves weight loss in women with type 2 diabetes. Diabetes Care. 2007; 30(5):1081–7.
32. Wing RR, Lang W, Wadden TA, Safford M, Knowler WC, Bertoni AG, et al. Benefits of modest weight loss in improving cardiovascular risk factors in overweight and obese individuals with type 2 diabetes. Diabetes Care. 2011;34(7):1481–6.
33. Pi-Sunyer X, Blackburn G, Brancati FL, Bray GA, Bright R, Clark JM, et al. Reduction in weight and cardiovascular disease risk factors in individuals with type 2 diabetes: one-year results of the look AHEAD trial. Diabetes Care. 2007;30(6):1374–83.
34. Vasankari T, Fogelholm M, Kukkonen-Harjula K, Nenonen A, Kujala U, Oja P, et al. Reduced oxidized low-density lipoprotein after weight reduction in obese premenopausal women. Int J Obes Relat Metab Disord. 2001;25(2):205–11.
35. Brown JD, Buscemi J, Milsom V, Malcolm R, O'Neil PM. Effects on cardiovascular risk factors of weight losses limited to 5-10. Translational behavioral medicine. 2016;6(3):339–46.

Experiencing integration: a qualitative pilot study of consumer and provider experiences of integrated primary health care in Australia

Michelle Banfield[1*], Tanisha Jowsey[2], Anne Parkinson[3], Kirsty A. Douglas[4] and Paresh Dawda[5]

Abstract

Background: The terms integration and integrated care describe the complex, patient-centred strategies to improve coordination of healthcare services. Frameworks exist to conceptualise these terms, but these have been developed from a professional viewpoint.
The objective of this study was to explore consumers' and providers' concepts, expectations and experience of integrated care. A key focus was whether frameworks developed from a professional perspective are effective models to explore people's experiences.

Methods: A qualitative pilot study was undertaken at one Australian multidisciplinary primary health care centre. Semi-structured interviews were conducted with consumers ($N = 19$) and staff ($N = 10$). Data were analysed using a framework analysis approach.

Results: Consumers' experience of integrated care tended to be implicit in their descriptions of primary healthcare experiences more broadly. Experiences related to the typologies involved clinical and functional integration, such as continuity of providers and the usefulness of shared information. Staff focused on clinical level integration, but also talked about a cultural shift that demonstrated normative, professional and functional integration.

Conclusions: Existing frameworks for integration have been heavily influenced by the provider and organisational perspectives. They are useful for conceptualising integration from a professional perspective, but are less relevant for consumers' experiences. Consumers of integrated primary health care may be more focussed on relational aspects of care and outcomes of care.

Keywords: Integration, Primary health care, Consumer experience

Background

When planning and describing desired health service provision, we often find the terms 'integration' and 'integrated care' used interchangeably. However, Kodner and colleagues have pointed out that 'integration' refers to structures and processes, while 'integrated care' is more concerned with the patient experiences and outcomes of such processes [1]. Despite this distinction, confusion remains in the literature, which others have noted [1–4]. This is largely due to the complexity with which integration and integrated care engage; operating on different levels of health systems, both horizontally and vertically [1, 5]. Kodner ([6], p.12) provides a useful definition of integrated care that further demonstrates the complexity:

> [a] multi-level, multi-modal, demand driven and patient-centred strategy designed to address complex and costly health needs by achieving better coordination of services across the entire care continuum. Not an end in itself, integrated care is a means of optimizing system performance and attaining quality patient outcomes.

* Correspondence: Michelle.Banfield@anu.edu.au
[1]Centre for Mental Health Research, Research School of Population Health, The Australian National University, 63 Eggleston Rd, Acton ACT 2601, Australia
Full list of author information is available at the end of the article

Given there is no recognised common model of integrated care, a conceptual framework is needed to better understand integrated care and guide empirical research [2, 3, 7–10]. As Goodwin recently argued, we lack the means to effectively measure and monitor outcomes in integrated care, 'particularly in terms of understanding improvements in the user experience'[11].

A useful starting point for demonstrating integration as a process (and for illustrating its complexity) may be the framework developed by Fulop et al. [12], which recognises the importance of process and cultural changes in addition to structures and governance. They identify six dimensions necessary for effective integration (see Table 1).

Also relevant is the taxonomy of integrated care that Valentijn and colleagues [3, 10, 13, 14] have developed, which uses a theory-driven mixed methods approach. The taxonomy, recently referred to as the Rainbow Model of Integrated Care [10] organises the six dimensions into the level of the system at which they operate (macro: systemic; meso: organisational and service/professional; and micro: clinical), with normative and functional integration described as enablers that operate across all levels. The model further identifies care as person- or population-focused and describes 21 key characteristics identified as necessary for achieving integrated care in a primary care setting (see Table 2) [3, 10, 13, 14]. However, as Valentijn and colleagues point out, not all stakeholders were engaged in their research, which consisted of Delphi studies with experts. For example, consumers were not included in the expert group, leaving the utility of these features for consumers unknown [13, 14].

The objective of the present study was to explore the perspectives of consumers and providers on integrated care within a newly-opened multidisciplinary primary healthcare centre. Of interest was how consumers with chronic illness and health care providers conceptualise integration, what they expect in terms of integrated care and what they experience. A key focus was whether the Fulop et al. model [12] and/or the Valentijn et al. taxonomy of features [13] could be effective modes through which people's perspectives may be explored and analysed.

Table 1 Fulop et al.'s six necessary dimensions for effective integration

Necessary dimensions for effective integration[a]	Details
Organisational integration	How the organisation is formally structured
Functional integration	How the non-clinical support and back-office processes are integrated
Service integration	How the clinical services are integrated
Clinical integration	How clinical team level care pathways are organised
Normative integration	The role of shared values
Systemic integration	The coherence of policies across organisational levels.

[a]Adapted from Fulop et al. [12]

Table 2 Key characteristics of integrated primary health care (adapted from Valentijn et al. [13])

Dimensions	Characteristics
Scope of care	
Person-focused care	1. Centrality of client needs
Population based care	2. Centrality of population needs
Dimensions and level of system	
Clinical integration (micro)	3. Case management
	4. Continuity
	5. Interaction between professional and client
	6. Individual multidisciplinary care plan
Service/Professional integration (meso)	7. Inter-professional education
	8. Agreements on interdisciplinary collaboration
	9. Value creation for the professional
Organisational integration (meso)	10. Inter-organisational governance
	11. Inter-organisational strategy
	12. Trust
System integration (macro)	13. Alignment of regulatory frameworks
	14. Environmental climate
Enablers of integration	
Functional integration	15. Learning organisations
	16. Information management
	17. Regular feedback of performance indicators
Normative integration	18. Shared vision
	19. Reliable behaviour
	20. Visionary leadership
	21. Linking cultures

Methods

The ethical aspects of the research were approved by The Australian National University Science and Medical Delegated Ethics Review Committee (protocol number 2014/651). All participants provided written consent to participate in the study and for interviews to be audio-recorded.

The research was developed and conducted according to a flexible participatory research model [15]. The research team included health professionals, consumer leaders and researchers from various disciplinary backgrounds. The team worked closely with a reference group throughout the project, comprising two consumer representatives, a General Practitioner (GP), an allied health professional, a nurse and a senior manager with the provider organisation. The reference group provided feedback on the research protocols, facilitated data collection and contributed to analysis and reporting of results.

The current study was part of a pilot project to explore methods of investigating integrated primary healthcare, including through clinical records (see McRae et al. [16]), a patient experience survey (unpublished data) and testing the utility of professionally-developed frameworks for consumer and provider experiences of integrated care (current study). As a pilot, participant numbers and the setting were purposely limited. Findings from the pilot study will be used to inform the design of broader-ranging studies of integrated primary healthcare, including different models and locations.

Data collection was conducted at a large, urban, multidisciplinary primary healthcare centre in Australia between April and August 2015. The centre had been in operation for approximately 15 months and had been funded under an Australian government program (GP Super Clinics) widely publicised in the media that aimed to promote co-location and integration of general practice with allied health and other service providers in order to more effectively support those with, or at risk of, chronic disease. The GP Super Clinics program provided infrastructure funding for more than 60 clinics, but did not fund service provision [17]. The program claimed not to prescribe a particular model of service delivery, but key objectives included patient-centred care and effective use of information technology, and key features included co-location of services such as allied health and diagnostic imaging [17]. At the time of the Super Clinic program, Australia was already experiencing a rapid shift in the mode of general practice from small privately owned 2–4 doctor practices to much larger group practices run by health service delivery organisations, with other subcontracted diagnostic services being housed in a single location or building. Multidisciplinary services at the centre in the current study were provided by health professionals with a direct contractual relationship with the medical centre operator as well as more broadly by services with a subcontracting relationship. At the time of the study, the practice consisted of 12 doctors, 6 practice nurses, 11 administrative staff and 9 allied health professionals with a direct contractual relationship with the medical centre operator. An additional 5 services were provided under subcontracting arrangements. Professionals with a direct contractual relationship could access the shared practice management system and patient records, whereas subcontractors managed their own systems and communicated via traditional referral and communication systems such as letter and phone.

Consumers were recruited through the practice nurses, who were asked to identify people with chronic conditions who had seen more than one health professional at the centre. Nineteen consumer interviews were conducted, recruited in two cohorts to participate in different aspects of the overall project. Cohort one ($n = 10$) was recruited for an interview to explore their experiences only. This was a convenience sample recruited by the senior practice nurse and it was observed that this resulted in participants who had seen the same two doctors and a limited range of other health professionals at the centre. Cohort two ($n = 9$) was originally recruited for the patient experience survey testing, but to extend the scope of interview data, were asked to also complete an interview on their experiences. To diversify the sample, consecutive consumers attending a nurse clinic were invited to participate in cohort two. The recruitment for both cohorts was undertaken by practice staff. The number of people who declined to participate was not recorded.

Ten interviews were also conducted with health professional and management staff at the healthcare centre. Staff were invited to participate at a staff meeting attended by the researchers. To provide a range of views in the limited time period available, a purposive sample of GPs, nurses, allied health professionals and managers was subsequently recruited with assistance of the Practice Manager. Sampling was designed to include both male and female GPs and with various lengths of employment at the centre, and we aimed to recruit at least one staff member with experience in the nursing, administrative and allied health aspects of the practice. No participants withdrew from the study before or after completion of an interview.

All interviews were guided by semi-structured protocols: the broad questions are presented in Table 3. The protocols were developed by the research team and reference group to encourage participants to volunteer their own perceptions and understanding of primary health care integration, with prompts related to the dimensions of the typologies [12, 13] used where necessary to more fully explore the existing theoretical basis for the project, including key features such as continuity, information sharing and organisational culture. Due to the time-limited nature of the pilot study, interviews were conducted by three researchers to maximise efficiency in data collection. These interviewers each had qualitative data collection experience, an interest in consumer experience and knowledge of the integration framework (AP, JG and MB). Interviewers discussed the study and the questions beforehand and agreed to adhere closely to the protocols to minimise variations in style during data collection in order to ensure comparability of data. No moderator was present during the interviews. The lead investigator (MB) reviewed audio files for consistency and

Table 3 Broad interview questions

Consumers
1. [This practice] is set up as an integrated primary health care centre. When I say "integrated primary health care", what sort of things come to mind for you?
2. What are your expectations of [this practice] for care for your chronic condition?
3. Can you tell me about your experiences with [practice] services?
4. We are particularly interested in the effect of integrated health care on the time people spend looking after their health. Can you talk about that?
Providers/managers
1. [This practice] is set up as an integrated primary health care centre. When I say "integrated primary health care", what sort of things come to mind for you?
2. What are your expectations of working in an integrated primary health care centre?
3. Can you tell me about your experiences with providing services/working at [this practice]?
4. How does [this practice] compare with other general practices where you've worked in the past?

debriefed interviewers during the during data collection period.

Interviews were held in a private consultation room at the healthcare centre: discussions with the reference group identified this as likely to be the most convenient and comfortable location for both consumers and health professionals due to its familiarity and the ability to schedule interviews around appointments. Interviews were digitally audio-recorded and with both groups lasted between five and 25 minutes (average approximately 10 minutes for consumers and 11 minutes for staff). All three interviewers conducted interviews of shorter and longer duration. The interviewers had no relationship or contact with participants prior to the interviews.

Analysis

The digital audio recordings were transcribed by an external transcribing service and the transcripts reviewed for accuracy by the research team. De-identified transcripts are available in The Australian National University Data Commons [18]. Data were managed using QSR NVivo10 software and were first analysed separately by three members of the research team (MB, TJ and AP). The coding frame presented in Table 4 was finalised by agreement; findings were also discussed with the reference group prior to drafting of publications.

A framework approach [19] combining both independent inductive development of themes and interrogation for the dimensions and characteristics of integration identified in the typologies was used for analysis. Several features of the current study, including the short timeframe, multidisciplinary research team and the need for answers to specific applied questions made the study a good fit with Ritchie and Spencer's suggested application of framework analysis [19]. As the objective of the study was primarily contextual, concerned with understanding people's experiences, attitudes and the nature of the system [19], the inductive approach kept a close focus on people's experiences, ideas and practices, in the context of an integrated health care service. Through an iterative process, experiences were organised into themes generated from the data: as the coding framework developed, earlier transcripts were re-examined to ensure the framework was representative of experiences across interviews [19]. Data were examined for both positive and negative accounts of phenomena. All interviews, regardless of length, were included in the analysis. Data saturation was reached by the twelfth consumer participant in the inductive analysis.

In addition to the inductive analysis, one researcher (MB) also mapped the data against the 21 features and six dimensions of the typologies (see Tables 1 and 2). In the final interpretative phase of analysis, data were organised into broad thematic areas, some with subthemes, based on the inductive analysis and intersections with features of the theoretical typologies identified (Table 4).

Interviews were numbered sequentially within their group (consumer, health professional or manager). Participant quotes used within findings are identified only by their group and number.

Results

Consumer experiences

Characteristics of participants

Consumer participants in the first interview cohort were not specifically asked for demographic details. All identified as having at least one chronic condition and during the course of the interview, four mentioned that they were retired. Six of the first cohort of consumer participants were female. The second cohort of consumer participants provided demographic details in the patient experience survey completed in addition to the interview. Participants were aged between 54 and 81 years and reported between three and twelve chronic conditions. Six of the participants in cohort two were male, the majority were retired or on disability, had at least some tertiary education and described themselves as financially comfortable.

Table 5 presents the health professionals and services within the health centre building accessed by participants in each cohort. Services offered by providers with a direct contractual relationship with the medical centre operator are marked with an asterisk. Other services were co-located but subcontracted. For the first cohort,

Table 4 Summary of major themes, subthemes and dimensions of integration

Theme	Subtheme	Dimensions of integration from typologies
Consumers		
Making meaning from the term integration		-
Experience at the healthcare centre		Person-focused care
	1. Access to services	Clinical integration
	2. Care continuity	Clinical integration
	3. Performing above expectations	Clinical integration
	4. Staff availability and competence	Functional integration
	5. Appointments/services running on time	Functional integration
	6. Friendly staff	Functional integration
	7. Shared attitude	Normative integration
Staff		
Making meaning from the term integration		Person-focused care
Experience at the healthcare centre		-
A cultural shift towards teamwork and care integration		Normative integration Clinical integration Professional/service integration Functional integration

services used were explored in the course of the interview and this information extracted and summarised. Participants in the second cohort indicated the services they had accessed in the patient experience survey. Participants in both cohorts were also questioned about their intentions to use other services within the building in future.

Almost all consumers had a usual GP and regularly saw the practice nurses. They also accessed a range of other services available in the building, particularly pathology and pharmacy. Many commented that they would make greater use of the on-site services such as physiotherapy when the need arose.

Perceptions, expectations and experiences

Participant experiences of health care, as reported in this study, were overwhelmingly positive. One participant summarised this: "But you know our health system here in Australia is way ahead of America, England, anywhere I've been. So I'm always very happy to be sick here" (Consumer 19).

Table 5 Health services accessed by consumers

Services accessed	Number of consumers $N = 19$
Practice Nurse*	17
Pathology	8
Pharmacy	7
Radiology	5
Dietician*	2
University training physio clinic	2
Specialist*	1
Physiotherapy*	1
Psychology*	1
Diabetes educator*	1
Sleep clinic	1

*Services offered by providers with a direct contractual relationship with the medical centre operator are marked with an asterisk

Making meaning from the term integration

Many consumers had not heard the phrase "integrated primary health care"; despite this, all participants were able to describe what they thought the term meant in ways that were consistent with definitions. Given the Super Clinic setting and the publicity that had surrounded this program, a particular focus of perceptions for consumers was that integration was increased through co-location. Consumers frequently used the term "one-stop shop" a phrase that had been used by the Health Minister promoting the original program to illustrate their experiences of integration.

> "'Integrated' to me indicates that it's not just a minor health centre where you go and see the GP for minor ailments and things like that but there are other treatments and things available where you can be interviewed for various other things besides just ordinary medical issues, like physiotherapies and things like that. I've noticed some of the signs around, you have a chemist available in the building and the X-ray facilities are also integrated into the building as well which makes it a very good medical centre to visit, in my opinion." (Consumer 01).

> "it [integrated primary health care] includes doctors, nurses, so I can get all my shots and my blood and everything done in the one spot, that I can get my X-rays… it's like a kind of one-stop shop." (Consumer 02).

Experience at the healthcare centre
Several consumer participants reported that they had followed their GP of 20+ years to the healthcare centre because they were satisfied with the quality of care offered by that particular GP and were motivated to seek continuity of care. Whilst not directly examples of integrated care, these comments illustrated the importance of retaining established relationships and the adaptations they were prepared to make.

> "Well based on long experience with certain doctors here [laughs] we just mentioned that we've known [doctor] for 35 years plus and some of his staff are also here now. I have full confidence in the resources of [healthcare centre]. ... the same people and the same good care." (Consumer 05).

> "I want to see the same doctor, because he's had, I don't know, 25, 30 years of contact with me, he's quite a busy man and so instead of being able to see him tomorrow, I might have to wait a few days. But I must say, the girls at the front are very good at fitting you in." (Consumer 19).

When asked to assess their experiences of the healthcare centre, and to compare with healthcare experiences they had elsewhere, participants overwhelmingly reported satisfaction. Many of the comments reflected **person-focused care** and related to **clinical level** features of integration such as continuity and case management, framed as consumers experience these elements as follows.

Access to services Consistent with their perception of integration as a "one-stop shop," many participants described the ease of access to multiple services offered by the centre and the concomitant increase in likelihood of them following up on referrals to these services as a result.

> "There's more nurses and that they can fit you in just for a flu shot whenever, or if I needed to have something else done they can fit you in straightaway which is great, and the fact that I can go downstairs and have bloods done if [name] says, you need bloods, and there's no waiting or expecting for me to go elsewhere, but compared to having to go to [other practice] one time it's more friendly, everyone's personable, everyone knows everyone, which is what I like." (Consumer 02).

> "... they said, oh well you need to go to a physio, you should see a physio, well – and this is what happened with the dietician with me, like, I probably honestly would not have got around to ringing up the dietician, to making the appointment, when someone had said – but I walked out the door and said, he wants me to see so-and-so, and she said, I'll make the appointment for you now." (Consumer 07).

> "... you've pretty much got the one stop place where you can come, see your GP, if you need a referral to go and do something you can just go downstairs or up, wherever you need to go and it's good because for people like me [with multiple sclerosis]. ... I think your energy levels get worse and you just don't have time and the energy to be going to three different places when you could be coming to one and go, I can do everything in the one hit here and it's done." (Consumer 10).

However, some participants felt the transport and parking were not ideal. Limited disabled parking and bus schedules that were difficult to follow meant that some people did not find getting to the centre very easy, but they still appreciated having multiple services in one location once they accessed it.

Another participant was concerned at the cost of multiple visits, which they believed should be free since the visits were part of a care plan. This may be interpreted as an example of poor communication between health care practitioners and patient:

> "When you're on the health care plan you're supposed to have access to certain other medical people like physio or whatever free. It's not free. ... I've got appointments with a physio coming up and it's going to cost me $300 for five visits and then hello here I'm on a pension only, I don't have other income and that was just, why do they keep saying you get access to these people [for] free. Five visits a year when it's *not* free, it costs. I can just phone up and make an appointment with a physio and it costs me the same amount." (Consumer 08).

Care continuity Consumers also expressed confidence in the continuity of care offered by the centre, including the completeness of records. Their comments reflected the importance of having one professional with knowledge of their entire history when dealing with chronic conditions.

> "I know that they always send [a] report – even, like, the eye specialist and that who'd been recommended by or referred by here, they all send letters back to the doctor so I know that all the things are going onto my file. Yeah, so she would be my [laughs] primary source of

information if anybody needed to know my whole history. I'm fairly confident that most of the stuff that I talk to with the other people actually do all get back to her in the end, yeah." (Consumer 07).

Performing above expectations Person-focused care was reflected in several descriptions of additional efforts by staff to accommodate specific consumer needs, including protecting vulnerable people from risk in the waiting area and avoiding unnecessary consultations for repeat prescriptions.

"... they've gone out of their way to make me kind of comfortable. I've been going through chemotherapy and when I've been here at that time when I'm susceptible to infection I've asked about going into – rather than being in an ordinary – this is just an example of the cooperation – rather than being in the waiting room with all the other patients I've been allocated my own room there for isolation, to protect me from infection there." (Consumer 05).

"I forgot to get a prescription repeat for whatever particularly, like, [nurse] and [nurse] and all of those who've known me for a long time, they'll just look up my record and go, oh it's this one, and they'll double-check it and go, OK I'll get [doctor] or [doctor] to write you out a script for that." (Consumer 10).

Descriptions of **person-focused care** also often included experiences with staff and healthcare organisation consistent with elements of **functional integration,** particularly their experience of service management.

Staff availability and competence Many consumers praised the responsiveness of the administrative staff, who they felt did their best to accommodate consumers' needs and provide information.

"They'll give me a choice of times, which is very good ... There's always someone who can answer the phone when you ring to make an appointment or a query, and they've always got the information available, which is very good." (Consumer 01).

"If I walk in, and [receptionist] always knows, or [receptionist] knows...when have you got to come back. Oh gee, that's going to be difficult, but we'll find a spot for you, hang on. And they take the time. And they know when you go to the counter, OK, he's coming in, he needs to see the clinic, or he needs to see the doctor, or he needs... and nothing's a problem." (Consumer 18).

However, not all experiences with availability were positive. One participant believed that the move to a large centre had made it more difficult to get appointments.

"I ring up one day and I say I want an appointment for the current [day], no, we can't do it. I said, you know, just make an appointment. But you've got... she's this and that, and we have a few spots that we save through the day, and you've got to ring at 7 o'clock in the morning, on the day, and see if we've got... if we can slot you in. Because she only works 'till lunch time, right. And I was on the phone for 20 minutes the other morning before somebody answered. And I thought, well this is just hopeless you know." (Consumer 15).

Appointments/services running on time Consumers' opinions were divided on whether the time management at the centre was effective. Some described the centre as efficient, with little evidence of extended waiting times.

"I'm very impressed that everything seems to run on time, it's efficiently run, which is a bonus, not sitting for hours and waiting. Whether that'll continue or not I know, hopefully will, but that's my first impression of – it's very well run." (Consumer 08).

"[doctor] is very quick, and likes to be on time, and we like that. We don't like waiting two hours, where we used to at a previous doctor." (Consumer 14).

Some participants also reported feeling that they had enough time in appointments (which could come at a cost to services running on time):

"I never feel rushed with [doctor] or any of the other doctors. They're prepared to listen to either [name] or I with our medical problems and advise us what to do." (Consumer 09).

"... she'll exhaust every avenue until the appointment's finished, so no I never feel – and even when I've seen [doctor] – never feel rushed, just do what I've got to do and that's that, so it's good." (Consumer 10).

However, not all participants shared these feelings. Some reported feeling rushed and guilty about the amount of time they took with the doctor.

"I know that whenever I get out and I go to make my next appointment the receptionist staff is constantly asking, do you need a double appointment, do you need a double appointment, and it's all, no I don't.

Like, it's done, and that kind of makes me feel like, oh have I been in there too long, have I – do you know what I mean? It makes me feel like I've done something wrong. Yeah, that makes me feel a bit – that makes me feel more rushed, actually being in with the doctor." (Consumer 06).

Friendly staff Participants reported that they appreciated feeling known by staff and they perceived staff within the centre as friendly. This included the GPs, receptionists, nurses, pharmacists and even the café personnel. The café personnel were considered by some to be equally important to their general feeling of 'being known';

"Respondent: ... now they've got the chemist downstairs, and a coffee shop ..., so I think you're pretty much covered in most of your...
Interviewer: Cover your caffeine as well as your meds [laughs].
Respondent: Yeah especially depending on the appointment yeah [laughs].
Interviewer: They make a good coffee, too, I had a couple this morning [laughs].
Respondent: Oh they're fabulous and the guy there's really lovely, I like him, so he's good value, so...
Interviewer: Yeah seems like a nice guy.
Respondent: Yeah that makes it nice too especially if you're feeling a bit stressed or something, you just need a friendly face to have a bit of a laugh." (Consumer 10).

Shared attitude Consumer participants had a sense of the collective attitude, trust and collaboration indicative of **normative integration**. One participant commented that this difference might even be overwhelming for new people, suggesting they felt it to be a strength of the healthcare centre.

"I think someone new coming in would find the experience almost overwhelming, it's all here, and if they actually get the care and treatment that makes it even better. And I think it's important they're all on that... the wavelength of wanting to help people." (Consumer 18).

Participants reported that they were so satisfied with the health service that they recommended it to family members and friends.

"I've certainly brought my mother – like, my mother had to have some imaging things done and she's going ... cause [other clinic] is such a pain to, you know, go to as well. There's one at [healthcare centre] so I've made sure she came here and things like – because of the convenient parking and the, you know, cause it's closer proximity and yeah. Mainly the parking has a lot to do with that." (Consumer 07).

Staff experiences

Ten staff participated in interviews: four GPs, one practice nurse, two managers, and three allied health professionals. To maintain confidentiality, no demographic details were recorded for the staff participants.

Making meaning from the term integration

When asked to describe integration, staff participants described it in terms of diverse services being co-located, patient-centric, and optimising continuity of care. They also described integration in terms of care providers having ready access to other care providers in order to seek advice or manage individual case needs (**person-focused care**). Staff participants said:

"Integrated primary health care should be where there's good co-ordination between allied health and medical practitioners and nursing staff, working towards the better health of patients." (Health professional 01).

"... communication, liaison, the ability to not just send emails, and it's to actually to be able to verbally communicate via telephone, or even walking into each other's rooms. And that's... what I see from that, patient coming in with a complaint or a condition, it's not just handled by one person, and then have to either (a) not contact the other person at all and just feed through the patient, but rather the patient can turn up to the clinic and go, "Does the physiotherapist know all my background," and the idea is, yes, because all the information that we store between the physio, the doctor, the podiatrist, and even the dietician, is all stored on our system, and therefore we've got a good rounding knowledge about what it is that this patient's complaint is, and we can also liaise quite easily on our same system, and through other physical means, of how we can interact around their care." (Health professional 02)

Experiences at the healthcare centre

Some staff members had specifically chosen to work at the healthcare centre because it was a GP Super Clinic. Despite this, both the health professionals and managers interviewed did not offer much information on what they expected of this type of centre. In addition to shared information and a high standard of care, one staff member suggested that they expected improved working conditions, such as backups/locums for doctors. Other staff members expected to provide more holistic care in an integrated centre, but suggested this may come with a need for wider knowledge.

> "Just you know broader range of knowledge. I've learnt a lot since I've been here about the different you know areas of health and things like that." (Manager 01).

> "... that's a very important part of I think integrated health, that you've got a team of people that the patients feel connected with, that they can ask for advice from, and get different levels of expertise and in different areas." (Health professional 01).

One staff participant described their motivation to join the healthcare centre in terms of the needs of patients not being met in a small general practice. By moving, they said, "We've lost the intimacy of a little private practice, but there's been so much more to gain" (Health professional 03).

A cultural shift towards teamwork and care integration

Staff experiences provided a strong sense of the collective attitude and collaboration underpinning **normative integration** as an enabler of integrated care. Elements of **clinical, professional** and **functional integration** were all clearly identifiable contributors to a culture of integration as reported by GPs, allied health professionals and managers alike.

A sense of teamwork and holistic care was reported as being an important element in the healthcare centre, one that staff participants had either not experienced in previous settings or had experienced but to a lesser degree.

> "Yeah, definitely the communication channel is a lot more open. Not only the... can you knock on the door, or go and talk to another health professional directly, but we have on the computer system all the patient notes available, we can send... you know request to have meetings with other health professionals to set up more... more flexibility I guess with catching up with people ... I think the whole philosophy here is so embraced by all the staff members. Everyone is so helpful and welcoming. I think it's the culture of what [the practice] is trying to promote really does resonate with everyone that works here. I think it's a very supportive environment not only for the clients, but also for the staff members." (Health professional 04).

Staff participants described a desire to see a real cultural shift in the sharing of information between practitioners of different modalities. They saw the healthcare centre as being a trailblazer towards this shift.

> "I think GPs and Allied Health sometimes struggle with the concept, and they need to just be open to the thoughts of their files being shared, their clinical notes being shared. Generally a GP initially shares clinical notes with ... their colleagues, not with external providers such as Allied Health, so I think the knowledge basis of what integration can do, can be improved." (Manager 02).

Key to the success of such cultural shifting, they explained, was communication. Formal modes of communication, such as writing clear and structured patient notes and sharing them, were described. Of equal value to the cultural shift was informal communication and developing a sense of friendship and community with staff of different modalities using the space.

> "Communication, it has to be strong, and it's time consuming. And obviously communication can be taken, especially written communication, can be taken in many ways, so just being careful of how things are communicated, to what extent, what detail." (Manager 02).

> "I found that obviously as physios we have our own acronyms, and I think GPs have their own acronyms, so I think it's something that I try to portray to the other physios here too, because this is the first time they've worked in this environment. If they write TVA, or if they write FIS, ... FIS for a doctor could mean FIS differently to what we think. So we're starting to write flexion standing, rather than FIS." (Health professional 05).

One staff participant explained that although the ideology of sharing information between practitioners to optimise patient care was generally held by staff at the healthcare centre, and that it was facilitated by the shared electronic information system, that difficulties arose in relation to sharing mental health information, which was partially addressed by psychologists providing notes that staff could read that were different from the patient notes.

> "... someone having counselling, that they may disclose something that they would never have told me, you know, or... yeah. And that's a difficulty of how much. And I'm not sure with the psychologist here how much... I think she keeps a lot of her own

records, so I've never looked to see. But I know the physio does put records in, and I know he looks at what we've got as well, too, to help him, and I'm the same. So they can look, and for instance the dietician can look and see what the latest cholesterol was, and you know things like that that are very useful to be... so it's just when you get that sort of super confidential bit of information, and that's probably more policies and procedures. ... they will give us a summary, or you know when there's times that we've got to perhaps do a referral to a psychiatrist, and give us some information there. But they actually keep totally separate notes." (Health professional 01).

Also key to the cultural shift toward integration, was the way space was used. Room sharing and communal areas were described as facilitating communication and care integration.

"I love the communication here. I love the fact that like in our section there, we're all... like the room that we're in right now it's an Allied Health room, which means everyone's to work as a team. It's not like the physiotherapist's room, or like the podiatrist's room, it's the Allied Health room, so it's got a really strong outlook in that getting everyone on board." (Health professional 05).

"[we do] A lot of horse trading in the corridors and tearooms. ... it's quite... a bit of a different flavour to what people are willing to type as opposed to as what they're willing to say" (Health professional 06).

When describing the value of the cultural shift, one participant summed it up in the following way: "I've seen the lot, as in solo practice with no nurses, no practice manager, and I wouldn't go back to that system by choice again." (Health professional 06).

Discussion

The healthcare centre was still relatively new and growing, but the interviews provided evidence that many dimensions of integration were already becoming established and consumers were experiencing integrated care. Consumers' experience of integrated care tended to be implicit in their descriptions of primary health care experiences more broadly. Their comments that could be related to the typologies [13, 14] were primarily about clinical and functional integration, particularly their experiences of continuity of providers, the usefulness of the shared information systems and the helpfulness of front desk staff. Staff had a strong focus on clinical level integration, but also talked about a cultural shift that demonstrated normative, professional and functional integration. Across all groups, discussion of normative integration was primarily in terms of a sense of collective attitude. There was very little discussion of organisational or system level integration.

Some specific issues arose that may be important to investigate in the implementation of integrated primary healthcare more broadly. Consumers and staff both liked the ease of communication and continuity provided by the shared record system. Consumers liked the idea that their entire medical history and notes from other providers may be in one place and available to their GP and other treating professionals in the centre. In contrast, some allied health professionals suggested that sensitive information should not necessarily be available to all providers accessing the system. This suggests shared records may have an important part to play in facilitating integrated care, although careful consideration may need to be given to restricting access to potentially sensitive details in consultation with the preference of the consumer. The availability of effective and compatible computer technology to facilitate these functions is also important for informing the extent to which information is shared electronically for integrated care [20–22].

Work specifically investigating the role of information systems in continuity and integration, both in the current study and previous research, has found that factors such as inconsistent record-keeping and terminology undermine their utility [16, 23]. It is therefore not surprising that both consumers and providers spoke extensively about the value of the familiarity between professionals enabled by co-location as an important feature of the healthcare centre. Interaction with people from other services, often in the staff tearoom, helped to establish relationships and build trust which then translated to comfort with recommending these services to consumers. Medical and allied health professional staff enjoyed the informal consultations with each other and the ability to "stop by" and discuss things without the need for formal referral or response letters when they were not appropriate. Consumers spoke of the convenience of having services all in one building, many able to be booked through the same reception staff as their GP. Consumers' descriptions conveyed a confidence in the services associated with their GP, especially where they had a long-standing relationship that pre-dated the creation of the Super Clinic.

Overall, this meant that not only was there evidence of the more "practical" elements of integration such as information flows, there was evidence of the development of a shared culture, noticeable to the consumers as well as staff. Rather than a focus on more business-like concepts such as coherence of polices and management, integration was described in terms of the way people interacted with one another and the ease of navigating healthcare. The value of relationships and the influence of co-location on their development and maintenance will be an important focus of broader work on models of integrated primary healthcare.

An investigation of overall coding patterns across all consumer and staff interviews against Fulop et al's [12] typology and Valentijn et al's [13, 14] key features suggested that these frameworks may be useful for capturing the way people in service provision, especially health professionals, describe integration, but less useful for consumers' experience of integrated care. Staff described a sense of collective attitude indicative of normative integration, underpinned by examples of clinical, professional and functional integration such as holistic care, improved communication and teamwork. Their responses tended to be framed similarly to the descriptors included in the Valentijn et al. [13] taxonomy, which was developed from a professional perspective. Clinical and functional dimensions were evident in the way consumers described their experiences of care such as continuity of providers, the usefulness of the shared information and the importance of administrative staff. They also reported a sense of collaboration characteristic of normative integration. However, dimensions that operate at the meso and macro level (professional, organisational and systemic integration) were absent from consumers' data and much of the way they framed their experiences fell outside the framework descriptors, focusing instead on elements of quality health care more broadly, such as access. Valentijn et al. [13] acknowledged that their Delphi process did not involve some key stakeholders, including consumers, suggesting work in local settings may further refine understanding of key features across groups. The current study provides evidence that work is still needed on the key concepts of quality integrated primary health care from the consumer perspective. A potential area of focus may be the intersection of integrated primary health care with dimensions of consumer experiences of health care more broadly [24].

Limitations

As a study pilot, there are a number of limitations to acknowledge. The study was conducted at one healthcare centre, constructed and promoted as part of a government program, the GP Super Clinic Program. It is not known whether findings would generalise to other GP Super Clinics or to other types of integrated primary healthcare centres. Consumer participants were also recruited by practice nurses, with interviews for cohort one arranged and scheduled by one nurse with whom many consumers had a long-term relationship. This may have biased the findings on the importance of continuity. Interviews were conducted by three researchers which may have affected the consistency of questioning and rapport with participants. The short duration of interviews and the small numbers of participants may also have affected data saturation and representativeness, particularly for health professionals. Finally, demographic information was not collected for most participants, limiting the conclusions that could be drawn regarding diversity of the sample.

Conclusion

Existing frameworks for integration have been heavily influenced by the provider and organisational perspectives. They are useful for conceptualising integration from a professional perspective, but are less relevant for consumers' experiences. Consumers of integrated primary health care may be more focussed on relational aspects of care and outcomes of the care with less focus on the organisational or structural processes necessary to produce them. Despite this, as proposed by previous authors [3, 12–14], the feature that unifies experiences of both providing and receiving integrated care is a sense of collective attitude. Thus, consistent with Kodner and colleagues' [1] distinction between integration as a process and integrated care as an outcome, future research into these concepts should focus on the area salient to each group and the influence of a shared culture for both.

Abbreviations

GP: General practitioner

Acknowledgements

The research team gratefully acknowledge the cooperation and assistance provided by the Ochre Health group and particularly the staff of Ochre Health Medical Centre Bruce. We also thank Laurann Yen and the project reference group for thoughtful insights into project design, processes, materials and findings. Thanks also to John Gosling, who assisted with interviews.

Funding

This research is a project of the Australian Primary Health Care Research Institute, which is supported by a grant from the Australian Government Department of Health. The information and opinions contained in it do not necessarily reflect the views or policy of the Australian Primary Health Care Research Institute or the Australian Government Department of Health. MB is supported by Australian Research Council Discovery Early Career Researcher Award (DE150100637). The funding bodies played no part in study design, implementation, analysis or the production of the manuscript.

Authors' contributions

MB contributed to the study design, collected and analysed data and drafted the manuscript. TJ contributed to study design, analysed data and edited the manuscript. AP contributed to study design, collected and analysed data and edited the manuscript. KD contributed to study design and edited the manuscript. PD conceived the study, contributed to study design and data analysis, and edited the manuscript. All authors approved the final manuscript.

Competing interests

Author PD is the Medical Director of the centre in which the study was conducted.

Author details
[1]Centre for Mental Health Research, Research School of Population Health, The Australian National University, 63 Eggleston Rd, Acton ACT 2601, Australia. [2]Centre for Medical and Health Sciences Education The University of Auckland, Auckland City Hospital, Building 599, Level 12, Auckland 1023, New Zealand. [3]Department of Health Services Research and Policy, Research School of Population Health, The Australian National University, 63 Eggleston Rd, Acton ACT 2601, Australia. [4]ANU Medical School, Canberra Hospital, Bldg 4, Level 2, Garran ACT 2605, Australia. [5]Ochre Health Medical Centre, Cnr Allawoona Street & Ginninderra Drive, Bruce ACT 2617, Australia.

References

1. Kodner DL, Spreeuwenberg C. Integrated care: meaning, logic, applications, and implications–a discussion paper. Int J Integr Care. 2002;2:e12.
2. What is the evidence on the economic impacts of integrated care? Policy summary 11. [http://www.euro.who.int/en/about-us/partners/observatory/publications/policy-briefs-and-summaries/what-is-the-evidence-on-the-economic-impacts-of-integrated-care]. Accessed 31 Aug 2015.
3. Valentijn PP, Schepman SM, Opheij W, Bruijnzeels MA. Understanding integrated care: a comprehensive conceptual framework based on the integrative functions of primary care. Int J Integr Care. 2013;13:e010.
4. Armitage GD, Suter E, Oelke ND, Adair CE. Health systems integration: state of the evidence. Int J Integr Care. 2009;9:e82.
5. Integrated Care: What Policies Support and Influence Integration in Health Care in Australia [http://www.phcris.org.au/researchevidence/item.php?id=8413&spindex=14]. Accessed 29 Sept 2015.
6. Kodner DL. All together now: a conceptual exploration of integrated care. Healthc Q 2009, 13 Spec No:6–15.
7. Goodwin N. Annual Conference Supplement 2010: Integrated care as a scientific discipline: the need for more theory and new analytical methods. Int J Integr Care 2010, 10(Suppl). doi: http://doi.org/10.5334/ijic.589.
8. Axelsson R, Axelsson SB. Integration and collaboration in public health–a conceptual framework. Int J Health Plann Manage. 2006;21(1):75–88.
9. Kodner DL, Kyriacou CK. Fully integrated care for frail elderly: two American models. Int J Integr Care. 2000;1:e08.
10. Nurjono M, Valentijn PP, Bautista MAC, Lim YW, Vrijhoef HJ. A prospective validation study of a rainbow model of integrated care measurement tool in Singapore. Int J Integr Care. 2016;16(1):1.
11. Goodwin N. How should integrated care address the challenge of people with complex health and social care needs? Emerging lessons from international case studies. Int J Integr Care 2015, 15(3). doi: http://doi.org/10.5334/ijic.2254.
12. Building integrated care: Lessons from the UK and elsewhere [http://www.nhsconfed.org/~/media/Confederation/Files/Publications/Documents/Building%20integrated%20care.pdf]. Accessed 31 Aug 2015.
13. Valentijn P, Vrijhoef H, Ruwaard D, Boesveld I, Arends R, Bruijnzeels M. Towards an international taxonomy of integrated primary care: a Delphi consensus approach. BMC Fam Pract. 2015;16(1):64.
14. Valentijn PP, Boesveld IC, Van der Klauw DM, Ruwaard D, Struijs JN, Molema JJ, Bruijnzeels MA, Vrijhoef HJ. Towards a taxonomy for integrated care: a mixed-methods study. Int J Integr Care. 2015;15:e003.
15. Banfield M, Yen L, Newby L. Stakeholder involvement in primary health care research. Report and recommendations. In. Canberra: Australian Primary Health Care Research Institute; 2011.
16. McRae I, Dawda P, Banfield M, Parkinson A. Can we measure integration of health care from administrative and clinical records? Aust Fam Physician. 2016;45(9):672–5.
17. About the GP Super Clinics Programme [http://www.health.gov.au/internet/main/publishing.nsf/Content/pacd-gpsuperclinic-about]. Accessed 29 Sept 2016.
18. Banfield M, Parkinson A, Dawda P, Jowsey T, Douglas K, Cox D, McRae I, Strazdins L. Consumer and provider experiences of integrated primary health care. In. The Australian National University Data Commons; 2016
19. Ritchie J, Spencer L. Qualitative data analysis for applied policy research. In: Bryman A, Burgess B, editors. Analyzing qualitative data. London: Routledge; 1994. p. 174–93.
20. Christensen T, Grimsmo A. Instant availability of patient records, but diminished availability of patient information: a multi-method study of GP's use of electronic patient records. BMC Med Inform Decis. 2008;8(1):12.
21. Henderson J, Britt H, Miller G. Extent and utilisation of computerisation in Australian general practice. Med J Australia. 2006;185(2):84.
22. Ludwick D, Doucette J. Adopting electronic medical records in primary care: lessons learned from health information systems implementation experience in seven countries. Int J Health Inform. 2009;78(1):22–31.
23. Banfield M, Gardner K, McRae I, Gillespie J, Wells R, Yen L. Unlocking information for coordination of care in Australia: A qualitative study of information continuity in four primary health care models. BMC Fam Pract. 2013;14:34.
24. Wong S, Haggerty J. Measuring patient experiences in health care: A review and classification of items and scales used in publicly-available questionnaires. In. Vancouver: Centre for Health Services Research and Policy Research, University of British Columbia; 2013.

22

How do population, general practice and hospital factors influence ambulatory care sensitive admissions

John Busby[1*], Sarah Purdy[2] and William Hollingworth[2]

Abstract

Background: Reducing unplanned hospital admissions is a key priority within the UK and other healthcare systems, however it remains uncertain how this can be achieved. This paper explores the relationship between unplanned ambulatory care sensitive condition (ACSC) admission rates and population, general practice and hospital characteristics. Additionally, we investigated if these factors had a differential impact across 28 conditions.

Methods: We used the English Hospital Episode Statistics to calculate the number of unplanned ACSC hospital admissions for 28 conditions at 8,029 general practices during 2011/12. We used multilevel negative binomial regression to estimate the influence of population (deprivation), general practice (size, access, continuity, quality, A&E proximity) and hospital (bed availability, % day cases) characteristics on unplanned admission rates after adjusting for age, sex and chronic disease prevalence.

Results: Practices in deprived areas (at the 90th centile) had 16% (95% confidence interval: 14 to 18) higher admission rates than those in affluent areas (10th centile). Practices with poorer care continuity (9%; 8 to 11), located closest to A&E (8%; 6 to 9), situated in areas with high inpatient bed availability (14%; 10 to 18) or in areas with a larger proportion of day case admissions (17%; 12 to 21) had more admissions. There were smaller associations for primary care access, clinical quality, and practice size. The strength of associations varied by ACSC. For example, deprivation was most strongly associated with alcohol related diseases and COPD admission rates, while continuity of primary care was most strongly associated with admission rates for chronic diseases such as hypertension and iron-deficiency anaemia.

Conclusions: The drivers of unplanned ACSC admission rates are complex and include population, practice and hospital factors. The importance of these varies markedly across conditions suggesting that multifaceted interventions are required to avoid hospital admissions and reduce costs. Several of the most important drivers of admissions are largely beyond the control of GPs. However, strategies to improve primary care continuity and avoid unnecessary short-stay admissions could lead to improved efficiency.

Keywords: Primary health care, General practice, Ambulatory care, Patient admission

* Correspondence: john.busby@qub.ac.uk
[1]Centre for Public Health, Queen's University Belfast, BT12 6BA, Belfast, UK
Full list of author information is available at the end of the article

Background

Unplanned admissions place a tremendous strain on UK healthcare resources, accounting for 67% of hospital bed days, costing £12.5bn annually [1] and disrupting elective care [2]. In England, they have increased by 47% over the last 15 years [1] with some arguing that their continued rise threatens to bankrupt the National Health Service (NHS) [3]. Reducing the number of unplanned admissions is a key priority [4], but is challenging due to complex hospital admission pathways.

Ambulatory care sensitive conditions (ACSCs) account for one in five unplanned admissions [5]. ACSCs are conditions where improved primary and community care could potentially prevent the need for hospital admission [6]. Substantial unexplained geographic variation in ACSC admission rates [7, 8] suggests reductions might be possible, however it remains uncertain how these can be achieved. Knowledge of how population (e.g. deprivation), general practice (e.g. quality) and hospital (e.g. bed availability) characteristics influence admission rates could aid the identification of poorer quality care, help redesign services, develop admission avoidance interventions, and yield financial savings for the NHS. However, currently this evidence is only available for a minority of ACSCs and is often impaired by poor generalisability, a lack of case-mix adjustment and other methodological weaknesses [9, 10].

In this paper we use routine data from English hospitals to examine the relationship between unplanned ACSC admission rates and several population, general practice and hospital characteristics. We determine if these factors have a differential impact across conditions.

Methods

Data source and preparation

Our study was set in the English NHS. The NHS is comprised of three broad sectors; primary care (e.g. general practitioners, pharmacists, community care), secondary care provided in hospitals, and specialist tertiary care. Primary care doctors are paid by the NHS though a weighted capitation method (based on the number and complexity of the patients under their care) with additional payments dependant on achieving quality targets through the Quality and Outcomes Framework (QOF). Hospital treatment is generally reimbursed by the NHS on a fixed payment system. Almost all services are free at the point of access.

We used the Hospital Episode Statistics (HES) admitted patient care dataset to identify admissions for 28 common (i.e. >3,000 admissions annually) ACSCs between 1st April 2011 and 31st March 2012 using ICD diagnosis codes from previous work (Additional file 1) [6]. We aggregated admissions to the level of the general practice and excluded practices with a registered population smaller than 1,000 ($n = 68$; 0.8%), as these are likely to represent atypical practices, or with missing covariate data ($n = 26$; 0.3%) leaving 8,029 practices, with over 55 million registered patients, in the final analysis. Practices were located within all 151 Primary Care Trusts (PCTs) that, at the time of the study, commissioned care for their local populations. We investigated the effect of population (deprivation), general practice (size, access, continuity, quality, A&E proximity) and hospital (bed availability, percentage day cases) characteristics on unplanned admission rates. Further details on the variables used within the analysis, including their potential weaknesses, are provided in Additional file 2.

Association with practice and hospital characteristics

We described the demographics of patients admitted for each condition. We estimated the relationship between unplanned ACSC admission rates and population, practice and hospital characteristics using two-level multivariate negative binomial regression models. These models include random PCT-effects which appropriately account for the clustering of practices within PCTs, adjust for latent PCT-level characteristics which could affect the demand for hospital admission, and allow the association of practice-level (e.g. access) and PCT-level (e.g. inpatient bed availability) characteristics to be estimated simultaneously. Each independent variable was scaled by the difference between a high (90th centile) and low (10th centile) practice or PCT to improve comparability across covariates (see Additional file 2 for further details).

We adjusted for differences in practice populations using a two-step process. First, we calculated the expected number of admissions using indirect standardisation (using quinary age groups and gender) and national data [11] to account for differences in the size and age-sex composition of practice populations (Additional file 3). We used negative binomial regression, and data from the QOF [12], to adjust for disparities in chronic disease prevalence among practices (atrial fibrillation, asthma, cancer, CKD, COPD, dementia, epilepsy, heart failure, hypertension, learning disability, mental health problems, obesity and stroke). Exploratory analysis revealed a non-linear relationship with A&E proximity for several conditions, so this were modelled using quartiles.

Results

Descriptive statistics

There were 1.77 million admissions for ACSCs accounting for 10.9 million bed days during 2011/2 (Table 1). Many admitted patients were older (mean age 56 years old), lived in more deprived communities (27% lowest quintile), had at least one comorbidity recorded (58%) and were admitted through A&E (75%). These overall results concealed substantial variation between conditions (Table 2), for example, over 30% of iron-deficiency anaemia and

Table 1 Admission details for all ACSCs admissions

Characteristics	Count (%)
Number of Admissions	1,767,550
Bed Days	10,903,662
Day Cases	443,760 (25.1)
Mean Age	55.6
0–19	264,541 (15.0)
20–39	207,032 (11.7)
40–59	338,316 (19.1)
60–79	512,017 (29.0)
80+	445,644 (25.2)
Male	844,537 (47.8)
Ethnicity	
White	1,495,974 (84.6)
Asian	100,486 (5.7)
Black	41,879 (2.4)
Mixed	14,623 (0.8)
Missing	114,588 (6.5)
Deprivation	
0 (Most Deprived)	477,437 (27.0)
1	387,099 (21.9)
2	339,554 (19.2)
3	302,310 (17.1)
4 (Least Deprived)	261,150 (14.8)
Comorbidities	
Any	1,032,628 (58.4)
Chronic obstructive pulmonary disease	465,731 (26.4)
Diabetes	288,168 (16.3)
Congestive heart failure	194,692 (11.0)
Cerebrovascular disease	185,824 (10.5)
Renal disease	133,975 (7.6)
Admission Source	
The usual place of residence	1,671,614 (94.6)
Other	94,806 (5.4)
Admission Method	
Emergency: via accident and emergency	1,326,882 (75.1)
Emergency: via general practitioner	290,218 (16.4)
Other	150,450 (8.5)
Discharge Destination	
The usual place of residence	1,597,060 (90.4)
Patient died	80,371 (4.6)
Nursing home	35,425 (2.0)
Other	54,694 (3.1)

ENT infection admissions originated from a GP referral, while this was the case for less than 5% of schizophrenia and alcohol-related disease admissions.

Association between unplanned ACSC admission rates and practice characteristics

For all ACSCs combined, practices located in deprived areas (at the 90th centile) had 16% (95% CI: 14, 18) higher admission rates than those situated in affluent localities (at the 10th centile, Table 3). The quartile of practices closest to A&E had 8% (95% CI: 7, 10) higher admission rates than those in the furthest away quartile. Practice admission rates were highly dependent on these characteristics. For example, after adjusting for age and sex, 83% of practices based in the most deprived quartile of areas had admission rates above the national average compared to only 15% in the least deprived areas (Fig. 1). Practices with poor care continuity (10th centile) had 9% (95% CI: 8, 11) more admissions than those with good continuity (90th centile, Table 3). Practices located in PCTs with more hospital beds had higher (12%, 95% CI: 8, 17) admission rates, as did those with a larger proportion of day case admissions (17%, 95% CI: 12, 22). The association between admission rates and primary care access, clinical quality, and practice size was much smaller.

The strength of associations varied substantially across ACSCs (Table 3, Fig. 2, Additional file 4). For example, admission rates for alcohol-related diseases and COPD were more than a third higher among patients registered at practices in deprived areas while differences of less than 8% were found for several ACSCs including hypertension and migraine / acute headache. Improved continuity of primary care was most strongly associated with lower unplanned admission rates for chronic conditions such as hypertension, COPD, peripheral vascular disease and iron-deficiency anaemia. Proximity to A&E was most strongly associated with high admission rates for mental-health conditions, alcohol-related diseases, and several conditions where patients were regularly admitted for less than a day (e.g. dental conditions, asthma, constipation).

Areas with increased bed availability had particularly high admission rates amongst conditions where very short hospital stays are commonplace (e.g. alcohol-related diseases, ENT infection, dehydration and gastroenteritis). PCTs with a larger proportion of day cases had increased admission rates for most ACSCs; this was particularly pronounced for ENT infections where areas with a high proportion had 183% (95% CI: 149, 222) more admissions than those with a low proportion. Unplanned admission rates for some ACSCs appear to be much less sensitive to population, practice and hospital characteristics. For example, hip fracture and stroke admission rates had little association with continuity of GP care, A&E proximity or bed availability.

Table 2 Characteristics of admitted patients by condition

Condition	Mean Age	% Male	% Most Deprived Quintile	% Admitted From GP	% Day Case
Alcohol-related diseases	43.8	68.0	40.1	4.3	35.4
Angina	60.5	54.6	27.0	9.1	37.8
Asthma	31.2	42.9	32.9	16.1	27.1
Atrial fibrillation / flutter	56.3	40.7	21.4	12.6	41.0
Cellulitis	51.6	52.1	27.4	26.6	22.5
Congestive heart failure	78.5	51.6	22.9	19.8	6.9
Constipation	51.4	42.6	27.6	27.0	32.4
Convulsions and epilepsy	37.6	53.5	29.8	4.2	32.6
COPD	71.2	48.3	33.5	15.6	12.1
Dehydration and gastro	40.8	44.8	27.5	26.0	28.2
Dental condition	35.1	51.8	31.8	11.8	27.2
Diabetes complications	44.9	54.6	30.6	15.6	9.6
Dyspepsia / otr stomach function	40.5	50.2	27.6	21.7	50.2
ENT infection	10.2	52.9	30.8	34.2	53.0
Fractured proximal femur	80.8	26.9	18.1	1.0	0.5
Hypertension	60.9	41.3	25.7	26.3	35.5
Influenza and pneumonia	67.5	51.2	24.7	17.0	7.5
Iron-deficiency anaemia	65.0	38.8	25.8	37.0	20.0
Migraine / acute headache	42.2	35.6	26.6	23.3	37.5
Neuroses	47.6	44.0	31.2	7.4	30.6
Pelvic inflammatory disease	32.6	0.0	30.7	24.5	15.1
Perforated / bleeding ulcer	56.5	54.1	26.7	19.3	24.3
Peripheral vascular disease	69.1	53.3	26.0	31.7	22.5
Pyelonephritis	63.2	34.7	24.4	19.9	15.5
Ruptured appendix	36.2	58.1	18.9	28.0	0.3
Schizophrenia	42.5	63.0	45.3	2.6	4.8
Senility / dementia	83.6	38.5	22.0	11.4	14.7
Stroke	74.7	49.3	20.0	6.7	3.7

Discussion

Statement of principal findings

ACSCs accounted for 1.77 million admissions and 10.9 million bed days during 2011/12. Admission rates were higher in practices located in deprived areas, within close proximity to an A&E department, with poor continuity of GP care, and situated in areas with a high inpatient bed supply or proportion of day case admissions. There was little evidence that access to primary care, clinical quality, or practice size were important contributors to variation in unplanned admissions. The strength of associations differed markedly across conditions.

Strengths and weaknesses

This study is based on a large nationally representative dataset containing almost all unplanned admissions in England. Applying standardised and robust methodology to a broad range of ACSCs provides new evidence on the factors associated with admission rates, and allows identification of the characteristics that should be prioritised when redesigning services and developing admission avoidance interventions.

Our study is observational; although we have undertaken extensive case-mix adjustment it is still possible that our results are confounded by unmeasured factors. For example, it is possible that our finding of lower admission rates among practices with higher care continuity could be due, at least in part, to these practices better organising their care in other ways (e.g. support for self-care, specialist disease clinics). However, the negligible associations for conditions where admission is not usually avoidable (e.g. hip fracture) suggests that residual confounding is not solely driving our results. Some of the characteristics considered within our study may be poorly measured.

Table 3 Difference in unplanned admissions between a high (90th centile) and low (10th centile) practice for selected conditions[a]

	All ACSCs Combined	Alcohol- Related Diseases	COPD	Dehydration and Gastro	ENT Infections	Hypertension	Hip Fracture	Stroke
Practice characteristics								
Deprivation	16 (14,18)	44 (35,54)	36 (30,42)	8 (5,11)	7 (3,12)	7 (−5,20)	7 (3,11)	12 (8,16)
A&E Distance								
Furthest Away	Ref	Ref	Ref	Ref	Ref	Ref	Ref	Ref
2nd Quartile	5 (4, 6)	9 (3,15)	6 (2,10)	8 (5,10)	4 (0, 7)	3 (−6,12)	−1 (−3, 2)	3 (0, 5)
3rd Quartile	7 (5, 8)	15 (8,23)	10 (6,14)	9 (6,12)	4 (0, 8)	8 (−2,19)	−1 (−4, 1)	1 (−2, 4)
Closest	8 (7,10)	21 (13,29)	10 (5,14)	14 (11,17)	11 (7,16)	12 (2,24)	−3 (−6,−0)	2 (−1, 5)
Continuity	−9 (−11,−8)	−7 (−11,−2)	−13 (−16,−10)	−7 (−9,−5)	−10 (−13,−7)	−20 (−26,−13)	−0 (−3, 3)	−2 (−5, 0)
Access	−1 (−2, 0)	1 (−3, 6)	−1 (−4, 2)	−2 (−4, 0)	−0 (−3, 2)	−2 (−9, 5)	1 (−1, 4)	2 (−1, 4)
Quality	−2 (−3,−1)	−4 (−7,−1)	−1 (−3, 1)	−1 (−3, 0)	−3 (−5,−1)	−4 (−10, 2)	1 (−1, 3)	−1 (−3, 1)
Size	−2 (−3,−1)	2 (−3, 6)	0 (−3, 3)	−1 (−3, 1)	1 (−2, 4)	−1 (−8, 6)	2 (0, 4)	0 (−2, 2)
PCT characteristics								
Bed Availability	12 (8,17)	39 (21,60)	16 (9,23)	24 (16,32)	25 (12,41)	24 (9,40)	−1 (−4, 2)	5 (1, 9)
% Day Cases	17 (12,21)	12 (−3,29)	9 (4,14)	28 (20,37)	183 (149,222)	1 (−11,14)	0 (−3, 3)	2 (−1, 6)

[a]After adjustment age, sex and chronic disease prevalence (atrial fibrillation, asthma, cancer, CKD, COPD, dementia, epilepsy, heart failure, hypertension, learning disability, mental health problems, obesity and stroke) and each of the factors listed in the table

Specifically, QOF clinical scores may not accurately reflect primary care quality [13], the IMD of a practice postcode may not accurately reflect the socioeconomic status of their registered patients [14], straight line distances to A&E departments may be a poor measure of travel times [15], and our survey-based estimates of primary care access and continuity may be imprecise. This measurement error is likely to have led us to underestimate the association between unplanned admission rates and each of the variables included within our analysis due to regression dilution bias [16].

Admission rates for mental health conditions may be inaccurate [17]. Although mental health trusts report data to HES, a range of community-based alternatives (e.g. crisis houses) may substitute for hospital treatment

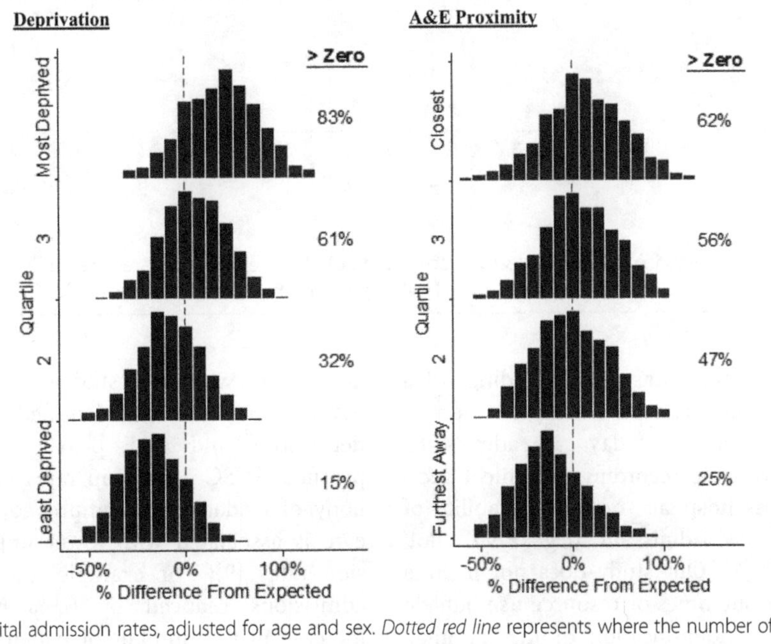

Fig. 1 Distribution of hospital admission rates, adjusted for age and sex. *Dotted red line* represents where the number of observed admissions matches the number that would be expected given the size and age-sex composition of the practice

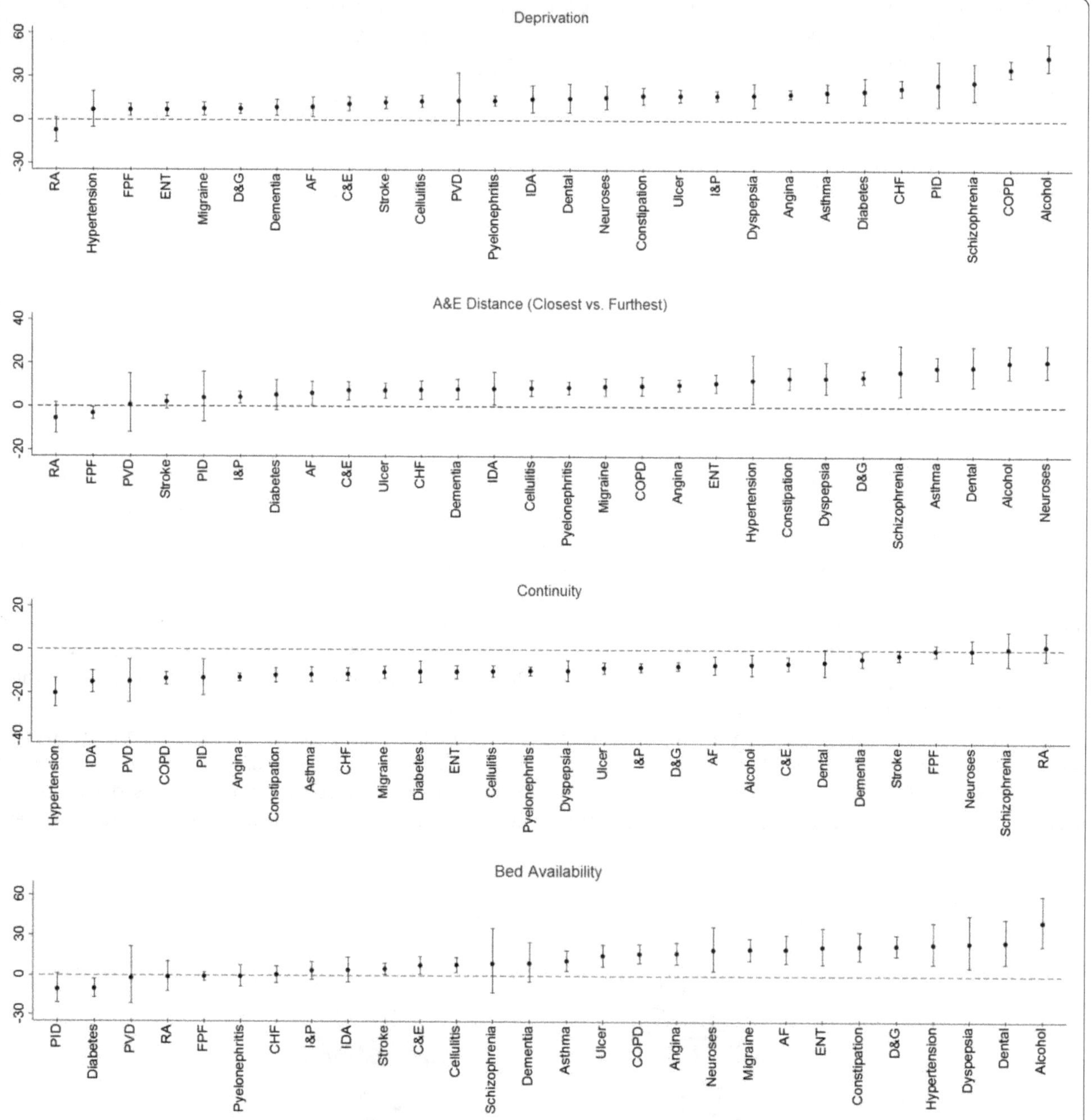

Fig. 2 Association of unplanned admission rates with selected practice and PCT characteristics. *Circles* represent the point estimate of the relative risk between the covariate and unplanned admission rates. Vertical lines represent 95% confidence intervals

and are not included in the dataset. Our findings of a very strong association between ENT infection admission rates and the proportion of day case admissions may be explained by variable recording of clinical decision unit activity across hospitals, or the availability of alternatives to short-stay admission (e.g. ENT 'hot' clinics) in some trusts [1]. Our study does not include information on patient outcomes or resource use outside hospital which prohibits identification of the 'optimal' admission rate.

Comparison with other studies

Several studies have identified the crucial role that deprivation and A&E proximity play in driving unplanned ACSC admission rates [9]. There is a growing body of evidence that improved continuity of primary care is associated with lower unplanned ACSC admission rates [9]. For example, one English study found admissions reduced by 0.5% per percentage point increase in the number of patients able to book with a specific GP [18]. Strong associations between inpatient bed availability and unplanned ACSC admission rates have been detailed elsewhere [10, 19], including in a UK study which found that patients resident in areas with the highest quintile of hospital beds had 13–15% higher respiratory disease admission rates than those within the lowest quintile [19].

A recent systematic review found little evidence of reduced unplanned ACSC admission rates among practices with better appointment availability within the UK or Europe [9]. Several studies investigating the association between QOF scores and unplanned admission rates have found little or no association except for a few specific conditions (e.g. COPD, CHD) [20]. There is negligible evidence that unplanned admission rates differ by general practice size [9].

Implications for clinicians and policymakers

Increasing unplanned admission rates are an important problem facing healthcare systems worldwide. Addressing the variance in continuity of GP care, finding and publicising convenient alternatives to admission for patients registered at practices closest to A&E, and reducing the number of short-stay admissions are potential components of successful admission avoidance interventions. Our results suggest that the success of each of these strategies is likely to vary by condition and that a multifaceted programme of interventions, tailored to local problems, is required to contain secondary care demand and reduce costs. Some of the characteristics investigated in this study are not readily modified (e.g. deprivation) or are largely beyond the control of GPs (e.g. local hospital bed availability, A&E proximity). Failure to account for these during routine audit or benchmarking could undermine efforts to detect and manage poorer quality primary care. Given the results of our study, it is likely that distinct adjustment models will be required for each condition to guard against residual confounding.

Continuity of care is an important facet of primary care, particularly for chronic conditions such as hypertension, COPD and CHF which often rely on frequent primary care management and co-occur with other morbidities. If the assocations observed in our study are causal, nearly 100,000 ACSC admissions could be avoided by practices annually through providing 'good continuity' care (defined being able to see or speak to their preferred GP 'Always,' Almost always' or 'A lot of the time' to the question) to 90% of their registered patients. Assuming an average ACSC admission cost of £1,739 [21], this would equate to hospital savings of around £170 million. Improved continuity would most obviously be attained through a growth in GP numbers, although this is likely to be challenging due to ongoing GP recruitment issues in many countries [22]. Other practice-level changes such as patient education, empowering patients to trade-off GP choice and speed of access, and better practitioner communication might be more easily achieved [23].

Our findings do not support recent UK government initiatives that focus on improvements in primary care access [24], particularly if these are implemented to the detriment of the continuity of care. A UK-based review investigating the link between primary care access and unplanned admission rates concluded that 'Existing evidence...is inadequate to inform national policy' [25]. Our results concur with this finding and suggest that a fuller investigation of the benefits and costs of increased access is required before implementation. The small and inconsistent association between clinical quality scores and admission rates suggests that this crude measure of primary care quality may not adequately encompass the most important aspects of GP care for averting unplanned ACSC admissions. The extent to which the care processes that the QOF incentivises lead to improvements in patient outcomes has generated substantial debate [26] and continues to evolve. The latest evidence suggests the QOF has been responsible for an 8% reduction in unplanned admission rates for incentivised ACSCs [27].

ACSC admission rates may be higher in some areas due to the increased frequency of very short admissions. Nationally, the number of short-stay admission has surged by 124% in the last 15 years [1] however our results suggest substantial geographic variation in their use. Some short hospital stays are clinically appropriate (e.g. severe exacerbations of asthma), however others may result from inappropriate referrals, limited community-based care options, patient confusion around out-of-hours care arrangements, or government targets (e.g. 4-hour A&E waits) [1]. Improved referral guidelines, enhanced community-based treatment options (e.g. telemedicine) or increased accessibility and awareness of alternatives to A&E attendance (e.g. walk-in clinics) might reduce these admissions, although there remains little research exploring their affect on overall healthcare outcomes and costs [28]. The strong influence exerted by inpatient bed availability and A&E proximity on admission rates suggests that some ACSC care may be 'supply sensitive' [29].

Unanswered questions and future research

Randomised controlled trials examining the effect of new interventions to improve the continuity of primary care are required. Evaluation of community-based interventions (e.g. improved self-management) aimed at preventing unnecessary hospital admissions are needed, particularly in deprived areas and those within close proximity to A&E.

Conclusions

Increasing unplanned hospital admissions is a key problem facing healthcare systems worldwide. The drivers of high unplanned ACSC admission rates are complex and include population (e.g. higher deprivation), practice (e.g. poor continuity of care) and hospital (e.g. increased inpatient bed availability) factors. The importance of these varies substantially across conditions suggesting multifaceted interventions are required to improve care and reduce costs. Several of the most important drivers of admissions are beyond the control of GPs. Strategies to increase the continuity of primary care and avoid unnecessary short-stay admissions could reduce admissions; however a fuller understanding of how these interventions affect aggregate healthcare costs and patient outcomes is required.

Additional files

Additional file 1: Included ACSCs and ICD-10 codes used to define them. List of ICD-10 codes used to identify admissions for each of the conditions used within the analysis.

Additional file 2: Independent variable description, potential weaknesses and source. Description of each independent variable used in the analysis.

Additional file 3: Calculation of age-sex specific GP population. Description of how the age-sex specific GP practice populations were determined.

Additional file 4: Association of unplanned admission rates with selected practice and PCT characteristics. Graphical representation of association between primary care access, primary care quality, practice size and percentage of day case admissions with unplanned ACSC admission rates.

Abbreviations

A&E: Accident and emergency; ACSC: Ambulatory care sensitive condition; CHD: Coronary heart disease; COPD: Chronic obstructive pulmonary disease; ENT: Ear, nose throat; HES: Hospital episode statistics; IMD: Index of multiple deprivation; NHS: National health service; PCT: Primary care trust; QOF: Quality and outcomes framework

Acknowledgements

None.

Funding

None to declare.

Authors' contributions

All authors conceived the study. JB conducted the analysis and drafted the manuscript. WH and SP critically revised the article for intellectual content. All authors read and approved the final manuscript. All authors had full access to the data in the study and can take responsibility for the integrity of the data and the accuracy of the data analysis.

Competing interests

The authors declare that they have no competing interests.

Consent for publication

Not applicable.

Author details

[1]Centre for Public Health, Queen's University Belfast, BT12 6BA, Belfast, UK. [2]School of Social and Community Medicine, University of Bristol, BS8 2PS, Bristol, UK.

References

1. Department of Health. Emergency admissions to hospital: managing the demand. London: Department of Health; 2013.
2. Caesar U, Karlsson J, Olsson LE, Samuelsson K, Hansson-Olofsson E. Incidence and root causes of cancellations for elective orthopaedic procedures: a single centre experience of 17,625 consecutive cases. Patient Saf Surg. 2014;8:24.
3. Robinson P. Are emergency admissions in England Out of control? 2010.
4. Quality Premium. http://www.england.nhs.uk/ccg-ois/qual-prem/. Accessed 21 Apr 2016.
5. Blunt I. Focus on preventable admissions. London: Nuffield Trust; 2013.
6. Purdy S, Griffin T, Salisbury C, Sharp D. Ambulatory care sensitive conditions: terminology and disease coding need to be more specific to aid policy makers and clinicians. Public Health. 2009;123(2):169–73.
7. Busby J, Purdy S, Hollingworth W. Using geographic variation in unplanned ambulatory care sensitive condition admission rates to identify commissioning priorities: an analysis of routine data from England. J Health Serv Res Policy. 2016;22:20–7.
8. Busby J, Purdy S, Hollingworth W. Opportunities for primary care to reduce hospital admissions: a cross-sectional study of geographical variation. Br J Gen Pract. 2017;67:e20–e8.
9. Huntley A, Lasserson D, Wye L, Morris R, Checkland K, England H, Salisbury C, Purdy S. Which features of primary care affect unscheduled secondary care use? A systematic review. BMJ Open. 2014;4(5):e004746.
10. Busby J, Purdy S, Hollingworth W. A systematic review of the magnitude and cause of geographic variation in unplanned hospital admission rates and length of stay for ambulatory care sensitive conditions. BMC Health Serv Res. 2015;15(1):1–15.
11. Numbers of Patients Registered at a GP Practice - April 2013. https://data.england.nhs.uk/dataset/numbers-of-patients-registered-at-a-gp-practice-april-2013. Accessed 21 Apr 2016.
12. Quality and Outcomes Framework. http://www.hscic.gov.uk/qof. Accessed 21 Apr 2016.
13. Langdown C, Peckham S. The use of financial incentives to help improve health outcomes: is the quality and outcomes framework fit for purpose? A systematic review. J Public Health (Oxf). 2014;36(2):251–8.
14. Strong M, Maheswaran R, Pearson T. A comparison of methods for calculating general practice level socioeconomic deprivation. Int J Health Geogr. 2006;5(1):1–5.
15. Haynes R, Jones AP, Sauerzapf V, Zhao H. Validation of travel times to hospital estimated by GIS. Int J Health Geogr. 2006;5(1):40.
16. Hutcheon JA, Chiolero A, Hanley JA. Random measurement error and regression dilution bias. BMJ. 2010;340:c2289.
17. White J, Gutacker N, Jacobs R, Mason A. Hospital admissions for severe mental illness in England: Changes in equity of utilisation at the small area level between 2006 and 2010. Soc Sci Med. 2014;120:243–51.
18. Bankart MJG, Baker R, Rashid A, Habiba M, Banerjee J, Hsu R, Conroy S, Agarwal S, Wilson A. Characteristics of general practices associated with emergency admission rates to hospital: a cross-sectional study. Emerg Med J. 2011;28(7):558–63.
19. Purdy S, Griffin T, Salisbury C, Sharp D. Emergency respiratory admissions: influence of practice, population and hospital factors. J Health Serv Res Policy. 2011;16(3):133–40.
20. Gillam SJ, Siriwardena AN, Steel N. Pay-for-performance in the United Kingdom: impact of the quality and outcomes framework: a systematic review. Ann Fam Med. 2012;10(5):461–8.
21. The Kings Fund. Data briefing: emergency hospital admissions for ambulatory care-sensitive conditions: identifying the potential for reductions. 2012.
22. Verma P, Ford JA, Stuart A, Howe A, Everington S, Steel N. A systematic review of strategies to recruit and retain primary care doctors. BMC Health Serv Res. 2016;16(1):126.
23. The Kings Fund. Continuity of care and the patient experience. 2010.
24. Seven-day a week NHS: Prime Minister's visit and speech. https://www.gov.uk/government/news/seven-day-a-week-nhs-prime-ministers-speech. Accessed 21 Apr 2016.

Multimorbidity, clinical decision making and health care delivery in New Zealand Primary care

Tim Stokes[1*], Emma Tumilty[1], Fiona Doolan-Noble[1] and Robin Gauld[2]

Abstract

Background: Multimorbidity is a major issue for primary care. We aimed to explore primary care professionals' accounts of managing multimorbidity and its impact on clinical decision making and regional health care delivery.

Methods: Qualitative interviews with 12 General Practitioners and 4 Primary Care Nurses in New Zealand's Otago region. Thematic analysis was conducted using the constant comparative method.

Results: Primary care professionals encountered challenges in providing care to patients with multimorbidity with respect to both clinical decision making and health care delivery. Clinical decision making occurred in time-limited consultations where the challenges of complexity and inadequacy of single disease guidelines were managed through the use of "satisficing" (care deemed satisfactory and sufficient for a given patient) and sequential consultations utilising relational continuity of care. The New Zealand primary care co-payment funding model was seen as a barrier to the delivery of care as it discourages sequential consultations, a problem only partially addressed through the use of the additional capitation based funding stream of *Care Plus*. Fragmentation of care also occurred within general practice and across the primary/secondary care interface.

Conclusions: These findings highlight specific New Zealand barriers to the delivery of primary care to patients living with multimorbidity. There is a need to develop, implement and nationally evaluate a revised version of *Care Plus* that takes account of these barriers.

Keywords: Multimorbidity, Primary care, General practice, Health services, Decision making

Background

Multimorbidity (the presence of two or more chronic conditions in a single patient) [1] is one of the biggest challenges facing health systems internationally as multiple disease care, not single disease care, becomes the norm in an aging society [2, 3] Multimorbidity is a major issue in primary care [4]. Recent epidemiological studies of chronic disease show that multimorbidity is the norm for people aged over 65 [5]. For example, a large Scottish primary care cross sectional study found that 23% of all patients were multimorbid with a prevalence rising to 65% in the 65-84 age group [6]. Multimorbidity leads to poorer health outcomes: it is associated with high mortality, reduced functional status and quality of life and increased use of inpatient and ambulatory health care [7, 8]. Research has identified that certain health care delivery interventions (e.g., enhanced multidisciplinary team care with structured visits) may improve health outcomes for older people with multimorbidity [9].

Chronic disease management is predominantly delivered using a traditional single disease model which means people with multimorbidity receive fragmented, inefficient and duplicate health care delivery [7, 8, 10]. There is therefore a need to develop new models of care to ensure integrated care for people with multimorbidity which is both effective and financially sustainable [3, 11]. A strong primary care health system is crucial to such integration and it is a central tenet of general practice care that it should be patient, not disease centred, and promote shared decision making [10, 12]. A recent

* Correspondence: tim.stokes@otago.ac.nz
[1]Department of General Practice and Rural Health, Dunedin School of Medicine, University of Otago, PO Box 56, Dunedin 9054, New Zealand
Full list of author information is available at the end of the article

qualitative synthesis of published studies exploring general practitioners (GPs') management of patients with multimorbidity found GPs faced a number of significant challenges delivering care to this group of which the disorganisation and fragmentation of health care, challenges in delivering patient centred care, inadequacy of clinical guidelines and barriers to shared decision making were key themes [13].

Multimorbidity research to date has largely been conducted in health systems outside of New Zealand (NZ). NZ has a strong first contact primary care health system (see Table 1). GPs are predominantly independent, self-employed providers with 50% of their funding coming from a capitated government-determined subsidy, paid through Primary Health Organisations (PHOs). The remainder of their funding comes from individual patient co-payments, which are set by each GP practice. The average patient co-payment for a GP consultation for an adult ranges from NZD15 to NZD45 (USD10–USD31) [14]. There is also a lower patient co-payment in general practices with "high needs"(>50% Māori; Pacific; lowest socioeconomic status) [15]. As with other similar health systems, the NZ health care system is struggling to cope with the rise in long term conditions as well as the increasing prevalence of multimorbidity [11, 16].

In 2004 the NZ Ministry of Health introduced *Care Plus*, an additional capitation based funding stream for primary care, which aims to "improve chronic care management, reduce inequalities, improve primary care teamwork and reduce the cost of services for high-need patients" [17–19]. *Care Plus* subsidises four extended consultations annually and its eligibility criteria [20] are presented in Table 2. A related payment stream is the provision of a High Use Health Card (HUHC), for which a patient must have received at least 12 health practitioner consultations within the last 12 months for a particular ongoing medical condition(s). *Care Plus* differs from the HUHC, however, in that it is intended to coordinate "a comprehensive approach to improve outcomes for people with chronic conditions, including lower cost access; whereas the HUHC is a subsidy approach tied to GP visits" [20]. The national *Care Plus* initiative has been complemented by regional health service initiatives. For example, in the Southern Health Region of NZ's South Island (Otago and Southland), the District Health Board (DHB) and PHO are working to further service integration through Alliance South [21], which is a contractual alliance between the two organisations aimed at improving care coordination and integration. Alliance South is developing a strategic health services plan in which better chronic disease management is a key priority [22]. If local health care services are to be redesigned to better meet the needs of patients living with multimorbidity then it is critical that this is informed by an understanding of the barriers and enablers to primary care's role in the management of such patients.

Table 1 The New Zealand Health System

New Zealand's 1938 Social Security Act was the world's first attempt to create a "national health service", but doctor resistance meant this was never achieved. A series of policy compromises mean that, today, public hospitals salary all staff and are free of patient charges. General Practitioners mostly practice privately and act as gatekeepers. They receive considerable government subsidies but charge most patients a fee per consultation, creating an access barrier [37]. There is a strong tradition of family practice and focus on primary care within the health system. Yet, the arrangements set down in the post-1938 compromise mean GPs and public hospitals work largely separately from one another. Government contributes around 80% of total health expenditure. Around 40% of public hospital specialists have a separate private practice. The parallel private system means patients of better means are able to circumvent public hospital waiting times when referred by their GP, or to access treatments considered to be lower priority in the constrained public sector [49].

Table 2 Eligibility criteria for Care Plus [20]

A general practice that is part of a PHO can enrol a patient in *Care Plus* if they are assessed by a doctor or nurse at the general practice as:

- being able to benefit from intensive clinical management in primary health care (at least 2 h of care from 1 or more members of the primary health care team over the following 6 months), and
- having 2 or more chronic health conditions, as long as each condition is one that:
- is a significant disability or has a significant burden of morbidity; and
- creates a significant cost to the health system; and
- has agreed and objective diagnostic criteria; and
- requires continuity of care and where a primary health care team approach has an important role in management; or
- requiring intensive clinical care because they:
- have a terminal illness (defined as someone who has advanced, progressive disease whose death is likely within 12 months); or
- have had 2 acute medical or mental health-related hospital admissions in the past 12 months (excluding surgical admissions); or
- have had 6 first-level service or similar primary health care visits in the past 12 months (including emergency department visits); or
- are on active review for elective services.

In this context, this study aimed to explore primary care professionals' - GP and primary care nurses (PCNs) (practice nurses and nurse practitioners) - accounts of managing multimorbidity in one NZ health region and the impact of this on clinical decision making and health care delivery.

Methods

Design and sampling

Semi-structured interviews were conducted between May and November 2015 with GPs and PCNs working in general practices throughout the Otago region. Otago, in the south of NZ's South Island, is the second-largest NZ region in terms of land area. It has a population of 202,467 (2013 NZ Census), being 4.8% of NZ's population

[23]. The city of Dunedin on the east coast is the regional centre. Otago overall has a much lower proportion of Māori (2.4%) than NZ as a whole (14.9%) [23] although it has areas with high Māori and Pasifika populations (e.g., South Dunedin). GPs and PCNs were sampled purposively in order to construct a maximum variation sample that reflected practice characteristics - such as number of GPs, level of deprivation and location (urban and rural) – that are related to practice organisation and chronic disease and multimorbidity prevalence [6].

Data collection

The interviews used a topic guide based on a literature review and discussions within the research team. The topic guide (see Additional file 1) covered: a) the organisation of local health care services and possible funding models for people with single conditions and multimorbidity; b) clinical management by GPs and PCNs (this was explored through participants describing situations where care for multimorbid patients was considered to have been delivered both well and poorly). The topic guide was used flexibly to allow participants to construct their accounts in their own terms, and was revised and refined throughout the interviewing process to reflect themes emerging from the concurrent data analysis. All interviews were digitally-recorded and transcribed verbatim.

Data analysis

A thematic analysis was conducted using the constant comparative method [24, 25]. A coding framework was developed from the initial interviews by ET, TS and FDN. Through an iterative process involving comparison across the transcripts, assisted by NVivo 10 qualitative analysis software, these descriptive codes were organized by ET into higher order thematic categories. TS and FDN independently assessed the plausibility and explanatory value of the categories against the transcripts, and also independently evaluated the assignment of a sample of the data to the categories. A reflexive diary of the analysis was maintained. This provided an 'audit trail' of the development of the framework and its categories and also promoted reflexive research practice. The consolidated criteria for reporting qualitative research (COREQ) (See Additional file 2) [26] were used to inform reporting of the findings.

Results

Twelve GPs and four PCNs were interviewed. All participants were involved in delivering chronic disease/long term condition management. The characteristics of participants and their general practices are shown in Table 3. Participants showed wide variation in terms of their personal characteristics and practice demography.

Table 3 Characteristics of GP and Primary Care Nurse (PCN) participants ($N = 16$) and of general practice demographics ($N = 15$)

Category	Participants, *n* (%)
GP and PCN participants	*16 (100)*
Profession:	
General Practitioner (GP)	12 (75)
Primary care Nurse (PCN)[a]	4 (25)
Sex:	
Female	7 (44)
Male	9 (56)
Ethnicity:	
New Zealand European	11 (69)
Other (including: Asian, Other European, African, etc.)[b]	5 (31)
Years in clinical practice:	
0–5 years	1 (6)
6–10 years	3 (19)
11–20 years	3 (19)
20 years +	9 (56)
General Practice demographics[c]	*15 (100)*
Practice Size:	
1–4 GPs	6 (40)
5–9 GPs	4 (27)
10+ GPs	5 (33)
Practice Location:	
Urban	9 (60)
Rural	6 (40)
Practice location New Zealand Deprivation Index	
1–3	4 (27)
4–7	10 (67)
8+	1 (6)

[a]Specific roles were: three nurses were based in general practice: nurse practitioner (1), practice nurse (2) and one was based in the relevant primary health organisation
[b]Non-New Zealand European categories were conflated to ensure participant anonymity
[c]One participant did not currently work in a general practice but within another local health organisation (primary health organisation)

We report here the themes that emerged from the interviews in terms of clinical decision making and health care delivery for patients with multimorbidity. Illustrative participant quotes are presented.

Clinical decision making

Complexity

All participants reported that lack of time within the NZ 15 min general practice consultation "standard" appointment length was an issue in terms of not only addressing a multimorbid patient's health needs, but also in communicating, prioritising, agreeing plans and endeavouring to get the patient engaged in self-management. Multimorbid patients were seen as complex:

That's a multi-morbidity, I can think of where there's a complex array of medical conditions which prevents that person from being able to cope alone at home, bringing on confusion with the number of medications that the person is on, and so on and so forth. It's like a big waterfall. (Participant 1 GP)

This complexity caused difficulty in managing care for patients with multimorbidity based on number of items on the patients' agenda to be addressed in the time available:

It's like people come in with their shopping list and they want a repeat of their 15 different interacting medications for their 6 six different pathologies. (...) (Participant 6 GP)

Further difficulty was experienced in trying to both negotiate with patients over their priorities and the ones the participants felt needed to be addressed that day. There was evidence of "safety netting" by participants, where GPs incorporate issues they felt needed attention in a consultation even if these were not a patient priority:

I think often they've got their agenda of what they want to talk about. You've got your idea that, okay, you want your prescriptions, but I also have to check a number of other things. Trying to focus on what they've actually come in for, which may not be the most urgent thing but is obviously the thing that's worrying them the most, and picking at there's nothing particularly dangerous that you're missing like the ones who at the end of the consult say, "Oh by the way, I've been having chest pain for the last six weeks." (Participant 2 GP)

While participants noted that the use of "catch up" time in the middle of their standard booked clinics allowed some flexibility to spend more time on individual patients this was constrained by financial cost (see health care delivery theme). Time limitations caused stress to both doctors and patients through regularly running behind time. In addition, participants mentioned patients changing GPs to see a doctor they perceived as giving patients more time could be stressful as this behaviour was noted to have wider ramifications:

Then of course you make a rod for your own back because I think by giving people more time and addressing more problems than you should, word gets around, people change to you because a friend recommends you. I've even had people change from doctors within the practice saying that they don't like Dr. So-and-So because he's always in such a hurry and so brusque and efficient, and your heart just sinks because you think, well yes, I will try and do a good job and give more time, but that comes at a cost to me and to my other patients, so you run later and later. (Participant 9 GP)

Inadequacy of single disease guidelines

Participants expressed concern about the use of clinical practice guidelines for people with multimorbidity, which are generally developed for single clinical conditions. They were felt as adding to the complexity of managing multimorbidity through the difficulty in applying multiple guidelines in a single patient:

Whereas if you have got one person with diabetes, it's fairly straightforward to follow the guidelines. People with multiple conditions, there are guidelines for each of them, and it's impossible..., it's not beneficial to the patient to stick to 4 guidelines for 4 conditions (Participant 7 GP).

Addressing clinical decision making in multimorbidity: "satisficing" and relational continuity of care

Participants reported two main strategies they used to address the problems of clinical decision making with a patient with multimorbidity: "satisficing" and relational continuity of care.

The first strategy, used in a single consultation, was that of squaring the need to deliver optimal disease management and patient-centred care in a time-limited consultation. This strategy, termed "satisficing", can be defined as "settling for chronic disease management that was satisfactory and sufficient, given the particular circumstances of that patient" [27]. One commonly used approach was that of relaxing treatment targets to below those recommended by clinical guidelines:

I think, not perfectly managed, but managed well enough within that person's individual parameters. (Participant 6 GP)

Another approach was to negotiate a compromise with the patient over which aspects of a recommended management plan needed to be adhered to:

I think it comes down to agreed management plan and I think that's really the point. There's some things you're going to agree and some things you don't. I think that's probably the point. It's an agreed management system, which is again why the imposition of targets and the imposition of a certain way of doing chronic disease management doesn't work. (Participant 4 GP)

When the patient's multiple conditions were viewed as stable the emphasis from GPs was that this stability should be maintained, rather than constantly strive to implement guideline recommendations:

So, although, in an ideal world I would say he should lose 20 kg and be completely pain-free from his back problems and not take any painkillers and not take this group of several medications that he's on, I think it's not a bad situation in that we're managing it and it's stable and relatively well-managed. (Participant 9 GP)

The second strategy participants used was to harness the longitudinal nature of the patient-primary care practitioner encounter through the provision of relational (personal) continuity of care ("an ongoing therapeutic relationship between a patient and one or more providers") [28]. This was the predominant approach used by participants and allowed GPs to both establish an ongoing personal relationship with patients and to ensure problems identified but not addressed in a first consultation were dealt with at subsequent consultations. Thus, GPs would address the time limitations of the single consultation by negotiating a subsequent consultation, employing an "additive-sequential" [29] approach to clinical decision making:

Sometimes if they've got a whole list of things you have to just sort of divide the list up and say, "Look, we'll do this today and maybe we can, we need to do something about these things, but then you can come back and we'll do the other thing," (Participant 2 GP)

Over the course of a year, 3 or 4 follow up appointments with the same GP allowed these ongoing issues to be addressed sequentially:

... with the people with multimorbidity you see frequently it's not just one 15 min time slot, it's just carrying on from where you left off last time. You build and build and build on that. In the year, you've had an hour and probably more. (Participant 6 GP)

The use of relational continuity of care as a tool to address multimorbidity was not limited to GPs. PCNs stated that they had longer consultation time with patients than GPs which provided space to get to know patients and helped initiate and reinforce self-management behaviour in the long term management of a patient's condition:

I work kind of half hour appointment. I aim for the first 10 min to be the patient introduction ... you know let them talk about whatever they would like to talk about and then I would bring it round to the last 20 min to hone in on specifically what I would like, tied in with what they would like. But I do have a lot of time with my patients and that's [how] you know I get to know them, what they've been up to, has anything happened in their lives recently, what are they worried about, you know, "how is the pet?. So we cover the social aspect and we just gently move around to the diabetes side of things (Participant 8 PCN)

Like GPs, one way they achieved this was to utilise multiple consultations to allow this advice to be delivered sequentially over time:

It's repeating the message, but repeating it in different ways. Sometimes I'll dwell on the medication management, other times I might dwell on their lab results, another time ... well I always talk about the lifestyle really. Just putting the stress on different things and finding out what clicks to people. Trying to find something that's sort of like, you know what it's like yourself. People can tell you the same thing but in one day someone will say it slightly different and you think oh! (Participant 3 PCN)

Although relational continuity of care was the predominant approach utilised, one participant noted that patients in their practice were increasingly seeing several GPs in their practice as the GPs were all part-time and s/he that noted management continuity of care ("a consistent and coherent approach to the management of a health condition that is responsive to a patient's changing needs") [28] was becoming more important for their patients with multimorbidity.

Health care delivery

Primary care funding model

Participants felt that the current mixed capitation/co-payment model of NZ primary care was a barrier to the delivery care for patients with multimorbidity. The current level of capitation funding was considered too low and the 50/50 split between capitation and co-payments created a particular challenge for NZ primary care:

I think New Zealand is in many ways the most difficult [setting to practise GP] because you have two customers scrapping for the same amount of time thinking that they're your exclusive customer. You've got the funding from the ministry of health through the PHOs ... [who] are not going to pay you if you don't tick [their] boxes. You've got your patient with their A3 list, and both of them want 20 min at least of the 15 min appointment. There's 40 min. Two customers fighting for the same time window. (Participant 16 GP)

The need for patient co-payment was also identified by participants as a specific barrier to the employment of the "additive-sequential" approach to clinical decision making described above:

They [Patients] will say, "Oh, this, this, and this." I'll say, "Well look, we can deal with this and deal with this, but the other, that sounds really important and I don't want to dismiss it. You will need to make another appointment to come back." That's very difficult, because I'm very aware that we charge [NZD] $39 for a consultation. I am very aware that a significant number of people in our area, that's a big portion of the money that they're getting that week. It's not easy. It's not easy to do that. (Participant 10 GP)

Use of Care Plus

Participants reported that *Care Plus* funding was used flexibly and in three broad ways by general practices to provide care for patients with multimorbidity. The funding could be used to subsidise GP visits only; visits with both GP and PCN; and visits to the PCN only. Within each of these approaches various ways of delivering consults with patients were described. The predominant model described was one of having one extended review appointment with a PCN (either a practice nurse or nurse practitioner) and then three subsidised appointments with the GP:

Once they've registered with a nurse they then are entitled to three appointments with the GP for [NZD] $15.50 and they can use that as they choose. It has to be about their medical problem. (Participant 8 PCN)

One participant described their general practice utilising a specific PCN-led *Care Plus* scheme in which relational continuity of care was encouraged:

We've identified people in our practice who qualify under the Care Plus funding scheme or the High User Health Card, to have regular input free of charge to them. We use that money, we don't charge our patients and they get two hours of free nursing time a year. Usually in four half an hour visits, but we can tailor it to the individual needs. And they are assigned a specific nurse. We have a care plan screening questionnaire, a good assessment of them, where they're at and what their needs are and what help they've got. And the nurse assigned to that particular patient, the idea is that we build a relationship with them and if they have a hospital admission or their spouse has a hospital admission or one of them is ill, or the circumstances change, or just to support people better. (Participant 3 PCN)

This model, however, was not typical and other participants described resistance from individual GPs for shifting regular ("three monthly") reviews from GPs to PCNs for this group of patients.

There was no consensus among participants as to whether *Care Plus* had actually improved care for patients with multimorbidity. Two problems were identified. Firstly, it was seen as an "add on" capitation funding stream to subsidise a limited number (4) of consultations in "high needs" patients. In itself it was considered inadequate to allow a reorganisation of how NZ general practice delivers chronic disease management:

What we've been trying to do for years is actually use the Care Plus funding in some way, which is actually quite difficult, as you're probably aware .... rather than [it] just be ... an extra on top of people's care, to actually to use it to fund chronic disease management per se and to pull that in as a funding element for a new system ... But it didn't work, A) because that's an enormous task, and we didn't have the resources and the ability to do that, B) there was no direct funding for that [chronic disease management] (Participant 4 GP)

Secondly, participants considered that the *Care Plus* eligibility criteria meant that not all patients who met the criteria had complex health needs. It was not consistently delivered to patients with complex health needs (e.g., multiple long term conditions and polypharmacy) as defined in Ministry of Health guidance: [17]

Care Plus is a pretty crude tool. You only need two long-term health conditions. It could be hypothyroidism and hypertension, you know, pretty straightforward conditions, really, so you get these people who are basically well, coming in every three months for their pills, and then people with eight conditions, who really need it. (Participant 10 GP)

Participants also considered that some patients simply used *Care Plus* as a way to get their individual quota of subsidised annual appointments irrespective of clinical need to consult their GP more frequently. In other words, Care Plus was seen as a barrier to persuading patients to come back for another appointment, where a consultation had proven insufficient, because patients knew they had another subsidised appointment scheduled in three months' time:

For example, if I say, "Come back in two weeks to get your blood pressure checked," it's quite likely that they will just wait until the next routine visit, when their pills are running out, and then once again they'll use a Care Plus visit and get it cheaper. (Participant 9 GP)

Fragmentation of health care provision

Fragmentation of health care was identified by participants as occurring both within NZ general practice and across the primary/secondary care interface. Within the primary care team participants noted that there had been a development of PCN-led single disease management clinics however this had to date not addressed multimorbidity:

> *We had a blood pressure clinic and you [practice nurse] did your blood pressure. The respiratory clinic, and you did your respiratory, and so on. You only did a little bit of this, that, and the other. You didn't see the whole picture. (Participant 13 PCN)*

In order to develop a general practice team-based patient-centric model of care for people with multimorbidity participants noted that there was a need to fully implement chronic disease management models in primary care, something which required a culture shift:

> *I think the concept of chronic disease management is a laudable prospect that should be delivered in primary care should be supported. I think rolling more of those ancillary services that are really designed for chronic disease management ... needs to come into that area [primary care] ... we need a philosophical shift as well.." (Participant 4 GP)*
>
> *I think it's actually early days in the whole scheme of it [chronic disease management] - at the moment [we are] trying to change the culture of the separate conditions. (Participant 13 PCN)*

Participants described fragmentation across primary and secondary care as systemic and pervasive and the result of a model that was outdated in relation to the context it applied in (i.e., an ageing population with increasing prevalence of long-term conditions/chronic disease and multimorbidity). This fragmentation was seen as institutional, caused by the disconnect between primary and secondary care:

> *The trouble is at the moment there's no viable model about sharing which would allow us to proceed and obviously because we've got two different kinds of systems and not really kind of integrated so it's a difficult one. (...) The trouble is that specialist medicine doesn't appreciate a shared model of care really. (Participant 12 GP)*

Participants were keen to see secondary care and primary care working more closely together and emphasised the need for better communication. Reference was made to recent initiatives such as shared computer records, electronic patient referral systems and telehealth as promoting better integration, but no specific examples were given as to where these initiatives had improved the care of patients with multimorbidity in the NZ health system either nationally or locally.

Discussion

Statement of principal findings

This is the first NZ-based study to specifically explore primary care professional accounts of managing multimorbidity and its impact on clinical decision making and health delivery. Primary care professionals (GPs and PCNs) encountered challenges in providing care to patients with multimorbidity with respect to both clinical decision making and health care delivery. Clinical decision making occurred in time-limited consultations where the challenges of complexity and inadequacy of single disease guidelines were managed through the use of "satisficing" (care deemed satisfactory and sufficient for a given patient) and sequential consultations utilising relational continuity of care. The NZ primary care co-payment funding model was seen as a barrier to the delivery of care as it discourages sequential consultations, a problem only partially addressed through the use of the additional capitation based funding stream of *Care Plus.* Fragmentation of care also occurred within general practice in relation to the distribution of care between health professional roles, as well as across the primary/secondary care interface. This latter fragmentation was due in part to a lack of system supported relationships between primary and secondary care and good communication processes (e.g., shared information systems).

Strengths and limitations

This qualitative interview study utilised purposive sampling to enable a maximum variation sample in terms of characteristics of participants (sex, ethnicity and years in practice) and general practice demographics (practice size, location and level of socioeconomic deprivation). The choice of individual interviews was appropriate as we wished to focus both on individual clinical decision making and health care delivery issues: an approach utilised in similar research studies in the UK [29, 30] and Ireland [27]. We chose to focus on one NZ health region (Otago) as this work was intended to inform Southern Health Region health service development for people with multimorbidity and it was also a requirement of the research funder that the work was conducted in this region. The inclusion of both GPs and PCNs meant that we were able to gain insight into the varying ways their roles are enacted in different practice settings to manage multi-morbidity. We were able to recruit a maximum variation GP sample and achieve data saturation (no new emergent themes) for the GP interviews. Furthermore, the interviews and emergent themes were subject to ongoing discussion and refinement within the research team and we consider our results are conceptually (theoretically) generalizable [31].

It is accepted, however, that those who participated are likely to have a greater interest in the subject matter than those who declined to participate. In addition, we were not able to recruit any primary care professionals who were Māori or Pasifika. More generally, the choice to conduct this study in one defined geographical region limits the ability to fully explore potential variation in health care delivery for this group across NZ. While we had not set a fixed number of planned interviews for both GPs and PCN interviews we had difficulty recruiting PCNs and only managed to interview 4 in total. We do not consider we were able to fully explore PCN accounts of managing multimorbidity and further NZ research is required here. It is also important to note that in conducting interviews we collected situated accounts [31] from health care professionals, thus we have described what people say they do, not what they necessarily did. Finally, the accounts are from the health care professionals only and as such provide no information regarding the patient's perspective of care when managing multimorbidity. In other health systems, a key finding in a recent review of the patient experience literature on multimorbidity is lack of holistic care [32].

Comparison with existing literature

There is a limited NZ research literature on managing multimorbidity in primary care [33–35] and none addresses the specific aims of this study. The findings reported in the *clinical decision making* theme are, however, consistent with the challenges of managing multimorbidity reported by general practitioners [13, 27] and PCNs [30, 36] working in similar first contact primary care health systems. Specifically, a meta-ethnography (qualitative synthesis) of the research literature up to 2012 identified three areas of difficulty which are also described here: inadequacy of guidelines and evidence-based medicine, challenges in delivering patient-centred care and barriers to shared decision making [13]. In our study we specifically report an inadequacy of single disease guidelines theme and consider challenges relating to shared decision making across several of the other reported themes, notably the "complexity" theme. The concept of "satisficing", which was one of the two main strategies participants used to address the problems of clinical decision making was first used in the multimorbidity literature by Sinnott and colleagues in their qualitative study of Irish GPs and prescribing in multimorbidity [27]. In terms of the second strategy, relational continuity of care ("an ongoing therapeutic relationship between a patient and one or more providers") [28] has also been identified as being perhaps the most important facilitator of care in multimorbidity in primary care. Relational continuity of care allows primary care practitioners to "foster trust, anticipate preferences and empower their patients over time" [13].

It is in the *health care delivery* theme that NZ health system specific barriers and facilitators are reported. Thus while the NZ primary care professionals, like their UK equivalent, used the "additive-sequential" clinical decision making approach [29] they faced an additional issue not encountered in the UK: the NZ co-payment model. This co-payment model means that patients encounter a financial barrier to see their primary care practitioner for repeated consultations. Inability to access primary care in NZ due to financial barriers is widely reported in the NZ health literature. For example, in a 2009 NZ national survey [37] 15.5% of respondents reported that they had deferred seeing their doctor/s at least once during the preceding 12 months, because they could not afford the cost of a visit and the presence of more than two co-morbid diseases was independently associated with increased odds of deferring doctors' visits. This finding is also consistent with a recent Commonwealth Fund Survey, where NZ was rated third worst (behind Switzerland and US) of 11 countries for adults going without needed health care because of costs [38].

Internationally, the most common model of chronic disease/long term condition management that underpins models of multimorbidity care, including NZ's *Care Plus* [17] is Wagner's chronic care model [39–41]. One key aspect of this model, the core approach of NZ's *Care Plus* - that of enabling delivery of extended appointments to people with multimorbidity – has also been used in other health systems [41] and is a key component of an ongoing Scottish multimorbidity complex intervention evaluation [42]. NZ *Care Plus* has, however, not been the subject of an independent evaluation of its effectiveness or cost effectiveness in spite of it being in operation since 2004. To date, its evaluation has been local (North Island PHO) and has focussed on exploring primary care practitioners' perceptions [43]. Our final finding, that of fragmentation of care, is also reported in the international literature [13]. The NZ health system, including the Southern Health region, [44] compares unfavourably with other health systems in terms of the degree of care fragmentation [11, 45].

Implications for clinical practice, health policy and research

The NZ GPs and PCNs in this study utilised a clinical decision making approach for patients with multimorbidity consistent with that used in other health systems with strong primary care: [10] that of "satisficing" [27] and relational continuity of care (delivered through an "additive-sequential" [29] model of consecutive consultations). It therefore adds to the evidence base on how primary care practitioners make clinical decisions for this group of patients and also suggests that recent evidence-based guidance on the clinical management of multimorbidity developed by the National Institute for Health and Care Excellence (NICE) for the UK National Health Service is likely to be generalizable to, and therefore implementable in, NZ primary care [46].

This study has also identified three key barriers to the delivery of health care to patients with multimorbidity in NZ: the primary care funding model, the variable interpretation and implementation of the *Care Plus* scheme by NZ general practices and the fragmentation of health care within general practices and across the health system. While all three elements will need to be addressed by NZ health policy makers if NZ is to have an equitable and integrated health care system there is a clear opportunity to review and revise *Care Plus* so it better meets its stated objectives in relation to long term conditions [17]. A key finding from this study is that simply focussing on "adding on" additional capitation for patients with multimorbidity without addressing the need to redesign primary and secondary health care delivery around their health needs [9] may lead to little or no health gain. One way forward would be to develop a more structured approach to *Care Plus* that specifically ensures it addresses all components of chronic disease management [39] – key elements will be a clear operational definition of who is eligible for the scheme, sufficient funding of extended and review consultations (so enabling relational continuity of care), training and support for general practices to deliver a structured approach to identifying patients' priorities for care and supporting patient self management. It will also be important to develop a model that is responsive to the range of health and social care needs of people with multimorbidity and recognises the high prevalence of multimorbidity in the population, as opposed to only focussing on the smaller group of patients with complex health care needs (e.g., frail elderly at risk of repeated readmission to hospital) [47]. Finally, there is an important need for NZ health research funders to commission independent research to evaluate at a national level the effectiveness and cost effectiveness of this revised *Care Plus* model of care delivery compared to usual care – as has been recommended [46] and commissioned [48] in other comparable health systems.

Conclusions

This study highlights specific New Zealand barriers to the delivery of primary care to patients living with multimorbidity: primary care professionals encounter challenges in providing care to patients with multimorbidity with respect to both clinical decision making and health care delivery. A key finding is that the New Zealand primary care co-payment funding model is seen as a barrier to the delivery of care as it discourages sequential consultations, a problem only partially addressed through the use of the additional capitation based funding stream of *Care Plus*. There is a need to develop, implement and nationally evaluate a revised version of *Care Plus* that takes account of these barriers.

Abbreviations

DHB: District health board; GP: General practitioner; HUHC: High user health card; NZ: New Zealand; PCN: Primary care nurse; PHO: Primary Health Organisation

Acknowledgements

The authors would like to thank Wellsouth Primary Healthcare Organisation (PHO), Healthcare Otago Charitable Trust and the GPs and PCNs who gave their time for interviews.

Funding

Healthcare Otago Charitable Trust.

Authors' contributions

TS conceived and designed the study with input from FDN and RG. ET conducted the GP and practice nurse interviews and led on the data analysis with input from TS and FDN. TS drafted the manuscript. All authors read, provided critical review and approved the final manuscript.

Competing interests

The authors declare that they have no competing interests.

Author details

[1]Department of General Practice and Rural Health, Dunedin School of Medicine, University of Otago, PO Box 56, Dunedin 9054, New Zealand. [2]Otago Business School, University of Otago, Dunedin, New Zealand.

References

1. Valderas JM, Starfield B, Sibbald B, Salisbury C, Roland M. Defining comorbidity: implications for understanding health and health services. Ann Fam Med. 2009;7(4):357–63.
2. Mangin D, Heath I, Jamoulle M. Beyond diagnosis: rising to the multimorbidity challenge. BMJ. 2012;344:e3526.
3. Goodwin N, Dixon A, Anderson GF, Wodchis W. Providing integrated care for older people with complex needs Lessons from seven international case studies. London: King's Fund; 2014. (http://www.kingsfund.org.uk/publications/providing-integrated-care-older-people-complex-needs). Accessed 22 February 2017.
4. Mercer SW, Smith SM, Wyke S, O'Dowd T, Watt GC. Multimorbidity in primary care: developing the research agenda. Fam Pract. 2009;26(2):79–80.
5. Violan C, Foguet-Boreu Q, Flores-Mateo G, Salisbury C, Blom J, Freitag M, Glynn L, Muth C, Valderas JM. Prevalence, determinants and patterns of multimorbidity in primary care: a systematic review of observational studies. PLoS One. 2014;9(7):e102149.
6. Barnett K, Mercer SW, Norbury M, Watt G, Wyke S, Guthrie B. Epidemiology of multimorbidity and implications for health care, research, and medical education: a cross-sectional study. Lancet. 2012;380(9836):37–43.
7. Wolff JL, Starfield B, Anderson G. Prevalence, expenditures, and complications of multiple chronic conditions in the elderly. Arch Intern Med. 2002;162(20):2269–76.
8. Salisbury C, Johnson L, Purdy S, Valderas JM, Montgomery AA. Epidemiology and impact of multimorbidity in primary care: a retrospective cohort study. Br J Gen Pract. 2011;61(582):e12–21.

9. Smith SM, Wallace E, O'Dowd T, Fortin M. Interventions for improving outcomes in patients with multimorbidity in primary care and community settings. Cochrane Database Syst Rev. 2016;3:CD006560.
10. Starfield B, Shi L, Macinko J. Contribution of primary care to health systems and health. Milbank Q. 2005;83(3):457–502.
11. Mays N: Reorienting the New Zealand health care system to meet the challenge of long-term conditions in a fiscally constrained environment. In: Paper prepared for New Zealand Treasury Long-term Fiscal External Panel, November 2012, and Chair of Public Finance, Victoria University of Wellington and New Zealand Treasury conference, Affording our Future, Wellington, 10-11 December 2013. (http://www.hiirc.org.nz/page/37816). Accessed 22 February 2017.
12. McWhinney IR, Freeman T. Textbook of Family Medicine. New York: Oxford University Press, Inc; 2009.
13. Sinnott C, Mc Hugh S, Browne J, Bradley C. GPs' perspectives on the management of patients with multimorbidity: systematic review and synthesis of qualitative research. BMJ Open. 2013;3(9):e003610.
14. Gauld R. The New Zealand Health Care System. In: Mossialos E, Wenzl M, Osborn R, Sarnak D, editors. 2015 International Profiles of Health Care Systems. New York: Commonwealth Fund; 2016. (http://www.commonwealthfund.org/~/media/files/publications/fund-report/2016/jan/1857_mossialos_intl_profiles_2015_v7.pdf). Accessed 22 February 2017.
15. Ministry of Health (MoH). Very Low Cost Access Scheme (VLCA). Wellington: MoH; 2016. [http://www.health.govt.nz/our-work/primary-health-care/primary-health-care-subsidies-and-services/very-low-cost-access-scheme]. Accessed 22 February 2017.
16. Carryer J, Doolan-Noble F, Gauld R, Budge C. New Zealand patients' perceptions of chronic care delivery. J Integr Care. 2014;22(2):71–80.
17. Ministry of Health. Care Plus: An Overview. Wellington: MoH; 2004. (http://www.health.govt.nz/publication/care-plus-overview). Accessed 22 February 2017.
18. CBG Health Research Limited. Care Plus Formative Report Prepared for Ministry of Health. Wellington: MoH; 2003. (http://www.health.govt.nz/our-work/primary-health-care/research-and-evaluation-primary-health-care-initiatives#eval-careplus). Accessed 22 February 2017.
19. CBG Health Research Limited. Care Plus Process Report Prepared for Ministry of Health. Wellington: MoH; 2004. (http://www.health.govt.nz/our-work/primary-health-care/research-and-evaluation-primary-health-care-initiatives#eval-careplus). Accessed 22 February 2017.
20. Ministry of Health. Eligibility for Care Plus. Wellington: MoH; 2015. (http://www.health.govt.nz/our-work/primary-health-care/primary-health-care-subsidies-and-services/care-plus). Accessed 22 February 2017.
21. Gauld R. What should governance for integrated care look like? New Zealand's alliances provide some pointers. Med J Aust. 2014;201(3 Suppl):S67–68.
22. Southern District Health Board. Southern Strategic Health Plan Piki te Ora. Dunedin: Southern District Health Board; 2015. (http://www.southerndhb.govt.nz/pages/sshp/). Accessed 22 February 2017.
23. 2013 New Zealand Census QuickStats about a place: Otago Region (http://www.stats.govt.nz/Census/2013-census/profile-and-summary-reports). Accessed 22 February 2017.
24. Braun V, Clarke V. Using thematic analysis in psychology. Qual Res Psychol. 2006;3(2):77–101.
25. Glaser BG. The constant comparative method of analysis. Soc Probl. 1965;12:436–45.
26. Tong A, Sainsbury P, Craig J. Consolidated criteria for reporting qualitative research (COREQ): a 32-item checklist for interviews and focus groups. Int J Qual Health Care. 2007;19(6):349–57.
27. Sinnott C, Hugh SM, Boyce MB, Bradley CP. What to give the patient who has everything? A qualitative study of prescribing for multimorbidity in primary care. Br J Gen Pract. 2015;65(632):e184–191.
28. Haggerty JL, Reid RJ, Freeman GK, Starfield BH, Adair CE, McKendry R. Continuity of care: a multidisciplinary review. BMJ. 2003;327(7425):1219–21.
29. Bower P, Macdonald W, Harkness E, Gask L, Kendrick T, Valderas JM, Dickens C, Blakeman T, Sibbald B. Multimorbidity, service organization and clinical decision making in primary care: a qualitative study. Fam Pract. 2011;28(5):579–87.
30. O'Brien R, Wyke S, Guthrie B, Watt G, Mercer S. An 'endless struggle': a qualitative study of general practitioners' and practice nurses' experiences of managing multimorbidity in socio-economically deprived areas of Scotland. Chronic Illn. 2011;7(1):45–59.
31. Murphy E, Dingwall R, Greatbatch D, Parker S, Watson P. Qualitative research methods in health technology assessment: a review of the literature. Health Technol Assess. 1998;2(16):iii–ix. 1-274.
32. Van der Aa M, Van den Broeke JR, Stronks K, Ploch T. Patients with multimorbidity and their experiences with the healthcare process: a scoping review. J Comorbidity. 2017;7(1):11–21.
33. Doolan-Noble F, Gauld R, Waters DL. Are nurses more likely to report providing care plans for chronic disease patients than doctors? Findings from a New Zealand study. Chronic Illn. 2015;11(3):210–7.
34. Ailabouni NJ, Nishtala PS, Mangin D, Tordoff JM. General practitioners' insight into deprescribing for the multimorbid older individual: a qualitative study. Int J Clin Pract. 2016;70(3):261–76.
35. McKinlay E, Graham S, Horrill P. Culturally and linguistically diverse patients' views of multimorbidity and general practice care. J Prim Health Care. 2015;7(3):228–35.
36. Jowsey T, Jeon YH, Dugdale P, Glasgow NJ, Kljakovic M, Usherwood T. Challenges for co-morbid chronic illness care and policy in Australia: a qualitative study. Aust N Z Health Policy. 2009;6:22.
37. Jatrana S, Crampton P. Primary health care in New Zealand: who has access? Health Policy. 2009;93(1):1–10.
38. Osborn R, Squires D, Doty MM, Sarnak DO, Schneider EC. In New Survey Of Eleven Countries, US Adults Still Struggle With Access To And Affordability Of Health Care. Health Aff. 2016;35(12):2327–36.
39. Wagner EH, Austin BT, Von Korff M. Organizing care for patients with chronic illness. Milbank Q. 1996;74(4):511–44.
40. Bodenheimer T, Wagner EH, Grumbach K. Improving primary care for patients with chronic illness: the chronic care model, Part 2. JAMA. 2002; 288(15):1909–14.
41. Stokes J, Man, MS., Bower, P., Guthrie, B., Mercer, C., Salisbury, C. : Models of Primary Care for Chronic Conditions and Multimorbidity: Comparing current approaches North American Primary Research Group (NAPCRG). Colorado Springs; 2016. (http://www.napcrg.org/Conferences/PastMeetingArchives/2016AnnualMeetingArchives). Accessed 22 February 2017.
42. Mercer SW, Fitzpatrick B, Guthrie B, Fenwick E, Grieve E, Lawson K, Boyer N, McConnachie A, Lloyd SM, O'Brien R, et al. The CARE Plus study - a whole-system intervention to improve quality of life of primary care patients with multimorbidity in areas of high socioeconomic deprivation: exploratory cluster randomised controlled trial and cost-utility analysis. BMC Med. 2016;14(1):88.
43. Eggleton K, Kenealy T. What makes Care Plus effective in a provincial Primary Health Organisation? Perceptions of primary care workers. J Prim Health Care. 2009;1(3):190–7.
44. Doolan-Noble F, Gauld R, Walters DL, de la Barra SL. New Zealand health professional and patient perceptions of chronic illness care. Eur J Person Centered Healthc. 2015;3(1):4–10.
45. Ham C. The ten characteristics of the high-performing chronic care system. Health Econ Policy Law. 2010;5(Pt 1):71–90.
46. National Guidelines Centre. Multimorbidity: clinical assessment and management [NICE Clinical Guideline NG56]. London: National Guidelines Centre on behalf of the National Institute for Health and Care Excellence (NICE); 2016. (https://www.nice.org.uk/guidance/ng56/evidence/full-guideline-2615543103). Accessed 22 February 2017.
47. Ministry of Health. Self-management Support for People with Long-term Conditions. 2nd ed. Wellington: Ministry of Health; 2016. (http://www.health.govt.nz/publication/self-management-support-people-long-term-conditions). Accessed 22 February 2017.
48. Mann C, Shaw A, Guthrie B, Wye L, Man MS, Hollinghurst S, Brookes S, Bower P, Mercer S, Salisbury C. Protocol for a process evaluation of a cluster randomised controlled trial to improve management of multimorbidity in general practice: the 3D study. BMJ Open. 2016;6(5):e011260.
49. Gauld R. Questions about New Zealand's health system in 2013, its 75th anniversary year. N Z Med J. 2013;126(1380):68–74.

Permissions

All chapters in this book were first published in FP, by BioMed Central; hereby published with permission under the Creative Commons Attribution License or equivalent. Every chapter published in this book has been scrutinized by our experts. Their significance has been extensively debated. The topics covered herein carry significant findings which will fuel the growth of the discipline. They may even be implemented as practical applications or may be referred to as a beginning point for another development.

The contributors of this book come from diverse backgrounds, making this book a truly international effort. This book will bring forth new frontiers with its revolutionizing research information and detailed analysis of the nascent developments around the world.

We would like to thank all the contributing authors for lending their expertise to make the book truly unique. They have played a crucial role in the development of this book. Without their invaluable contributions this book wouldn't have been possible. They have made vital efforts to compile up to date information on the varied aspects of this subject to make this book a valuable addition to the collection of many professionals and students.

This book was conceptualized with the vision of imparting up-to-date information and advanced data in this field. To ensure the same, a matchless editorial board was set up. Every individual on the board went through rigorous rounds of assessment to prove their worth. After which they invested a large part of their time researching and compiling the most relevant data for our readers.

The editorial board has been involved in producing this book since its inception. They have spent rigorous hours researching and exploring the diverse topics which have resulted in the successful publishing of this book. They have passed on their knowledge of decades through this book. To expedite this challenging task, the publisher supported the team at every step. A small team of assistant editors was also appointed to further simplify the editing procedure and attain best results for the readers.

Apart from the editorial board, the designing team has also invested a significant amount of their time in understanding the subject and creating the most relevant covers. They scrutinized every image to scout for the most suitable representation of the subject and create an appropriate cover for the book.

The publishing team has been an ardent support to the editorial, designing and production team. Their endless efforts to recruit the best for this project, has resulted in the accomplishment of this book. They are a veteran in the field of academics and their pool of knowledge is as vast as their experience in printing. Their expertise and guidance has proved useful at every step. Their uncompromising quality standards have made this book an exceptional effort. Their encouragement from time to time has been an inspiration for everyone.

The publisher and the editorial board hope that this book will prove to be a valuable piece of knowledge for researchers, students, practitioners and scholars across the globe.

List of Contributors

Agnès Oude Engberink
Department of General Medicine, University of Montpellier, Montpellier, France CEPS Platform, University of Montpellier, Montpellier, France
Epsylon EA4556, Dynamic of Human Abilities and Health Behaviors, University of Montpellier, Montpellier, France
Centre de Médecine Générale, 2 rue IBN Sinai dit AVICENNE, Cabestany 66330, France

Grégory Ninot
CEPS Platform, University of Montpellier, Montpellier, France
Epsylon EA4556, Dynamic of Human Abilities and Health Behaviors, University of Montpellier, Montpellier, France
SIRIC Montpellier Cancer, Institut Régional du Cancer de Montpellier (ICM), Montpellier, France

Pierre Senesse
Epsylon EA4556, Dynamic of Human Abilities and Health Behaviors, University of Montpellier, Montpellier, France
SIRIC Montpellier Cancer, Institut Régional du Cancer de Montpellier (ICM), Montpellier, France
Department of Clinical Nutrition and Gastroenterology and supportive Care, Institut Régional du Cancer de Montpellier (ICM), Montpellier, France

Joanna Norton
Inserm U1061, Montpellier, France
Université de Montpellier, U1061, Montpellier, France

Simon M. Collin and Esther Crawley
School of Social and Community Medicine, University of Bristol, Oakfield House, Oakfield Grove, Bristol BS8 2BN, UK

Inger J. Bakken
Norwegian Institute of Public Health, 0403 Oslo, Norway

Irwin Nazareth
Primary Care and Population Science, UCL Department of Primary Care and Population Health, UCL Royal Free Campus, Rowland Hill Street, London NW3 2PF, UK

Peter D. White
Psychological Medicine, Wolfson Institute of Preventive Medicine, Barts, London School of Medicine and Dentistry, Queen Mary University of London, London, UK

John Busby
Centre for Public Health, Queen's University Belfast, BT12 6BA, Belfast, UK

Sarah Purdy and William Hollingworth
School of Social and Community Medicine, University of Bristol, BS8 2PS, Bristol, UK

Juan Jose Rodriguez-Cristobal
Centre Atenció Primària Florida Sud. Direcció Atenció Primària Costa de Ponent-ICS. L'Hospitalet, Institut Universitari d'Investigacióen Atenció Primària Jordi Gol (IDIAP Jordi Gol), Barcelona, Spain

Carlos Alonso-Villaverde
Cardiovascular Research Center, CSIC-ICCC, Hospital de la Santa Creu i Sant Pau (UAB), IIB-Sant Pau, Barcelona, Spain

Esther Peña
Cardiovascular Research Center, CSIC-ICCC, Hospital de la Santa Creu i Sant Pau (UAB), IIB-Sant Pau, Barcelona, Spain
Cardiovascular Research Center, Hospital de la Santa Creu I Sant Pau, C/Sant Antoni Ma Claret, 167 08025 Barcelona, Spain

Jose Ma Panisello
FUFOSA (Fundación Fomento Salud), Barcelona, Spain

Pere Travé-Mercade
Univestitat de Barcelona, Facultad de Farmacia, Barcelona, Spain

Francisca Rodriguez-Cortés
Unitat de Salut Mental Collblanc, L'Hospitalet del Llobregat, Barcelona, Spain

Josep Ramon Marsal
Cardiovascular Department, Epidemiology Unit, University Hospital Vall d'Hebron. Lleida Research Support Unit, Primary Care Research Institut (IDIAP) Jordi Gol, Autonomus University of Barcelona, Barcelona, Catalonia, Spain

John Wakerman, Lisa Sparrow and Susan L Thomas
Flinders Northern Territory, Casuarina, Australia
Centre for Research Excellence in Rural and Remote Primary Health Care, Flinders University, Bedford Park, South Australia 5042, Australia

John S Humphreys
School of Rural Health, Monash University, Melbourne, Australia
Centre for Research Excellence in Rural and Remote Primary Health Care, Flinders University, Bedford Park, South Australia 5042, Australia

Mike Jones
Psychology Department, Macquarie University, Sydney, Australia
Centre for Research Excellence in Rural and Remote Primary Health Care, Flinders University, Bedford Park, South Australia 5042, Australia

Géraldine Tournu,
General practice department, University Paris Diderot, F-75018 Paris, France

Laurent Abramowitz
AP-HP and GREP; Gastroenterology and proctology unit, Bichat University hospital, Paris, France

Camille Couffignal
INSERM, IAME, UMR 1137, F-75018 Paris, France
University Paris Diderot, IAME, UMR 1137, Sorbonne Paris Cité, F-75018 Paris, France
AP-HP, Bichat hospital, Biostatistics unit, F-75018 Paris, France

Frédéric Juguet
Tivoli Ducos Clinic, Bordeaux, France

Agnès Sénéjoux
Proctology unit, Private hospital, Saint Grégoire, France

Stéphane Berger
Montigny les Cormeilles, France

Anne-Laure Wiart
Bordeaux, France

Marc Bernard
Cadaujac, France

Françoise Provost
Rennes, France

Hélène Pillant-Le Moult
Blomet Clinic, Paris, France

Dominique Bouchard
Proctology unit, Bagatelle hospital, Talence, France

Jean-Pierre Aubert
Sorbonne Paris Cité, General practice department, University Paris Diderot, F-75018 Paris, France; REMES, F-75018 Paris, France

Michelle DiGiacomo, Anna Green, Patricia Delaney and John Delaney
University of Technology Sydney, Faculty of Health, Broadway, Sydney, NSW 2007, Australia

Patrick Patradoon-Ho
Blacktown and Mt Druitt Hospitals, Western Sydney Local Health District, Blacktown Road, Blacktown, NSW 2148, Australia
Western Sydney University, Penrith, NSW 1797, Australia

Patricia Mary Davidson
University of Technology Sydney, Faculty of Health, Broadway, Sydney, NSW 2007, Australia
Johns Hopkins University, School of Nursing, 525 N. Wolfe Street, Baltimore, MD 21205, USA

Penelope Abbott
Western Sydney University, Penrith, NSW 1797, Australia

Elisabeth Björk Brämberg
Unit of Intervention and Implementation Research for Worker Health, Institute of Environmental Medicine, Karolinska institutet, 171 77 Stockholm, Sweden
Närhälsan Eriksberg Primary Health Care Centre, Sjöporten 4, 417 64 Göteborg, Sweden

Jarl Torgerson
Department of Psychosis, Sahlgrenska University Hospital, 431 80 Mölndal, Sweden

Anna Norman Kjellström
Department of Data Management and Analysis, Head Office, Region Västra Götaland, 541 80 Skövde, Sweden

Peder Welin
Centre for Equity in Health, Region Västra Götaland, Regionens Hus, 405 44 Göteborg, Sweden

Marie Rusner
Department of Research, Södra Älvsborgs Hospital, Brämhultsvägen 52, 501 82 Borås, Sweden
Institute of Health and Care Sciences, Sahlgrenska Academy, University of Gothenburg, 405 30 Gothenburg, Sweden

J. A. Wildeboer
VU University Amsterdam, De Boelelaan 1105, 1081 HV Amsterdam, Netherlands

A. R. T. van de Ven
St. Anna Hospital, Bogardeind 2, 5664 EH Geldrop, Netherlands

D. de Boer
NIVEL, Otterstraat 118-124, 3518 CR Utrecht, Netherlands

Zahirah Tharek
Discipline of Primary Care Medicine, Faculty of Medicine, Universiti Teknologi MARA (UiTM), Selayang Campus, Jalan Prima Selayang 7, 68100 Batu Caves, Selangor, Malaysia

Anis Safura Ramli
Discipline of Primary Care Medicine, Faculty of Medicine, Universiti Teknologi MARA (UiTM), Selayang Campus, Jalan Prima Selayang 7, 68100 Batu Caves, Selangor, Malaysia
Institute of Pathology, Laboratory and Forensic Medicine (I-PPerForM), Universiti Teknologi MARA (UiTM), Sungai Buloh Campus, Jalan Hospital, 47000 Sungai Buloh, Selangor, Malaysia

David Leonard Whitford
Department of General Practice, Royal College of Surgeons in Ireland (RCSI), Mercer Building, Noel Purcell Walk, Dublin, Republic of Ireland

Zaliha Ismail
Discipline of Population Health and Preventive Medicine, Faculty of Medicine, Universiti Teknologi MARA (UiTM), Sungai Buloh Campus, Jalan Hospital, 47000 Sungai Buloh, Selangor, Malaysia

Maryam Mohd Zulkifli
Department of Family Medicine, School of Medical Sciences, Universiti Sains Malaysia (USM), 16150 Kubang Kerian, Kelantan, Malaysia

Siti Khuzaimah Ahmad Sharoni
Department of Nursing, Faculty of Health Sciences, Universiti Teknologi MARA (UiTM), Puncak Alam Campus, 42300 Bandar Puncak Alam, Selangor, Malaysia

Asrul Akmal Shafie
Discipline of Social and Administrative Pharmacy, School of Pharmaceutical Sciences, Universiti Sains Malaysia (USM), 11800 Penang, Malaysia

Thevaraajan Jayaraman
Discipline of Medicine, Faculty of Medicine, Universiti Teknologi MARA, Sungai Buloh Campus, Jalan Hospital, 47000 Sungai Buloh, Selangor, Malaysia

Anita Kärner Köhler and Tiny Jaarsma
Department of Social and Welfare Studies (ISV/OMV), Linköping University, Norrköping, Sweden

Pia Tingström
Department of Medical and Health Sciences (IMH), Linköping University, Linköping, Sweden

Staffan Nilsson
Department of Medical and Health Sciences (IMH), Linköping University, Linköping, Sweden
Primary Health Care, Region Östergötland, Linköping, Sweden

Linda Sheiban
School of Public and Health and Health Systems, University of Waterloo, Waterloo, Ontario, Canada
Schlegel Centre for Advancing Seniors Care, Conestoga College, Kitchener, Ontario, Canada

Paul Stolee
School of Public and Health and Health Systems, University of Waterloo, Waterloo, Ontario, Canada
Schlegel-UW Research Institute for Aging, Kitchener, Ontario, Canada

Veronique Boscart
School of Public and Health and Health Systems, University of Waterloo, Waterloo, Ontario, Canada
Schlegel Centre for Advancing Seniors Care, Conestoga College, Kitchener, Ontario, Canada
Schlegel-UW Research Institute for Aging, Kitchener, Ontario, Canada

Carrie McAiney
Department of Psychiatry and Behavioural Neurosciences, McMaster University, Hamilton, Ontario, Canada

Fiona von Buedingen, Marc S. Hammer, Ferdinand M. Gerlach and Christiane Muth
Institute of General Practice, Johann Wolfgang Goethe University, Theodor-Stern-Kai 7, 60590 Frankfurt, Main, Germany

Andreas D. Meid
Department of Clinical Pharmacology and Pharmacoepidemiology, University of Heidelberg, Im Neuenheimer Feld 410, 69120 Heidelberg, Germany

Walter E. Müller
Pharmacological Institute for Natural Scientists, Johann Wolfgang Goethe University, Max-von-Laue-Str. 9, 60438 Frankfurt am Main, Germany

Pasqualina Santaguida
Department of Health Research Methods, Evidence and Impact, McMaster University HSC 3N50-G, 1280 Main Street West, Hamilton, Ontario L8S 4L7, Canada

Larkin Lamarche
Department of Family Medicine, DBHSC, McMaster University, 5th Floor 100 Main St West, Hamilton, ON L8P 1H6, Canada

Lisa Dolovich
Department of Family Medicine, DBHSC, McMaster University, 5th Floor 100 Main St West, Hamilton, ON L8P 1H6, Canada
Leslie Dan Faculty of Pharmacy, University of Toronto, Toronto, Ontario M5S 3M2, Canada

Doug Oliver
Department of Family Medicine, DBHSC, McMaster University, 3rd Floor, 100 Main St West, Hamilton, ON L8P 1H6, Canada

Anne Gilsing
Department of Health Research Methods, Evidence and Impact, McMaster University, 175 Longwood Rd. S. Suite 207A, Hamilton, ON L8P 0A1, Canada

Lauren E. Griffith
Department of Health Research Methods, Evidence and Impact, McMaster University, 175 Longwood Rd. S. Suite 309A, Hamilton, ON L8P 0A1, Canada

Julie Richardson
School of Rehabilitation Sciences, McMaster University, 1400 Main St. W. IAHS 443, Hamilton, ON L8S 1C7A, Canada

Mangin
Department of Family Medicine, DBHSC, McMaster University, 5th Floor, 100 Main St West, Hamilton, Ontario L8P 1H6, Canada

Monika Kastner
Institute of Health Policy, Management and Evaluation, University of Toronto, 155 College Street, Toronto, ON M5T 3M6, Canada

Parminder Raina
Department of Health Research Methods, Evidence and Impact, McMaster University, 175 Longwood Rd. S. Suite 309A, Hamilton, ON L8P 0A1, Canada

Staffan Nilsson
Primary Health Care and Department of Medical and Health Sciences, Linköping University, Linköping, Sweden

Per O. Andersson
Primary Health Care and Department of Medical and Health Sciences, Linköping University, Linköping, Sweden

Sofia Sederholm Lawesson and Ingela Thylén
Department of Cardiology and department of Medical and Health Sciences, Linköping University, Linköping, Sweden

Jan-Erik Karlsson
Department of Internal Medicine, Region Jönköping County, Jönköping, and Department of Medical and Health Sciences, Linköping University, Linköping, Sweden

Bianca Lauria-Horner and Tara Beaulieu
Department of Psychiatry, Dalhousie University, Halifax, Nova Scotia, Canada

Stephanie Knaak
Opening Minds Anti-Stigma Initiative, Mental Health Commission of Canada, Ottawa, ON, Canada
University of Calgary, Calgary, Alberta, Canada

Rivian Weinerman
University of Bristish Columbia, Medical Staff Honorary Status Island Health Authority, Victoria, Canada

Helen Campbell
Department of Psychiatry, University of British Columbia, Vancouver, Canada

Scott Patten
University of Calgary, Calgary, Alberta, Canada

Elzbieta Kaszuba
Samaritens Primary Health Care Centre, 374 80 Karlshamn, Sweden
Department of Clinical Sciences in Malmö General Practice, Center for Primary Health Care Research, Lund University, 205 02, Malmö, Sweden

Håkan Odeberg, Lennart Råstam and Anders Halling
Department of Clinical Sciences in Malmö General Practice, Center for Primary Health Care Research, Lund University, 205 02, Malmö, Sweden

Andrée-Anne Paré-Plante
Département de Médecine de Famille et de Médecine d'Urgence de l'Université de Sherbrooke, Campus de Longueuil, 150 place Charles-Le Moyne, 9e étage, Longueuil J4K 0A8, Canada
Centre de recherché Charles-Le Moyne - Saguenay-Lac-Saint-Jean sur les innovations en santé, Campus de Longueuil, 150 place Charles-Le Moyne, 9e étage, Longueuil J4K 0A8, Canada

Djamal Berbiche and Mylaine Breton
Centre de recherché Charles-Le Moyne - Saguenay-Lac-Saint-Jean sur les innovations en santé, Campus de Longueuil, 150 place Charles-Le Moyne, 9e étage, Longueuil J4K 0A8, Canada
Département des Sciences de la Santé Communautaire de l'Université de Sherbrooke, Sherbrooke, Canada

Maryse Guay
Centre de recherché Charles-Le Moyne - Saguenay-Lac-Saint-Jean sur les innovations en santé, Campus de Longueuil, 150 place Charles-Le Moyne, 9e étage, Longueuil J4K 0A8, Canada
Département des Sciences de la Santé Communautaire de l'Université de Sherbrooke, Sherbrooke, Canada
Direction de Santé Publique, CISSS de la Montérégie-Centre, Longueuil, Canada

Antoine Boivin
Département de Médecine de Famille et Médecine d'Urgence de l'Université de Montreal, Montreal, Canada
Centre de Recherche du Centre Hospitalier de l'Université de Montréal, Montreal, Canada
Institut de Recherche en Santé Publique de l'Université de Montréal, Montreal, Canada

R. Allison, D. M. Lecky and C. A. M. McNulty
Primary Care Unit, National Infection Service, Public Health England, Microbiology Dept, Gloucestershire Royal Hospital, Great Western Road, Gloucester GL1 3NN, UK

K. Town, K. A. Folkard and J. K. Dunbar
HIV/STI Department, Centre for Infectious Disease Control and Surveillance, Public Health England, London, UK

C. Rugman
Formerly Public Health England, Primary Care Unit, Microbiology Dept., Gloucester GL1 3NN, UK

E. J. Ricketts
Formerly Public Health England, Primary Care Unit, Microbiology Dept., Gloucester, now Derriford Hospital, Derriford Road, Plymouth, UK

N. Ockendon-Powell
Formerly Public Health England, Primary Care Unit, Microbiology Dept., Gloucester, now Biotechnology and Biological Sciences Research Council (BBSRC), Polaris House, North Star Avenue, Swindon, UK

Mélanie Badin, Philippe Serayet, Sylvain Pavageau and François Lucas
Department of General Medicine, University of Montpellier, Montpellier, France

Gérard Bourrel
Department of General Medicine, University of Montpellier, Montpellier, France CEPS Platform, University of Montpellier, Montpellier, France
Epsylon EA4556, Dynamic of Human Abilities and Health Behaviors, University of Montpellier, Montpellier, France

Catalina Martinez, Gonzalo Grandes, Alvaro Sanchez, Haizea Pombo and Paola Bully
Primary Care Research Unit of Bizkaia, Basque Healthcare Service - Osakidetza, BioCruces Health Research Institute, Luis Power 18 4th floor, Bilbao 48014, Spain

Gonzalo Bacigalupe
University of Massachusetts Boston, College of Education and Human Development, 100 Morrissey Bvld, Boston, MA 02125, USA

Michelle Banfield
Centre for Mental Health Research, Research School of Population Health, The Australian National University, 63 Eggleston Rd, Acton ACT 2601, Australia

Tanisha Jowsey
Centre for Medical and Health Sciences Education The University of Auckland, Auckland City Hospital, Building 599, Level 12, Auckland 1023, New Zealand

Anne Parkinson
Department of Health Services Research and Policy, Research School of Population Health, The Australian National University, 63 Eggleston Rd, Acton ACT 2601, Australia

Kirsty A. Douglas
ANU Medical School, Canberra Hospital, Bldg 4, Level 2, Garran ACT 2605, Australia

Paresh Dawda
Ochre Health Medical Centre, Cnr Allawoona Street and Ginninderra Drive, Bruce ACT 2617, Australia

Josep M. Cortada
Deusto Primary Health Care Center. Bilbao-Basurto Integrated Care Organisation. Basque Healthcare Service - Osakidetza. BioCruces Health Research Institute, Luis Power 18, Bilbao 48014, Spain

Nerida Volker, Thomas Cochrane, Tanya Clancy and Rachel C. Davey
Health Research Institute, Centre for Research and Action in Public Health, University of Canberra, College Road, Bruce, Canberra, ACT 2601, Australia

Lauren T. Williams
Health Research Institute, Centre for Research and Action in Public Health, University of Canberra, College Road, Bruce, Canberra, ACT 2601, Australia
Menzies Health Institute of Queensland, Griffith University, Parklands Drive, Southport, QLD 4222, Australia

Tim Stokes, Emma Tumilty and Fiona Doolan-Noble
Department of General Practice and Rural Health, Dunedin School of Medicine, University of Otago, Dunedin 9054, New Zealand

Robin Gauld
Otago Business School, University of Otago, Dunedin, New Zealand

Index

www.ingramcontent.com/pod-product-compliance
Lightning Source LLC
LaVergne TN
LVHW080908210926
848485LV00004B/612
* 9 7 8 1 6 3 9 2 7 4 4 6 8 *